Psychopharmacology

FROM THEORY TO PRACTICE

Canst thou not minister to a mind diseas'd,

Pluck from the memory a rooted sorrow,

Raze out the written troubles of the brain,

And with some sweet oblivious antidote

Cleanse the stuff'd bosom of that perilous stuff

Which weighs upon the heart?

Macbeth (V. iii. 40-45)

Psychopharmacology

FROM THEORY TO PRACTICE

EDITORS

Jack D. Barchas, M.D.
Philip A. Berger, M.D.
Roland D. Ciaranello, M.D.
Glen R. Elliott, Ph.D.

DEPARTMENT OF PSYCHIATRY AND BEHAVIORAL SCIENCES
STANFORD UNIVERSITY SCHOOL OF MEDICINE

NEW YORK
OXFORD UNIVERSITY PRESS
1977

LIBRARY OF CONGRESS CATALOGING IN PUBLICATION DATA
Main entry under title:

Psychopharmacology.

 Bibliography: p.
 Includes index.
 1. Psychopharmacology. I. Barchas, Jack D.
RM315.P7534   615'.78   76-57489
ISBN 0-19-502214-9
ISBN 0-19-502215-7 pbk.

Printed in the United States of America

Foreword

In history, let alone in evolution, a quarter century is a brief moment of time. Yet this remarkable book could not, in any useful sense, have been written a quarter century ago. At that time, we lacked the fundamental knowledge base, the well-designed clinical research, the abundant clinical experience, and the interdisciplinary cooperation to make such a book possible.

But now we have it. A group of dedicated and well-informed authors, based firmly on the ground of first-rate scientific training, abundant research accomplishment, and rich clinical experience, have assembled an exceedingly valuable guide to the new territory of psychopharmacology.

The volume takes advantage of recent developments in knowledge of neuroregulators and mechanisms involving neuroregulators, to provide a framework in which the action of the various drugs can be viewed. There is extensive discussion of the probable mechanisms of the various disorders; that information is related to the nature of the drugs used in treatment. Extensive coverage of the actual use of drugs is provided in a practical way. Although the volume is basically concerned with neurochemical approaches, the authors are alert to the importance of psychosocial approaches, and these are discussed where appropriate.

It is a fairly large book because the field is growing rapidly, not only in quantity but also in quality. There is much here by way of intellectual stimulation, a sense of the moving frontiers of research, and clinical acumen. There is much that will be helpful to today's patients, and even more that bodes well for tomorrow's patients. Here is an area of immense human suffering in which the burden is ,beginning to be lifted.

It is a heartening prospect for today's students to have such a penetrating book at their disposal. It is more heartening still to know that the field is producing young leaders of the ability and integrity of these authors.

For those who care deeply about human suffering, and who believe that science can help, this is your book.

David A. Hamburg

Preface

The fundamental concerns of this text are the major psychiatric disorders and the manner in which the science of pharmacology may be applied, either immediately or ultimately, to their amelioration. Every book has a set of intellectual themes, the expression of which is the dream of those responsible for it. Our dream has been to integrate the basic science and clinical aspects of psychopharmacology in a single text comprehensive enough for those who will be responsible for treating psychiatric patients, yet not too long to be read through. Although several excellent texts are already available, their approaches have been primarily to concentrate on patient management or to provide detailed descriptions of drug classes or to summarize drug efficacy studies or to review classifications of psychiatric illnesses. We have endeavored first to explain clearly the scientific principles behind psychopharmacology and then to demonstrate their relevance to the use of psychopharmacological agents in good patient care.

In the following chapters, we have described some biological aspects of the psychiatric disorders in which psychopharmacology currently plays a role. We have discussed the major biological hypotheses involving the various disorders and the presumed mechanisms of action of the drugs that are used in their treatment—two important levels of knowledge that complement each other. In the belief that a full understanding of the actions of psychopharmacological agents requires multiple levels of analysis, we have supplemented biochemical approaches, where possible, with other scientific perspectives. In presenting material, albeit limited, on the psychological and sociological aspects of psychopharmacological agents, we hope to emphasize their importance. It is clear that the serious psychiatric disorders reflect an interplay between biological and behavioral factors.

One central theme of this text is the importance of neuroregulators. As described in Chapter 1, these are compounds that function either as transmitters between nerve cells (neurotransmitters) or as modulators of neuronal action (neuromodulators). A remarkable amount has been learned about these compounds in the past few years, and it has been amply demonstrated that they are profoundly affected by pharmacological agents. Thus, a recognition of the interrelationships between pharmacological agents, neuroregulators, and behavior has become essential for those involved in helping individuals who have psychiatric disorders.

The criteria for linking one or more neuroregulators to a specific psychiatric disorder include the following:

- Each neuroregulator must be an endogenously formed substance for which receptors exist in the brain or which alters normal neuronal transmission.
- A characteristic pattern of neuroregulator activity should occur in relation to the psychiatric disorder.
- Alteration of the activity of neuronal systems involving one or more neuroregulators or alteration of the balance between them should alter the psychiatric disorder.
- The psychiatric disorder should be induced by appropriate manipulation of the neuroregulator system or systems.
- Unless the process is irreversible, restoration of normal neuroregulator activity or balance should ameliorate the psychiatric disorder.

There is strong evidence that links neuroregulators to behavior and thereby to normal as well as to abnormal processes. The diversity of regulatory mechanisms offers multiple sites for alteration or stress beyond normal limits. The resulting changes in behavior might contribute to an "abnormality" designated as a psychiatric disability.

While one can speculate about the mechanisms by which behavioral processes alter biochemical mechanisms and vice versa, another exciting level of inquiry deals with their reciprocal interactions over time. For example, in what ways does behavior alter biochemistry and the altered biochemistry then change subsequent behavior? Such an approach suggests a constant dynamic process. One could well imagine that effects of early experience on subsequent behavior—a notion important to many conceptualizations in psychiatry—might be reflected in biochemical changes which could alter neurotransmission later in life. In this view, within limits set by genetic factors, behavioral processes may influence the setting of "regulostats," biochemical mechanisms in which there may be plasticity. Genetic, developmental, behavioral, and neurochemical interactions would thus be important areas for continued study of neuroregulators, and such studies should have clear relevance to our understanding of psychiatric disorders.

There are a variety of complex behavioral processes in humans that may have biochemical concomitants. One can imagine, for instance, that in susceptible individuals certain types of psychological stress might lead to an alteration of neuroregulatory activity that would produce changes leading to disordered function, perhaps by a "locking in" of a biochemical process. Such mechanisms may pertain only to a certain proportion of individuals with psychiatric disorders. To give two examples of such possible effects, schizophrenic patients are particularly vulnerable to stress, including the stress of social interaction, while some depressed patients experience the disorder in reaction to life events involving loss.

A concern with the relationships between neuroregulators and psychiatric disorders does not preclude a recognition of the important role that psychological factors have in these states. Indeed, one could envision a spectrum of interactions between psychological and biochemical processes. Some illnesses probably involve both processes, while others may be primarily either biochemical or psychological. Thus, we believe in a variety of approaches growing out of relationships among psychopharmacology, behavioral neurochemistry, and psychiatry. Each area should be mastered by people who are involved in the treatment of psychiatric patients. We have tried to provide a knowledge base of psychopharmacology which not only will permit readers to be informed practitioners but will also enable them to evaluate new information as it becomes available.

Out of such convictions and concerns have come the themes and organization of this volume. The book is divided into five parts. The first reviews basic fields of study in psychopharmacology ranging from biochemical information on neuroregulators and drug mechanisms of action to aspects of the psychological and sociological effects of psychopharmacological agents. The second part describes the disorders that affect most patients who require psychiatric care. Part III deals with drugs of abuse. Not only do these compounds present a grave social problem, but their powerful psychopharmacological effects may shed light on the traditional psychiatric disorders and on normal brain function. Part IV is concerned with the treatment of the young and the elderly, two groups that are often overlooked in terms of psychopharmacology and whose proper care can differ markedly from that of adults. Finally, Part V deals with several special topics that are important in psychopharmacology, ranging from the psychiatric effects of nonpsychiatric drugs to the interactions of psychopharmacology and psychotherapy and the use of placebos. In addition to presenting the known psychopharmacology of each disorder, we have endeavored to make the treatment sections as practical as possible, covering both normal doses and side effects.

To the delight and sometimes the confusion of those within the field, psychiatry, more than any other specialty in medicine, utilizes a variety of treatment modalities. Many of these methods of treatment can give great aid to patients, and it is encumbent upon practitioners to view the discipline from an open perspective. A substantial body of information about psychiatric treatment has been acquired through great effort. This volume concentrates upon that portion relating to psychopharmacology. We believe that it provides the psychopharmacological information needed to facilitate the care of psychiatric patients, along with the bases from which this information was derived. We would welcome comments and suggestions from our readers.

Jack D. Barchas
Philip A. Berger
Roland D. Ciaranello
Glen R. Elliott

APRIL, 1977
NANCY PRITZKER LABORATORY OF BEHAVIORAL NEUROCHEMISTRY
AND PSYCHIATRIC CLINICAL RESEARCH CENTER
STANFORD, CALIFORNIA

Acknowledgments

As a result of the individual efforts of many investigators over the last two decades, we are already able to alleviate some of the pain caused by psychiatric disorders, and the field is on the verge of important discoveries. Those efforts which led to this base of practical knowledge depended upon support from various institutions and agencies and were greatly influenced by teachers, books, and colleagues. We, and everyone else, owe much to all who have helped to produce the body of information which is the heart of this volume.

There are many people who fill the role of teacher for the editors. One person who is specially singled out is Daniel X. Freedman, formerly of Yale and now of the University of Chicago. He recognizes multiple levels of dynamics in inquiry—as in all other parts of life. His valiant attempts to pass on his vision have had some effect, and we are grateful.

We wish Nicholas Giarman of Yale were here. His comments and gentle suggestions would have improved the book. We hope this volume meets standards he would have held for it.

For more than one of us, Dr. Julius Axelrod of the National Institute of Mental Health, Dr. Arvid Carlsson of Göteborg, and Dr. Seymour Kety of Harvard have had a major impact on our thinking about problems of psychopharmacology and have been a source of scientific excitement.

Few are gifted in creating conditions that permit endeavors—and people—to flourish. David Hamburg has that gift. In this instance, he created a department which promotes productive interactions among individuals of divergent backgrounds, beliefs, and approaches. We are deeply appreciative of his early recognition of the field and of his continuing support and encouragement.

It has been a pleasure to work with the contributors, both in the context of this book and in other ways. Each was associated with this department at the time of writing. In this, as in other activities, the department has been positive and encouraging and has fostered task-oriented interactions. We have felt a strong spirit of colleagueship.

The progress of the book has been greatly facilitated by our chairman, Dr. Thomas A. Gonda. His enthusiasm and concern for psychiatry, psychiatric care, and psychiatric science has guided his direction of the department, to the benefit of those in it.

Mr. Jeffrey House, our editor at Oxford Press, is the epitome of a professional: we don't know what troubles we might have had. He has amply earned this accolade by being, at each stage of the volume, thoughtful, responsive, and encouraging. Ellen Fuchs and the staff of Oxford University Press also were most helpful.

As it has affected our careers, and hence this volume, we would like to acknowledge the critical importance of the National Institute of Mental Health, which has profoundly influenced basic psychiatric research. The staff of the Extramural Research Branch has understood and, as far as they were able, has supported the basic thrust of the work of many investigators, thus contributing to the development of the body of knowledge which seems so near to fruition. From the Grant Foundation, the late Dr. Douglas Bond and Mr. Phillip Sapir made a major impact upon our ability to perform research with adults and children. That research ultimately led to our interest in preparing this volume. The Pritzker Foundation has graciously provided encouragement and support which should markedly facilitate our future efforts. The Commonwealth Fund was helpful to us at an early point in providing funds for a monograph.

A very special note of thanks is due to Mrs. Sue Poage, the manuscript typist who has worked with us for several years. Throughout that work she has demonstrated skill, care, thoughtfulness, concern, and an ability to work with tight deadlines. The illustrations were prepared by Charlene Levering and Linda Toda. The index, by Mrs. Sharon Willy.

Also, thanks to the residents who, over several years, have commented both on the course and on working versions of the text.

Lastly, we wish to thank our spouses and children: Patricia Barchas, Isaac Barchas; Deborah Berger, Tamara Berger, Cynthia Berger; Nancy Ciaranello, Andrea Ciaranello; and Janette Elliott.

CONTRIBUTORS

Huda Akil, Ph.D.: Special Research Fellow, Department of Psychiatry and Behavioral Sciences and Adjunct Assistant Professor, Department of Psychology, Stanford University.

Thomas F. Anders, M.D.: Director, Child Psychiatry Program and Associate Professor of Psychiatry and Behavioral Sciences, Stanford University.

Jack D. Barchas, M.D.: Director, Nancy Pritzker Laboratory of Behavioral Neurochemistry and Nancy Friend Pritzker Professor of Psychiatry and Behavioral Sciences, Stanford University.

Patricia R. Barchas, Ph.D.: Assistant Professor of Sociology and (by courtesy) Psychiatry and Behavioral Sciences, Stanford University.

Philip A. Berger, M.D.: Director, Psychiatric Clinical Research Center, Stanford University and Palo Alto Veterans Administration Hospital; and Assistant Professor of Psychiatry and Behavioral Sciences and Assistant Professor of Pediatrics, Stanford University.

Roland D. Ciaranello, M.D.: Director, Laboratory of Developmental Neurochemistry, Child Psychiatry Program, Department of Psychiatry and Behavioral Sciences, Stanford University.

Kenneth L. Davis, M.D.: Assistant Director, Psychiatric Clinical Research Center, Palo Alto Veterans Administration Hospital.

Emanuel De Fraites, M.D.: Formerly, Clinical Fellow, Department of Psychiatry and Behavioral Sciences, Stanford University. Currently, Clinical Associate, National Institute of Mental Health, Bethesda.

William C. Dement, M.D., Ph.D.: Director, Sleep Research Center and Professor of Psychiatry and Behavioral Sciences, Stanford University.

Burr Eichelman, M.D.: Formerly, Special Research Fellow, Department of Psychiatry and Behavioral Sciences, Stanford University. Currently, Assistant Professor of Psychiatry, University of Wisconsin, Madison.

Glen R. Elliott, Ph.D.: Assistant Director, Nancy Pritzker Laboratory of Behavioral Neurochemistry, Department of Psychiatry and Behavioral Sciences, Stanford University.

Floyd M. Estess, M.D.: Chief of Clinical Psychiatry, Psychiatry Service, Palo Alto Veterans Administration Hospital; and Professor of Clinical Psychiatry, Stanford University.

Thomas A. Gonda, M.D.: Chairman and Professor of Psychiatry and Behavioral Sciences, Stanford University.

George D. Gulevich, M.D.: Chief, Acute Psychiatric Inpatient Unit; and Associate Professor of Psychiatry and Behavioral Sciences, Stanford University.

Leo E. Hollister, M.D.: Director, Laboratory of Clinical Psychopharmacology, Palo Alto Veterans Administration Hospital; and Professor of Medicine and Professor of Psychiatry and Behavioral Sciences, Stanford University.

R. Bruce Holman, Ph.D.: Senior Research Associate, Department of Psychiatry and Behavioral Sciences, Stanford University.

Bert S. Kopell, M.D.: Director, Laboratory of Clinical Psychophysiology and Psychopharmacology and Chief, Psychiatry Service, Palo Alto Veterans Administration Hospital; and Professor of Psychiatry and Behavioral Sciences, Stanford University.

Helena C. Kraemer, Ph.D.: Associate Professor of Psychiatry and Behavioral Sciences, Stanford University.

Robert L. Patrick, Ph.D.: Senior Research Associate, Department of Psychiatry and Behavioral Sciences, Stanford University.

Adolf Pfefferbaum, M.D.: Director, Psychiatric Outpatient Clinic and Associate Director, Laboratory of Clinical Psychophysiology and Psychopharmacology, Palo Alto Veterans Administration Hospital; and Assistant Professor of Psychiatry and Behavioral Sciences, Stanford University.

Joachim Raese, M.D.: Special Research Fellow, Department of Psychiatry and Behavioral Sciences, Stanford University.

Jean Renson, M.D.: Special Research Fellow, Department of Psychiatry and Behavioral Sciences, Stanford University.

Walton T. Roth, M.D.: Chief, Psychiatric Consultation Service and Associate Director, Laboratory of Clinical Psychophysiology and Psychopharmacology, Palo Alto Veterans Administration Hospital; and Assistant Professor of Psychiatry and Behavioral Sciences, Stanford University.

Robert L. Sack, M.D.: Ward Chief, Psychiatric Intensive Care Unit,

Palo Alto Veterans Administration Hospital; and Assistant Professor, Department of Psychiatry, Stanford University.

Jared R. Tinklenberg, M.D.: Director of Training and Chief, Drug and Alcohol Treatment Programs, Psychiatry Service, Palo Alto Veterans Administration Hospital; and Associate Professor of Psychiatry and Behavioral Sciences, Stanford University.

Stanley J. Watson, Ph.D., M.D.: Special Research Fellow, Department of Psychiatry and Behavioral Sciences, Stanford University.

Vincent Zarcone, M.D.: Ward Chief, Drug Unit and Director, Sleep Research, Palo Alto Veterans Administration Hospital; and Associate Professor of Clinical Psychiatry and Behavioral Sciences, Stanford University.

Contents

Psychopharmacology

FROM THEORY TO PRACTICE

I | Central Mechanisms of Psychopharmacology

Part I offers a cross-section of the multiple levels at which drug effects can be viewed, ranging from subcellular control mechanisms to social groupings. Since it is impossible to describe all aspects of drug action that may be relevant to psychopharmacology, the following chapters concentrate on some of the major highlights of the relationships between neuroregulators and behavior. Chapter 1 examines general issues arising in studies of these interactions. It is followed by two chapters about neuroregulators which are believed to be particularly important in psychopharmacology. The catecholamines dopamine and norepinephrine present an opportunity to discuss neuronal systems about which a great deal is already known. As described in Chapter 2, many psychopharmacological agents, including the antidepressants and the antipsychotics, are thought to act upon these two transmitter systems. Chapter 3 considers other neuroregulatory substances, including 5-hydroxytryptamine (serotonin), acetylcholine, and γ-aminobutyric acid (GABA), that are also of current interest, even though their exact relationship to the actions of psychopharmacological agents is less clear.

While studies of cellular organization and biochemistry are one way to analyze the effects of drugs, another is neurophysiological investigations, in which activities of single cells or of cell groups are studied. Chapter 4 emphasizes that the actions of some drugs become clear only in light of their effects upon neuronal networks or upon select cells in specific brain regions. Furthermore, it describes some of the emerging technological and theoretical developments which are enabling investigators to examine neurophysiological mechanisms in humans. Potentially, such studies may offer a means for quicker assessment of the suitability of individual patients for drug treatments.

Surprisingly little is known about the psychological effects of psychopharmacological agents, although many of the tools needed for such analyses are now available. Knowing exactly what aspects of behavior are altered would be particularly helpful in evaluating a drug's mode of action and also in understanding psychological disorders. Chapter 5 describes some of the tremendous problems inherent in such studies and provides a brief survey of behavioral data already available for major classes of psychopharmacological agents.

Drugs also alter social behavior. Indeed, many drugs are taken specifically for their social effects. In addition, disturbances of social behavior are one of the most important aspects of the severe psychiatric disorders. As discussed in Chapter 6, the processes which make up social structure, including status, normative behavior, and conformity, offer still another level of analysis of the action of drugs and another way of understanding their use and abuse.

Each of the analytical approaches presented in the following chapters can be viewed as a separate tool. However, we believe that their greatest power emerges as they are used jointly. Even for the most thoroughly studied drugs, we have much to learn. Still, the information already at our disposal helps to provide a framework for understanding how many of the psychoactive drugs exert their effects. In that light, Part I may be viewed as an introduction to the rest of the book.

1 | Neuroregulators and Behavior

GLEN R. ELLIOTT, R. BRUCE HOLMAN, and

JACK D. BARCHAS

INTRODUCTION

The current formulation of brain function postulates that organized behavior results from impulse transmission through intricate networks of neurons. Interconnections among these neurons are extensive and consist primarily of chemical synapses, each of which offers a potential site for establishing or modifying a neuronal circuit (1). Subsequent chapters in this section will describe our current understanding both about the details of the events which occur at the synapse and about the internal and external processes which help to shape synaptic activity into organized behavior. This chapter will concentrate upon some of the complexities involved in attempting to combine the information gained from these two important levels of analysis.

We will be considering the role of compounds which act either as transmitters between nerve cells (neurotransmitters) or as modulators of neuronal function (neuromodulators). Collectively, these two classes of compounds may be referred to as neuroregulators. In the past several years, a remarkable amount has been learned about neuroregulators. Investigation of these compounds has been fostered not only by intellectual curiosity but also by the increasing evidence that they are relevant to understanding severe psychiatric disorders. Thus, it is vitally important to learn how information about neuroregulators may be applied to improving our ability to treat psychiatric patients with specific agents which have few undesirable side effects.

The step from studies of individual neuroregulators or of neuronal circuits to investigations of their relationships to behavior is an enormous one. Reis (2) has suggested one approach to defining the guidelines with which to establish a causative link between a specific neurotransmitter system and a given behavior (Table 1-1). Similar guidelines

TABLE 1-1.
CRITERIA FOR LINKING A NEUROTRANSMITTER TO A BEHAVIOR

Neurotransmitter must exist in the central nervous system.

Precursors and enzymatic machinery for synthesis and degradation must be present in association with the transmitter.

A characteristic pattern of transmitter release should occur in relation to the behavior.

Induction of that characteristic transmitter release should elicit the behavior.

Destruction of the involved neuronal system should both deplete the transmitter and abolish normal control of that behavior.

Increases or decreases in transmitter activity should have opposing behavioral effects.

Modified from Reis (2).

would apply for neuromodulators. Implicit within such criteria are at least three important assumptions: 1) neuroregulator activity has both synaptic and systemic components; 2) behavior can be identified as a discrete, reproducible phenomenon; and 3) a given behavior arises from characteristic patterns of neuroregulator activity. These assumptions set important, often unrecognized, expectations both for biochemical and neurophysiological and for behavioral studies of man and animals. In the following material, we will discuss some aspects of behavioral and biochemical processes which are important in evaluating relationships between neuroregulators and behavior.

HISTORY

The concept of chemical mediation of neuronal transmission is less than seventy-five years old (3). Its origins may be traced to work done in the late nineteenth century with several substances which were found to mimic the effects of normal neuronal activity. For example, in 1895, Oliver and Shafer demonstrated that adrenal extracts produced physiological effects which resembled those resulting from sympathetic nerve stimulation. Subsequently, epinephrine (adrenaline) was isolated from and identified as the active principle of these extracts by Abel, von Furth, Takamine, Stolz, and others. Similarly, muscarine, described by Schmledeberg and Koppe in 1869, was shown to mimic many of the effects of parasympathetic nerve stimulation. Pilocarpine also produced muscarine-like effects, as demonstrated by Langley in 1904. These observations were first formulated into an hypothesis of chemical transmission in 1905 by a Cambridge student, T. R. Elliott. Elliott suggested that nerve endings might release small amounts of a chemical substance, such as epinephrine, which could then act upon effector sites.

Much of the initial progress in proving the hypothesis of neurochemical transmission came from work on acetylcholine. In 1907, Dixon reexamined the physiological effects of muscarine and concluded that parasympathetic fibers might release a muscarine-like substance. That same year, Hunt published his studies of acetylcholine. During the next ten years, studies by Dale, Barger, and other coworkers led to the conviction that acetylcholine was involved in transmission in parasympathetic fibers. In fact, Dale proposed that these fibers be called "cholinergic" and that acetylcholine and similar drugs be called "parasympathomimetic." Similarly, he proposed that sympathetic fibers be called "adrenergic," with epinephrine-like drugs being "sympathomimetic."

The next major advance in our understanding of transmission in parasympathetic nerves came from the classical experiments of Loewi, beginning in 1921. Using isolated frog hearts connected by perfusion medium, Loewi found that vagus nerve stimulation of the first, innervated heart produced a substance—*vagusstoff*—which slowed the second, denervated one. Loewi and many subsequent investigators were able to show that *vagusstoff* was, in fact, acetylcholine. Subsequent discoveries about the many sites at which acetylcholine acts as a neurotransmitter are described in Chapter 3.

Interestingly, work begun in 1921 also signaled a breakthrough in our understanding of the transmitter for adrenergic, or sympathetic, nerves. In that year, Cannon and Uridil isolated "sympathin," a substance which was released upon stimulation of sympathetic nerves in the liver. Subsequent investigations demonstrated that sympathin was released by all sympathetic nerves. In addition, sympathin was shown to strongly resemble epinephrine, although the two substances were not identical pharmacologically. Absolute identification of sympathin proved to be difficult. As early as 1934, Bacq suggested that sympathin might be norepinephrine, the N-demethylated derivative of epinephrine; however, he maintained that epinephrine was the final mediator of nerve transmission. Positive identification of sympathin as norepinephrine was delayed until 1946, when von Euler used newly developed techniques for quantitative identification of small amounts of norepinephrine (4,5). As described in Chapter 2, studies of norepinephrine and other catecholamines have been tremendously influential in molding our concepts of synaptic activity for both peripheral and central nerves.

NEUROCHEMICAL AND NEUROPHYSIOLOGICAL CONSIDERATIONS

Research on the central nervous system (CNS) continues to enlarge our understanding of the brain at both cellular and multicellular levels. Synaptic regulation is being elucidated not only by isolating and characterizing synthetic and degradative enzymes but also by studying intact neurons with single-unit recordings and iontophoresis. Parallel investigations utilizing fluorescence histochemistry and autoradiography have led to the visualization and mapping of the cell tracts and interconnections which constitute neuronal networks. These simultaneous advances have greatly enhanced our appreciation of the role of individual cells as functional components of more complex systems.

Since many of the important parameters and available techniques for studying neuroregulator and electrical activity in the brain are described in the next three chapters, we shall mention them here only briefly. For the neuroregulators, measurement of content has been and continues to be an important part of studying relationships between specific compounds and behavior, both in man and in animals. Fortunately, the available arsenal of assay procedures has expanded rapidly in recent years and now permits the detection and quantitation of numerous brain substances and their precursors and metabolites. In addition, an improved understanding of basic regulatory mechanisms now permits inspection of those parameters upon which neuroregulator content depends. These include long- and short-term regulation of synthetic rate, utilization of storage mechanisms, and inactivation of transmitter activity through either sequestration or metabolic degradation. Recent advances have further extended our realm of investigation to the postsynaptic site, with studies of the receptor's role in recognizing and transmitting the chemical message. These topics are discussed more fully in Chapters 2 and 3 (cf. 6).

As described in Chapter 4, neurophysiologists have developed powerful techniques for assessing the chemical and electrical parameters of single cells and for monitoring spontaneous and event-related electrical activity of cell groups. Careful use of these methods can provide information about neuronal systems and interconnections and about the involvement of those systems with specific behaviors. The elucidation of a feedback loop between dopaminergic terminals in the caudate nucleus and cell bodies in the substantia nigra represents a particularly interesting example of the potential contributions of this approach. It offers important insight into one mechanism by which the brain maintains the intricate and delicate balance necessary for normal function.

There are two basic strategies for studying the biochemical and neurophysiological parameters of behavior: 1) manipulate the neurochemical and electrical activity of the brain and observe changes in behavioral initiation or execution or 2) observe the neurochemical and electrical changes which accompany various stages of a behavioral state. Available techniques for the first approach include lesions, electrical stimulation, and pharmacological treatments. These methods share the advantage of establishing tentative links between neuronal systems and behaviors, but they suffer both from being nonphysiological and from having variable specificity. The second approach is more recent and employs techniques such as cortical superfusion and ventricular and push-pull cannula perfusions, as well as single-cell, multicell, and scalp electrical recordings. The complexities of using these latter techniques are great, but they enable investigators to examine progressive stages of specific behaviors in conscious animals (7,8). Through the second approach, one would hope to gain information about patterns of neurochemical change which occur through time in relation to specific behaviors. Both approaches are essential in our continuing efforts to understand behavior.

BEHAVIORAL CONSIDERATIONS

In their desire to increase the precision and power of biochemical and neurophysiological measures, investigators often forget that their results are also affected by factors which influence the behavior they are studying. Since behavior involves both information processing and the translation of that information into a response, such factors can be quite complex. Good behavioral analyses require careful delineation and control of the environment. This can create a stable, ongoing response pattern, free of excessive variability, whether the behavior is unconditioned or conditioned. For example, in a carefully controlled environment, even normal activities such as locomotion, feeding, drinking, and sleeping become reliable, reproducible behaviors, since they all occur with relatively stable patterns over appropriate time periods. Alternatively, specific behavioral patterns can be established deliberately if the correct stimulus-response contingencies are chosen, as illustrated with reinforcement schedules. Under such conditions, if a defined stimulus elicits a desired response, the animal either receives a positive reinforcement or escapes or avoids a negative one.

An enormous literature exists about the uses and limitations of the many available testing procedures and reinforcement schedules in animals (9,10). An important theme in this literature is that even apparently minor changes in the testing conditions can produce marked differences in the outcome. Animal, apparatus, stimulus, task, reinforcement, and desired response pattern—all profoundly affect the final behavior (6). Similar variables are also extremely important in studies of the psychological functions of man (Chapter 5).

The correct perception of a stimulus and the strength of the coupling between stimulus and response are both intimately involved in the successful elicitation of a reinforced behavior. Thus, it is not surprising that even minor changes in the stimulus can affect behavior. Of potentially greater interest is the ability of internal alterations to induce similar effects (11). "State-dependent learning" is a classical example of this phenomenon. Thus, if rats learn to run a maze while intoxicated with pentobarbital, they show no familiarity with the maze when they are tested while in a drug-free state. Reintoxication restores prior training. Such effects have been demonstrated under a variety of conditions and with numerous drugs. State-dependent learning might also be of importance in clinical psychopharmacology. Harvey (12) has suggested that the combined use of drugs and psychiatric therapy might result in a coupling between the patient's improved mental condition and his drug state. If this occurred, cessation of drug treatment might also mean loss of the beneficial effects from psychiatric intervention.

MODELS IN BEHAVIORAL NEUROCHEMISTRY

It is tempting to conclude that all really crucial information about the human brain must be gained from studies on humans. And yet to date such studies have yielded conflicting or inconclusive data, both because the human brain is complex and because our most sophisticated technology is generally too destructive or too dangerous to use in such studies. Thus, crucial neurochemical and neurophysiological changes must be inferred from observations at distant sites with measures from urine, blood, or cerebrospinal fluid or with recordings on the scalp. These indirect data are subject to so many possible influences that precise interpretation is virtually impossible.

In light of these difficulties, investigators have sought analogous animal models, upon which they can impose better control of neurochemical and behavioral variables. Potentially, this approach offers a powerful tool for the elucidation of the underlying regulatory mechanisms of a specific behavior. However, a delicate balance exists between the need for good behavioral control and delineation and the danger of destroying the model's information value. For example, reserpine appears to induce behavioral depression in some normal humans and to exacerbate symptoms of depressed patients (Chapter 29). In animals, it decreases locomotor activity and body temperature. Animal studies have provided important information about the neurochemical systems involved in this hypomotility and hypothermia. Unfortunately, it is unclear whether these same neurochemical mechanisms are responsible for human depression (Chapter 10). Thus, the desire to isolate and study a particular aspect of a behavioral or pharmacological effect must be tempered by the need to understand its functional relevance to the total behavior.

One successful approach to developing animal models of human states utilizes data from clinical pharmacology. Animal studies may reveal the primary neurochemical actions of clinically effective agents, thus providing insight into drug mechanisms. This, in turn, may lead to an understanding of the involved neurochemical pathways. The dopamine theory of schizophrenia is an important example of this process (Chapter 8). Clinically, the phenothiazines and butyrophenones are effective antipsychotics; neurochemically, they are blockers of dopamine receptors. Indeed, their clinical efficacy may be directly correlated with their effectiveness as dopamine receptor blockers. Amphetamine can produce stereotypy in animals and a behavioral state in humans which resembles paranoid schizophrenia. Again, these behavioral effects have been linked to a change in the functional activity of dopaminergic systems (Chapter 21).

Despite the apparent success of this approach to animal models, it is not without problems. A crucial, often tacit, assumption of such a model is that the same neurochemical mechanism underlies both animal and human behavior. Unfortunately, such a connection is frequently impossible to prove. For example, as discussed in Chapter 8, the existence of symptoms which are common to schizophrenia and amphetamine-induced psychosis need not imply that the same neurochemical systems are involved. Investigators have only recently begun to design strict criteria for comparing animal models to human state. For example, Matthysse and Haber (13) have extracted several pharmacological criteria from the clinical effects of antipsychotic agents. Animal models of schizophrenia such as amphetamine-induced stereotypies, self-stimulation, operant-behavior tasks, arousal, and conditioned avoidance all failed to meet even half of these criteria. Thus, extrapolations from animal models to human conditions must be made cautiously.

Behavioral models are also complicated by the difficulties of distinguishing between primary and secondary effects. For example, eating is often taken as an index for hunger. Unquestionably, a change in hunger should appear as a change in eating patterns. The converse need not be true. Take, for example, the ability of hypothalamic lesions to

produce aphagia in rats. Animals with these lesions will eventually recover, if they are force fed for several weeks (14). Studies of these recovered animals reveal that they are much more sensitive to dilute
quinine solutions than are normal controls, suggesting that the aphagia
probably results from a secondary effect on eating, rather than from a
destruction of the "hunger drive." Such secondary effects can totally
invalidate investigations both of animal models and of human states
(cf. Chapter 5).

Similar difficulties can arise in neurochemical studies of behavior.
Although a biological change can elicit behaviors, behaviors can also
induce biological changes. This is a particular problem in human studies, in which manipulations are naturally minimized. For example, cerebrospinal fluid concentrations of the dopamine metabolite homovanillic
acid (HVA) increase during mania, suggesting a possible connection
between mania and increased dopaminergic activity (Chapter 10).
However, a similar increase in homovanillic acid has been seen with
depressed patients who merely mimicked manic hyperactivity (15).
Thus, the increased homovanillic acid appears more to result from
mania than to reflect a cause of it. However, despite such problems,
attempts to assess human functioning have a great deal to offer, particularly when both their clinical and their chemical aspects are carefully
considered.

CONCLUSION

The difficulties of understanding the functional interactions between
biological events in the brain and behavior activity are immense. And
yet, several developments in both biochemical and behavioral approaches to the brain offer particular promise.

It is becoming increasingly apparent that past efforts to associate a
given behavior with a single neurotransmitter are much too restrictive.
With the development of techniques which permit the simultaneous
measurement of numerous neuroregulators, scientists have begun to explore the possibilities of interactions among these substances. Furthermore, the ability to monitor the electrical and neurochemical activity

of the brain throughout a behavior promises to expand our understanding of temporal, as well as physical, interactions among neuroregulators and between neuroregulators and behavior.

Combinations of behavioral, neurophysiological, and neurochemical analyses are also essential. Many of the potential applications of neurophysiology are described in Chapter 4. Electrical recordings of brain activity cannot tell us what is happening at the synapse, but they may provide an important adjunct for comparing human and animal systems. They may also serve as excellent monitors of brain function during a behavior, offering a timeline upon which to mark changes in neuroregulator activity. In addition, our expanding knowledge of neuroregulators fosters the development of increasingly stringent criteria for comparing animal and human behaviors. Finally, the powerful genetic factors which appear to influence some neuroregulatory processes may also find important applications in developing and investigating animal models of human behavior (16,17).

Interactions between neuroregulators and behavior are the essence of psychopharmacology. Empirical observations that many psychoactive compounds interfere with or mimic normal neuronal function have repeatedly been instrumental in expanding our knowledge of brain mechanisms. As our understanding of these mechanisms has grown, so too has our ability to rationally develop better and more specific drugs with which to manipulate them. Many of those drugs have proven to be valuable not only to the basic scientist but also to the clinician.

REFERENCES

1. Roberts, E. and Hammerschlag, R. An overview of transmission, *In: Basic Neurochemistry*. R. W. Albers, G. J. Siegel, R. Katzman, and B. W. Arganoff, *eds.*, Boston: Little, Brown, 1972, pp. 83–88.
2. Reis, D. J. Consideration of some specific behaviors or disease. *J. Psychiatr. Res. 11*:145–148, 1974.
3. Koelle, G. B. Neurohumoral transmission and the autonomic nervous system. *In: The Pharmacalogical Basis of Therapeutics*, 5th ed. L. S. Goodman and A. Gilman, *eds.*, New York: Macmillan, 1975, pp. 404–444.
4. Axelrod, J. Neurotransmitters. *In: Progress in Psychobiology. Readings from Scientific American* Ser. R. F. Thompson, ed. San Francisco: Freeman, 1976, pp. 122–129.
5. Von Euler, U. S. Historical background for studies on neurotransmitter release. *In: Neurotransmitter Function: Basic and Clinical Aspects*. W. Fields, *ed.*, New York: Stratton Intercontinental, 1977, pp. 1–10.
6. Holman, R. B., Elliott, G. R., and Barchas, J. D. Perspectives in behavioral neurochemistry. *In: Essays in Neurochemistry and Neuropharmacology*. Vol. 2. M. B. H. Youdim and W. Lovenberg, *eds.*, London: John Wiley and Sons, in press.
7. Sparber, S. B. Neurochemical changes associated with schedule-controlled behavior. *Fed. Proc. 34*:1802–1812, 1975.
8. Holman, R. B., Elliott, G. R., and Barchas, J. D. Neuroregulators and sleep mechanisms. *Ann. Rev. Med. 26*:499–520, 1975.
9. Ferster, C. B. and Skinner, B. F. *Schedules of Reinforcement*. Irvington: Century Psychology Series, 1957.
10. Iversen, S. D. and Iversen, L. L. *Behavioral Pharmacology*. New York: Oxford University Press, 1975.
11. Overton, D. A. Drugs and learning. *In: Behavioral Analysis of Drug Action: Research and Commentary*. J. A. Harvey, *ed.*, Glenview: Scott, Foresman and Co., 1971, pp. 55–83.
12. Harvey, J. A. Complexities of drug analysis. *In: Behavioral Analysis of Drug Action: Research and Commentary*. J. A. Harvey, *ed.*, Glenview: Scott, Foresman and Co., 1971, pp. 114–115.
13. Matthysse, S. and Haber, S. Animal models of schizophrenia. *In: Model Systems in Biological Psychiatry*. D. J. Ingle and H. M. Shein, *eds.*, Cambridge: The MIT Press, 1975, pp. 4–25.
14. Teitelbaum, P. and Stellar, E. Recovery from the failure to eat produced by hypothalamic lesions. *Science 120*:894–895, 1954.
15. Post, R. M. and Goodwin, F. K. Simulated behavior states: an approach to specificity in psychobiological research. *Biol. Psychiatry 7*:237–254, 1973.
16. Barchas, J. D., Ciaranello, R. D., Dominic, J. A., Deguchi, T., Orenberg, E. K., Renson, J., and Kessler, S. Genetic aspects of monoamine mechanisms. *In: Neuropsychopharmacology of Monoamines and Their Regulatory Enzymes*. E. Usdin, *ed.*, New York: Raven Press, 1975, pp. 195–204.
17. Fieve, R. R., Rosenthal, D., and Brill, H. *Genetic Research in Psychiatry*. Baltimore: Johns Hopkins University Press, 1975.

2 | Catecholamine Neuroregulators

ROLAND D. CIARANELLO and

ROBERT L. PATRICK

AN OVERVIEW OF THE NEURON

Both this chapter and Chapter 3 rely heavily upon an understanding of current concepts about a "typical" neuron, an idealized model of which is illustrated in Figure 2-1. Although much of this picture has been constructed from work in peripheral sympathetic systems of animals, many of the general "features" appear to apply to neurons in human brains.

The cell body has the general function of maintaining neuronal integrity. Its nucleus contains DNA, in which is encoded information for all of the enzymes needed in normal cell function. Among the enzymes synthesized in the cell body are those involved in the synthetic and degradative pathways of the specific transmitter for that neuron. Cell bodies also contain mechanisms in their membranes to specifically take up the appropriate neurotransmitter precursor, such as tyrosine, choline, or tryptophan, from the surrounding milieu. Both precursor and enzymes are then transported down the axon to the nerve terminal. Specific transport systems are available for different materials. Thus, enzymes travel at rates which differ markedly from those for mitochondria or for amino acids. The transport systems require energy and can be blocked by colchicine and vinblastine—drugs which disrupt microtubular architecture.

All uptake, synthetic, degradative, and release processes occur at the nerve terminal. The synthetic enzymes may be either "soluble" in the cytoplasm or "insoluble" in association with membranes. The terminal contains structures, called vesicles or granules, which are specialized for the uptake, storage, and release of neurotransmitters. Terminal endings are also rich in mitochondria, which generate the metabolic energy required for these processes. In addition, mitochondria contain some important degradative enzymes, such as monoamine oxidase.

16

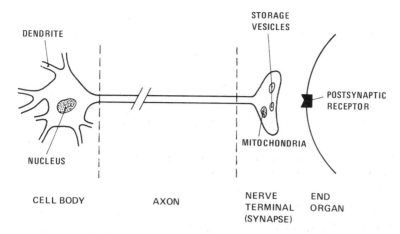

FIGURE 2-1. Schematic Representation of a Neuron

The cell body is the site of synthesis for synthetic and degradative enzymes and for storage vesicles. In addition, precursors are taken up into the cell from the surrounding milieu by specific uptake mechanisms. The axon transports enzymes, vesicles, and precursors from the cell body to the nerve terminals. In addition, it conducts electrical impulses of nervous transmission. The nerve terminal is the site of transmitter synthesis and storage. With electrical excitation, the transmitters are released into the synaptic cleft, where they activate the postsynaptic receptors. Transmitters are then degraded or taken back up into the nerve terminal by active reuptake mechanisms, thus ending the synaptic transmission.

Depolarization of the nerve cell membrane by an action potential results in changes in the flux of sodium, potassium, and calcium. Calcium appears to be critical in the transmitter release process. Following depolarization, the transmitter is released from its storage vesicle. Although precise release mechanisms have still not been entirely elucidated, the first step appears to involve fusion of the vesicle to the membrane of the nerve terminal. The vesicular contents are then extruded into the synaptic cleft by a process known as exocytosis. In addition to the neurotransmitter, other associated materials are also released. Thus, peripheral adrenergic nerves release norepinephrine, adenosine triphosphate (ATP), and dopamine-β-hydroxylase.

Once released, the neurotransmitter diffuses across the synaptic cleft, where it interacts with the postsynaptic receptor. Receptor dynamics are currently one of the most active and controversial areas of neurobiology, and our understanding of them is far from complete.

Receptor protein molecules are an intimate constituent of the cell membrane. Their structure is highly specific for a particular transmitter, and they bind the transmitter in a "lock-and-key" arrangement. Binding of the transmitter appears to alter the receptor conformation, resulting in changes in the membrane permeability for sodium and potassium, which permit propagation of the action potential. In addition, receptor-transmitter binding initiates a complex chain of intracellular reactions within the postsynaptic effector cell, probably mediated via adenylate cyclase and cyclic AMP, which stimulate the cell to carry out its particular function (Chapter 3).

The association of transmitter to receptor is an equilibrium process in which transmitter molecules are constantly dissociating from the receptor, freeing it to be restimulated. In the cholinergic system, neurotransmitter action is terminated at the postsynaptic membrane by acetylcholinesterase (Chapter 3). For catechol- and indoleamines, termination of transmitter action depends upon washout of the synaptic cleft by microcirculatory perfusion, postsynaptic degradation, or reuptake of the transmitter into the presynaptic neuron, the last being the most important. The reuptake process is highly dependent on sodium and is an active transport system which can be saturated by high concentrations of transmitter.

CATECHOLAMINE NEUROTRANSMITTERS

The catecholamines are important biological agents derived from the amino acid tyrosine. The principal members of this class of compounds are dopamine, norepinephrine, and epinephrine. In biological systems the catecholamines act both as hormones and as neurotransmitters. Although they are ubiquitously distributed, the catecholamines are manufactured primarily in the adrenal glands, the peripheral sympathetic neurons, and the brain (1,2).

The adrenal medulla synthesizes the bulk of the catecholamines which subserve hormonal roles. Embryologically, the adrenal gland consists of a glucocorticoid-secreting cortex of mesenchymal origin and a catecholamine-secreting medulla derived from the neural crest. The adrenal medulla receives input from the splanchnic nerves, which play a major role in regulating the levels of medullary catecholamines. The splanchnic axons have cell bodies in the lateral horn of the spinal cord and form cholinergic synapses directly onto the adrenal medullary chromaffin cells. Thus, the adrenal medulla is actually a modified sympathetic ganglion in which the medullary cells represent the sympathetic postsynaptic neurons. Epinephrine is the principal catecholamine synthesized in the adrenal medulla. Once synthesized, epinephrine is released via the adrenal venous effluent into general circulation. All of the epinephrine and a small portion of the norepinephrine found in the peripheral circulation comes from the adrenal medulla. Epinephrine has important hormonal actions on the heart, plays a major role in lipolysis and glycogenolysis, and interacts with the thyroid hormones to potentiate their action.

Dopamine and norepinephrine appear to function primarily as central and peripheral neurotransmitters. The peripheral sympathetic neurons synthesize norepinephrine for direct release onto the smooth musculature of blood vessels, digestive tract organs, various secretory glands, and structures in the face and head. Norepinephrine is the neurotransmitter in the sympathetic nervous system, where it facilitates smooth muscle contraction, leading to vasoconstriction, cardiac acceleration, and glandular secretion. Circulating norepinephrine is derived almost exclusively from peripheral sympathetic nerve terminals innervating the vasculature.

The brain synthesizes and degrades a substantial portion of the total body content of catecholamines. Catecholamines in the brain are synthesized mainly within central nervous system neurons, since the peripherally formed catecholamines cross the blood-brain barrier only to a limited extent. These central catecholamines, principally dopamine and norepinephrine, act as neurotransmitters.

SYNTHESIS

The metabolic pathways involved in catecholamine synthesis and degradation are shown in Figure 2-2. Catecholamines are derived from the amino acid tyrosine, which is taken up into the neuronal cell body. Tyrosine then undergoes a series of enzymatic transformations into active neurotransmitters. The enzymes catalyzing these reactions are found in the adrenal gland, in neurons of the sympathetic nervous system, and in adrenergic and dopaminergic neuronal tracts in the brain.

The first step in catecholamine biosynthesis is the conversion of tyrosine to dihydroxyphenylalanine (L-DOPA) by tyrosine hydroxylase (3,4). Tyrosine hydroxylase is found in the cytoplasmic and membrane fractions of the nerve cell. It is an iron-containing, mixed-function oxidase which utilizes tetrahyrobiopterin as its electron-donating cofactor. There is evidence that this enzyme is the rate-limiting step in the catecholamine biosynthetic pathway. L-DOPA is then converted to dopamine by the soluble enzyme, L-aromatic amino acid decarboxylase (5). This enzyme, which also converts 5-hydroxytryptophan to 5-hydroxytryptamine, requires pyridoxal phosphate as a cofactor. Despite its obvious significance as a common step in the biosynthesis of two neurotransmitters and its ubiquitous distribution and in defiance of an extensive investigational effort, little is known about the regulation of this enzyme. The conversion of dopamine to norepinephrine is catalyzed by dopamine-β-hydroxylase (6). This enzyme is found in both the soluble and the vesicular membrane fractions of the nerve cell. Like tyrosine hydroxylase, dopamine-β-hydroxylase is a mixed-function oxidase which utilizes ascorbic acid as its cofactor; it is a copper-containing enzyme. The conversion of norepinephrine to epinephrine occurs primarily in the adrenal medulla; a very limited amount of synthesis also occurs in discrete areas of the brainstem. The enzyme which catalyzes this reaction is phenylethanolamine N-methyltransferase, which utilizes S-adenosylmethionine as its methyl donor (7).

CATABOLISM

The inactivation of the catecholamines is carried out by several enzymes acting in an extensive pathway (Fig. 2-2) (1,2). Monoamine oxidase (MAO) is a mitochondrial enzyme which acts on a number of catechol- and indoleamine substrates. MAO is the principal route of inactivation of *intraneuronal* catecholamines; it is an oxidative deaminase which converts the catecholamine to its corresponding aldehyde. Catecholamines which have been O-methylated by catechol O-methyltransferase are also substrates for MAO. Catechol O-methyltransferase is a soluble, ubiquitously distributed enzyme which is present in high concentrations in liver and kidney. It utilizes S-adenosylmethionine as

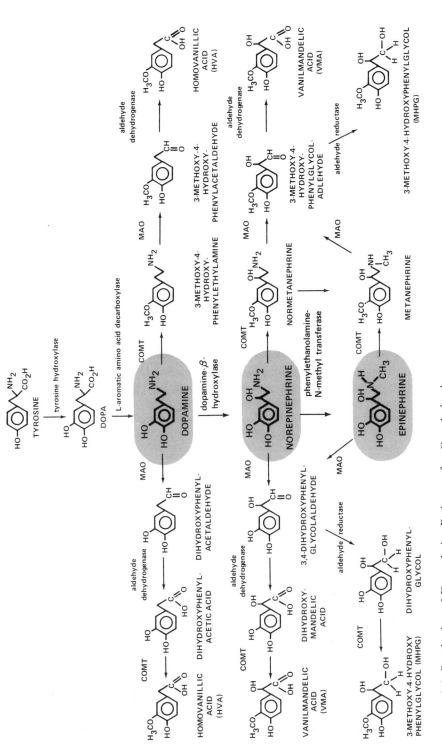

FIGURE 2-2. Synthetic and Degradative Pathways for Catecholamines

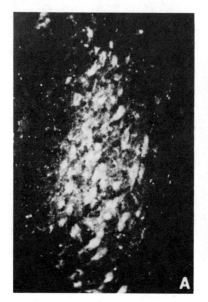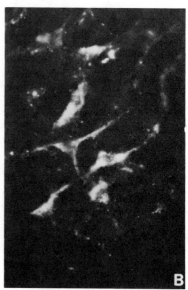

FIGURE 2-3. Catecholaminergic Cells in the Central Nervous System
Monoamine containing cells are usually localized in brainstem nuclei. The cells of the locus coeruleus (Fig. 2-3A, × 240) contain norepinephrine, and the cells of the substantia nigra area contain dopamine (Fig. 2-3B, × 760). Note that the locus coeruleus cells are relatively compact and that the dopamine cells have a nonfluorescent nucleus and multiple processes filled with transmitter. Typically, mono-

its methyl donor and is the principal *extraneuronal* route of catecholamine inactivation. Catechol O-methyltransferase acts on the catecholamines or their aldehydes, producing the corresponding O-methylated derivative.

The catechol aldehydes can undergo either oxidation or reduction to form the corresponding acid or alcohol. The relative formation of alcohol or acid derivatives appears to depend upon the precursor: β-hydroxylated catecholamines are metabolized to alcohols, while others are converted to the acid derivative. Thus, norepinephrine is metabolized primarily to its corresponding alcohol, 3-methoxy-4-hydroxyphenylglycol (MHPG), while dopamine is converted primarily to its acid derivative, homovanillic acid (HVA). The conversion to the alcohol (glycol) is catalyzed by aldehyde reductase; the formation of the acid is mediated by aldehyde dehydrogenase. The concentration of

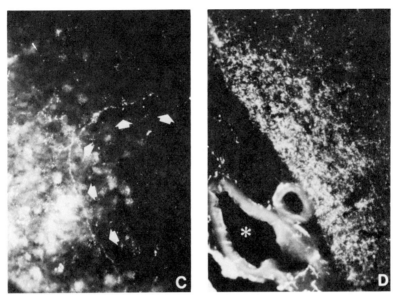

FIGURE 2-3 (con't.)
amine cell groups project through long axonal pathways into multiple brain areas. They terminate either in fine beaded axons (see arrows, Fig. 2-3C; cortex × 500) or in dense terminal ramifications. (Fig. 2-3C; olfactory tubercule × 450). Next to the fine punctate terminal area of Fig. 2-3D is a blood vessel with its peripheral sympathetic innervation. Sections were prepared by the glyoxylic acid-cryostat procedure (10).

the alcohol or acid end products is frequently the only index of catecholaminergic activity which can be measured in human clinical studies, so their metabolism is of obvious importance to investigators.

Any of the above reactions inactivates the catecholamine molecule. The alcohol and acid products are eliminated from the body after conjugation with sulfate, which further solubilizes them and promotes renal clearance.

ANATOMY OF CATECHOLAMINE PATHWAYS

Detailed information about the distribution of dopamine and norepinephrine comes primarily from histofluorescence procedures (8,9). Figure 2-3 shows catecholamine cells, axons, and terminals as visualized by the glyoxylic acid histofluorescence method (10). Recently it has been possible to clearly differentiate norepinephrine pathways from dopamine pathways, using specific antibodies against dopamine-β-hydroxylase (11). As illustrated in Figure 2-4, specific brainstem nuclei contain a particular transmitter. For example, norepinephrine is found in the cells of the locus ceruleus, while dopamine is present in the cells of the substantia nigra. Norepinephrine cells project caudally to the spinal cord; dorsally to the cerebellum; and rostrally to a wide variety of structures, including cortex, hippocampus, hypothalamus, and septum. Dopamine neurons project rostrally to the caudate-putamen and cortex and to limbic structures such as nucleus accumbens, olfactory tubercle, and septum.

REGULATION OF SYNTHESIS

Clearly, the rate at which catecholamine production and inactivation proceeds is a major factor in the regulation of catecholaminergic neuronal processes and, therefore, of behavior. Catecholamine synthesis can be modified in the following two ways: *activation* or *inhibition* of one or more of the biosynthetic enzymes, so that the reaction velocity is altered without a change in the number of enzyme molecules (12); and change in the *number* of molecules of one or more of the enzymes in the pathway (13). Both processes are extremely important in regulating catecholamine synthesis *in vivo*.

Certain drugs can affect the activity of the catecholamine synthesizing enzymes, thus modifying the rate of product formation. Activation or inhibition of the enzymes appears to permit short-term modulation of synthesis. This can involve a direct effect on the enzyme, as occurs with competitive inhibition by a substrate analogue. Alternatively, it can occur indirectly through end-product feedback inhibition. Such inhibition is a common process in multistep enzyme pathways and occurs when the final reaction product, e.g. norepinephrine, binds to or "feeds back on" one of the enzymes in the sequence, thus modulating its activity. Feedback regulation in multistep pathways can be either stimulatory or inhibitory. In the catecholamine pathway, norepinephrine inhibits tyrosine hydroxylase activity. Drugs which block intraneuronal catecholamine inactivation, such as the MAO inhibitors, cause a secondary increase in intraneuronal catecholamine concentration; the

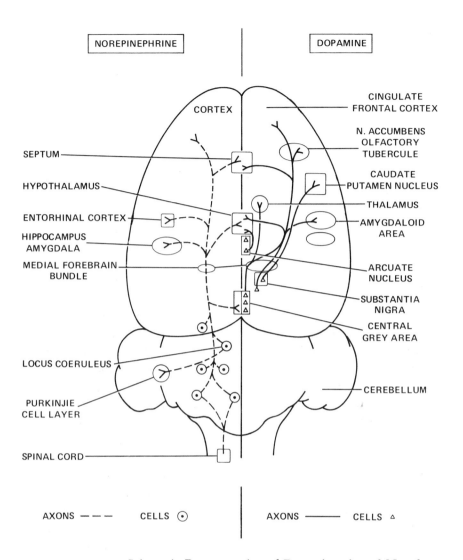

FIGURE 2-4. Schematic Representation of Dopaminergic and Noradrenergic Pathways in the Rat Brain

Norepinephrine pathways and cell bodies are indicated on the left side of the illustration, while dopamine projections are shown on the right side. We wish to thank Dr. Stanley J. Watson for supplying this drawing, adapted from Lindvall and Björklund (8) and Ungerstedt (9).

compensatory effect of this increase is a reduction in the rate of norepinephrine synthesis via feedback inhibition of tyrosine hydroxylase. Similarly, depletion of catecholamines and a compensatory increase in the rate of synthesis can occur after the administration of certain depleting agents. Such a regulatory process dampens the effect of environmental perturbations.

Changes in the number of enzyme molecules appear to involve long-term regulatory modulation. Chronic stress, or other situations calling for prolonged elevations of catecholamine formation, result in an increase in the tissue levels of the catecholamine synthesizing enzymes. These changes occur more slowly and are longer-lasting than are the transient effects of enzyme activation or inhibition. Powerful controls regulate the levels of the catecholamine synthesizing enzymes. In the adrenal medulla, steady-state levels of tyrosine hydroxylase, dopamine-β-hydroxylase, and phenylethanolamine N-methyltransferase are controlled by adrenal glucocorticoids. Reduction of glucocorticoids, as occurs with pituitary removal or destruction, profoundly reduces the levels of these three enzymes, possibly by accelerating their degradation by proteolysis (14). However, the glucocorticoids seem to control only steady-state enzyme levels, since neither exogenous administration of glucocorticoids nor excessive endogenous glucocorticoid production increase the level of the enzymes. Increases in enzyme levels are mediated via the splanchnic neuronal input to the medullary cell; increased neuronal activity enhances the rate of synthesis of the enzymes (13–15); this has been termed transsynaptic induction.

The role of glucocorticoids in regulating biosynthetic enzyme levels in the peripheral sympathetic neuron and in the brain is not well understood. There is some evidence that circulating glucocorticoids may play a role in maintaining tyrosine hydroxylase activity in sympathetic ganglia, but practically nothing is known about the importance of glucocorticoids to catecholamine synthesis in the brain. In these latter two systems, regulation of catecholamine synthesis is predominantly determined by activity of the nerves making synaptic formations with the catecholaminergic neurons. Increased presynaptic input induces the synthesis of tyrosine hydroxylase and dopamine-β-hydroxylase in peripheral sympathetic ganglia and in central adrenergic neurons.

INTERACTIONS OF DRUGS WITH THE CATECHOLAMINE SYSTEMS

From the description of the catecholamine systems given above, it is apparent that drugs can affect these systems in a variety of ways. In this section, we will describe some of the known effects of drugs on synthesis, storage, release, reuptake, inactivation and receptor interaction (Table 2-1). The primary emphasis will be on drugs which are commonly used in psychiatry and also upon agents whose psychoactive properties have caused them to be designated as drugs of abuse. Several of these drugs, including alcohol, opiates, amphetamines, cocaine, sedatives, and hallucinogens are treated separately in Section III and will not be discussed in detail here.

Drugs Affecting Catecholamine Synthesis

Catecholamine synthesis can be blocked quickly by administration of inhibitors of tyrosine hydroxylase. Tyrosine analogues such as α-methyl-p-tyrosine produce a rapid decline in tissue catecholamine content and are used experimentally to estimate the catecholamine turnover rate. Inhibition of tyrosine hydroxylase blocks the synthesis of both dopamine and norepinephrine. Specific inhibition of norepinephrine synthesis is seen after administration of dopamine-β-hydroxylase inhibitors such as fusaric acid and disulfiram (Antabuse). Fusaric acid has been tried in experimental clinical studies as an antihypertensive and as an antimanic agent (Chapter 12). Disulfiram also inhibits aldehyde dehydrogenase and is widely used as a deterrent in the treatment of chronic alcoholism (Chapter 23). Catecholamine formation may be increased by compounds which bypass the rate-limiting tyrosine hydroxylase step, such as L-DOPA. Parkinson's disease is apparently caused by damage to the nigrostriatal dopaminergic pathway. The symptoms of this disease are quite responsive to L-DOPA. Analogously, dihydroxyphenylserine (DOPS) has been suggested as a pharmacological precursor for norepinephrine; however, its conversion to norepinephrine may not occur in brain.

Certain drugs may alter the rate of catecholamine formation by affecting the number of molecules of transmitter-synthesizing enzymes. For example, after three days of reserpine treatment, the amount of tyrosine hydroxylase in the rat adrenal increases by threefold. This increase represents an induction of synthesis of new enzyme and is me-

TABLE 2-1.

EFFECTS OF VARIOUS DRUGS ON CATECHOLAMINERGIC FUNCTION

CLASS	PRIMARY EFFECT	SECONDARY EFFECT	CLINICAL ACTION
Antipsychotics	Dopamine receptor blockade	Increased dopamine synthesis	
Phenothiazines			Antipsychotic
Butyrophenones			Antipsychotic
Thioxanthines			Antipsychotic
Antimanics	Decreased membrane permeability; decreased transmitter release	Decreased catecholamine synthesis	
Lithium			Antimanic
Antidepressants			
Tricyclic antidepressants	Reuptake inhibition		Antidepressant
MAO inhibitors	Metabolic blockade		Antidepressant
Synthesis stimulators			
L-DOPA	Increased formation of dopamine		Antiparkinsonian
Synthesis blockers			
α-Methyl-*p*-tyrosine	Tyrosine hydroxylase inhibition		Under investigation
Fusaric acid	Dopamine-β-hydroxylase inhibition		Under investigation
Disulfiram	Dopamine-β-hydroxylase inhibition		Alcohol abuse deterrent*
Amine depleters and/or releasers			
Reserpine	Depletion of intraneuronal catecholamine stores via blockade of uptake into vesicle	Induction of enzyme synthesis	Antihypertensive
Amphetamine	Increased concentrations of catecholamines in the synaptic cleft via stimulation of release and/or inhibition of reuptake		Stimulant
Tyramine	Displacement of catecholamines from storage vesicles	Feedback inhibition of catecholamine synthesis	Vasopressor

* See Chapter 23.

diated via increased activity of the splanchnic nerves. Reserpine-induced increases in the synthesis of new tyrosine hydroxylase in the central nervous system have also been reported. It is possible, therefore, that drug administration in humans can produce profound alterations not only in the activity of the catecholamine synthesizing enzymes but also in the actual amount of enzyme.

Storage

Catecholamine-depleting agents markedly reduce the intraneuronal levels of transmitter. Reserpine reduces the catecholamine stores by preventing the uptake of catecholamines into the storage vesicles. In animals, this drug produces a marked sedation which can be antagonized by L-DOPA administration. In humans, reserpine administration may be associated with depressive syndromes (Chapter 29). One complication in interpreting the various effects of reserpine is that other biogenic amines are also markedly depleted by the drug. This is particularly true for the serotonergic system (Chapter 3). It therefore becomes difficult to determine exactly which system is responsible for a change seen after reserpine treatment. In animals, a more selective depletion of catecholamine stores can be achieved by direct administration of 6-hydroxydopamine into the central nervous system. This compound is concentrated in catecholamine neurons and chemically destroys them.

Release

Various drugs facilitate the release of catecholamines into the synaptic cleft. Amphetamine is one such agent (Chapter 21). The indirectly active sympathomimetic agents, such as tyramine, cause a displacement of catecholamines from their storage vesicles into the cellular cytoplasmic fraction, from which they can efflux to the cell exterior. The pressor action of tyramine does not occur in animals depleted of their catecholamine stores. The inhibition of catecholamine synthesis produced by tyramine is thought to result from the intracellular buildup of catecholamines. Electrically induced release of labeled catecholamines from rat brain tissue slices has been found to be inhibited by antipsychotics, prostaglandins, acetylcholine, ethanol, and morphine, demonstrating that the release process itself represents a sensitive site for drug-transmitter interaction. Lithium carbonate, the drug of choice for manic-depressive illness, also inhibits norepinephrine efflux from the nerve terminal (Chapter 12). This apparently results from a decrease in membrane permeability. Chronic lithium treatment also causes a decrease in dopamine synthesis in rat brain striatal slices.

Reuptake

The tricyclic antidepressants, such as imipramine (Tofranil), are very effective inhibitors of norepinephrine and 5-hydroxytryptamine reuptake in the central nervous system. They are relatively ineffective, however, in inhibiting dopamine uptake in the striatum. Recently, several compounds have been developed which offer a greater selectivity in specifically inhibiting either norepinephrine or 5-hydroxytryptamine uptake; this has been correlated, in part, with efficacy in treatment of different types of depressive disorders (Chapter 11). Amphetamine and cocaine also block catecholamine uptake (Chapter 21).

Inactivation

Attempts to alter catecholamine inactivation in psychiatric patients have centered around inhibition of MAO activity. As described in Chapter 10, this line of investigation stemmed from the discovery that iproniazid produced mood elevation and inhibited MAO. Other MAO inhibitors which have been utilized in the treatment of depression include nialamide (Niamid), phenelzine (Nardil), and tranylcypromine (Parnate). As with reuptake inhibitors, efforts have been made to develop MAO inhibitors which can selectively inhibit specific transmitter inactivation. Recent pharmacological evidence suggests that at least two types of MAO isoenzymes—designated Types A and B—can be identified in rat and human brain. Norepinephrine and 5-hydroxytryptamine are preferred substrates for the Type A isoenzyme, and clorgyline is a specific inhibitor. β-Phenylethylamine is a preferred substrate for Type B, and deprenyl is a selective inhibitor. Tyramine, tryptamine, and dopamine are good substrates for both forms of MAO.

Receptor Interaction

Antipsychotic drugs appear to block dopamine receptors (Chapters 8 and 9). Apomorphine is thought to produce a decrease in dopamine synthesis by activating dopamine receptors, causing neuronal feedback inhibition. This effect of apomorphine is blocked by the antipsychotics. Antipsychotics also block the ability of dopamine to activate striatal, dopamine-rensitive adenylate cyclase. The antipsychotics cause a marked increase in the rate of dopamine synthesis in areas of the brain such as the striatum and the nucleus accumbens—areas which are known to contain a high concentration of dopaminergic nerve terminals. This increase in synthesis is probably a secondary effect of receptor blockade.

REFERENCES

1. Molinoff, P. B. and Axelrod, J. Biochemistry of catecholamines. *Ann. Rev. Biochem. 40:*465–500, 1971.
2. Axelrod, J. The fate of noradrenaline in the sympathetic neurone. *Harvey Lectures, Series 67:*175–197, 1973.
3. Udenfriend, S. Tyrosine hydroxylase. *Pharmacol. Rev. 18:*43–51, 1966.
4. Musacchio, J. M. and Carviso, G. L. Properties of tyrosine hydroxylase. *In: Frontiers in Catecholamine Research.* E. Usdin and S. Snyder, *eds.,* New York: Pergamon, 1973, pp. 47–52.
5. Dairman, W., Christenson, J., and Udenfriend, S. Characterization of dopa decarboxylase. *In: Frontiers in Catecholamine Research.* E. Usdin and S. Snyder, *eds.,* New York: Pergamon, 1973, pp. 61–68.
6. Kaufman, S. Dopamine β-hydroxylase. *In: Catecholamines and Schizophrenia.* S. Matthysse and S. Kety, *eds.,* New York: Pergamon, 1973, pp. 303–316.
7. Ciaranello, R. D. Regulation of phenylethanolamine N-methyl transferase. *In: Frontiers in Catecholamine Research.* E. Usdin and S. Snyder, *eds.,* New York: Pergamon, 1973, pp. 101–107.
8. Lindvall, O. and Björklund, A. The organization of the ascending catecholamine neuron systems in the rat brain as revealed by glyoxylic acid fluorescence method. *Acta. Physiol. Scand., Suppl. 412:*1–18, 1974.
9. Ungerstedt, U. Stereotaxic mapping of the monoamine pathways in the rat brain. *Acta Physiol. Scand., Suppl. 367:*1–48, 1971.
10. Watson, S. J. and Barchas, J. D. Histofluorescence in the unperfused CNS by cryostat and glyoxylic acid: a preliminary report. *Psychopharmacol. Commun. 1:*523–531, 1975.
11. Hartman, B. R. Immunofluorescence of dopamine-β-hydroxylase: application of improved methodology to the localization of the peripheral and central noradrenergic nervous tissue. *J. Histochem. Cytochem. 21:*312–332, 1973.
12. Weiner, N., Bjur, R., Lee, F-L., Becker, G., and Mosimann, W. F. Studies on the mechanism of regulation of tyrosine hydroxylase activity during nerve stimulation. *In: Frontiers in Catecholamine Research.* E. Usdin and S. Snyder, *eds.,* New York: Pergamon, 1973, pp. 211–222.
13. Thoenen, H., Otten, U., and Oesch, F. Trans-synaptic regulation of tyrosine hydroxylase. *In: Frontiers in Catecholamine Research.* E. Usdin and S. Snyder, *eds.,* New York: Pergamon, 1973, pp. 179–186.
14. Ciaranello, R. D., Wooten, G. F., and Axelrod, J. Regulation of dopamine β-hydroxylase in rat adrenal glands. *J. Biol. Chem. 250:* 3204–3211, 1975.
15. Joh, T. H., Geghman, C., and Reis, D. Immunochemical demonstration of increased tyrosine hydroxylase protein in sympathetic ganglia and adrenal medulla elicited by reserpine. *Proc. Nat. Acad. Sci. 70:* 2767–2771, 1973.

3 | Indoleamines and Other Neuroregulators

GLEN R. ELLIOTT, ARTHUR M. EDELMAN,

JEAN F. RENSON, and PHILIP A. BERGER

INTRODUCTION

Numerous substances have been proposed as neurotransmitters and neuroregulators. The catecholamines were described in Chapter 2. Other substances, including 5-hydroxytryptamine, acetylcholine, and γ-aminobutyric acid (GABA) have also been implicated as neuroregulators which might be involved in the actions of psychoactive drugs. Generally, mechanisms which control the synthesis and inactivation of these compounds are still only poorly understood. However, recent advances in monitoring and manipulating individual cells in the brain, in measuring small amounts of neuroregulators and metabolites, and in visualizing specific compounds and enzymes in the brain have greatly increased our ability to obtain answers about important functional aspects of these other neuroregulators.

5-HYDROXYTRYPTAMINE

History

5-Hydroxytryptamine was first shown to be an endogenous component of the body through work by two independent investigators (1). In the early 1950's, Page and his colleagues were examining a substance in blood which produced vasoconstriction. They were able to isolate this substance, which they called serotonin, and to identify it as 5-hydroxytryptamine. At the same time, Erspamer and his co-workers in Italy were investigating enteramine, a substance from enterochromaffin cells of the intestine, which induced contraction of smooth muscles. Enteramine, too, proved to be 5-hydroxytryptamine.

Connections between 5-hydroxytryptamine and psychopharmacology came almost immediately after it was found in mammalian tissues. Lysergic acid diethylamide (LSD), which is structurally related to 5-hydroxytryptamine, had just been discovered to be a potent hallucinogen (Chapter 20); this was followed by demonstrations that LSD is a potent inhibitor of the effects of 5-hydroxytryptamine on smooth muscle and that 5-hydroxytryptamine is present in brain. These discoveries had a major impact upon investigations of schizophrenia (Chapter 8). In the intervening twenty years, 5-hydroxytryptamine has also been implicated in other aspects of physiology, including sleep, sexual behavior, pain sensitivity, thermoregulation, and control of pituitary hormones (2).

SYNTHESIS

The metabolic pathways of 5-hydroxytryptamine are summarized in Figure 3-1. Tryptophan is an essential amino acid, which means that it must be supplied by the diet. It is taken up into neuronal cells by an active process. The next step, hydroxylation of tryptophan by tryptophan hydroxylase, is the rate-limiting process in the synthesis of 5-hydroxytryptamine. This enzyme has recently been purified from mammalian brain (3). The purified enzyme requires both molecular oxygen and a pteridine cofactor, tetrahydrobiopterin, for activity. Studies of the enzyme kinetics with respect to substrate concentrations suggest that, with normal *in vivo* concentrations of tryptophan, the enzymatic activity is below maximum capacity. As discussed later, this may be an important mechanism for controlling the synthesis of 5-hydroxytryptamine. 5-Hydroxytryptophan, the product of tryptophan hydroxylation, is decarboxylated rapidly by L-aromatic amino acid decarboxylase (5-hydroxytryptophan decarboxylase). This latter enzyme is thought to be identical with DOPA decarboxylase (Chapter 2), although some investigators argue that they are similar but distinct (4).

CATABOLISM

As indicated in Figure 3-1, the major metabolic fate of 5-hydroxytryptamine is oxidation. The first step of this process is catalyzed by

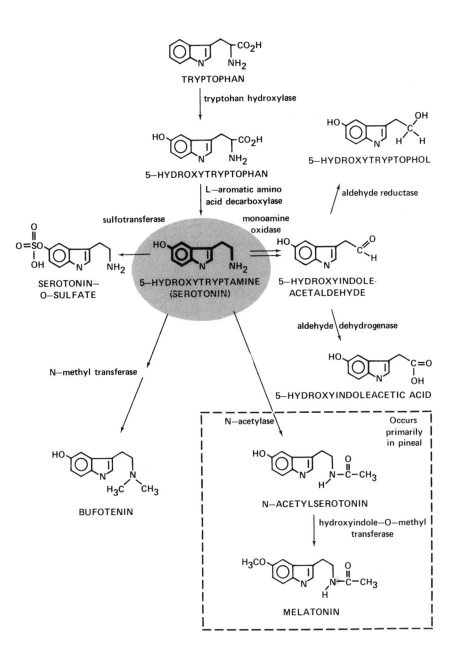

FIGURE 3-1. Synthetic and Metabolic Pathways for 5-Hydroxytryptamine

35

the mitochondrial enzyme monoamine oxidase (MAO), which has already been discussed as a metabolic enzyme for the catecholamines (Chapter 2). MAO exists in at least two forms, termed Types A and B. 5-Hydroxytryptamine is a better substrate for Type A.

The product of MAO, 5-hydroxyindoleacetaldehyde, is rapidly converted to either 5-hydroxytryptophol or 5-hydroxyindoleacetic acid, depending upon the relative abundance of the enzymatic cofactors NAD and NADH (4). Both the reductase and the dehydrogenase catalyze the conversion of a variety of aldehyde substrates. Under normal conditions, 5-hydroxyindoleacetic acid is the major product, and investigators often monitor its concentration in cerebrospinal fluid as a rough indication of serotonergic activity in the brain. There are some situations in which this metabolic pattern is shifted. For example, under conditions of high blood concentrations of acetaldehyde following ethanol consumption, urinary excretion of 5-hydroxytryptophol increases, while that of 5-hydroxyindoleacetic acid declines. These changes have not been seen in the central nervous system, and their significance is unknown (see Chapter 20).

Conjugation by a sulphotransferase may also be an important metabolic pathway, with serotonin-O-sulfate accounting for about 33 percent of urinary metabolites of 5-hydroxytryptamine (5). Although 5-hydroxytryptamine has also been reported to be N-methylated, both the importance and the enzymatic mechanism of this reaction are unknown (6). Discovery of this pathway produced tremendous excitement, since it suggested a mechanism by which endogenous psychotogens might be formed; however, no consistent links have been established between these compounds and schizophrenia (Chapter 8). In the pineal, 5-hydroxytryptamine undergoes two additional reactions to form melatonin, which may act as a hormone.

ANATOMY OF SEROTONERGIC PATHWAYS

To date, maps of the serotonergic systems have relied upon data from chemical and electrical lesions, which deplete 5-hydroxytryptamine when they interrupt a pathway, and fluorescence histochemical methods, which visualize 5-hydroxytryptamine directly (4,7). These methods are now being supplemented by immunocytochemical techniques, since antibodies to purified tryptophan hydroxylase can be used to localize that essential synthetic enzyme. A fairly consistent and reasonably complete picture is available for serotonergic pathways in the rat brain (Fig. 3-2). Serotonergic cells are located primarily in the raphé nuclei, from which they send ascending axons to a wide variety of structures, including the limbic system and cortical areas. Descending serotonergic systems innervate the medulla and spinal cord. The good separation between cell bodies and terminal fields has been of great aid to investigations of the electrical and pharmacological properties of the serotonergic neurons (cf. Chapters 4 and 22).

REGULATORY MECHANISMS

Remarkably little is known about the controls on the serotonergic system. Studies of *in vitro* preparations of serotonergic nerve terminals have not been successful in elucidating such controls. As yet it is unclear whether these failures reflect our inability to ask the right question in the right way or the importance of control mechanisms which require relatively intact neuronal systems.

Control of Synthesis

Tryptophan, oxygen, and a pteridine cofactor are all required for the synthesis of 5-hydroxytryptophan. In theory, changes in the concentrations of any one of these can alter the rate of synthesis. Methods for selectively manipulating the pteridine cofactor *in vivo* are not available, and this potentially important aspect of control remains to be studied. Increasing the tissue content of oxygen markedly enhances the synthesis of 5-hydroxytryptamine (4); however, mechanisms which control the availability of tissue oxygen to specific enzymes are entirely unclear. Changes in tryptophan concentrations also produce changes in brain concentrations of 5-hydroxytryptamine (10). The physiological importance of this phenomenon remains controversial. Tryptophan concentrations vary markedly even over a single day and depend primarily upon dietary intake. Many investigators find it difficult to conceive of a neuroregulator system which is subject to the vagaries of a changing food supply. Tryptophan hydroxylase has not been shown to be inhibited by physiologically relevant concentrations

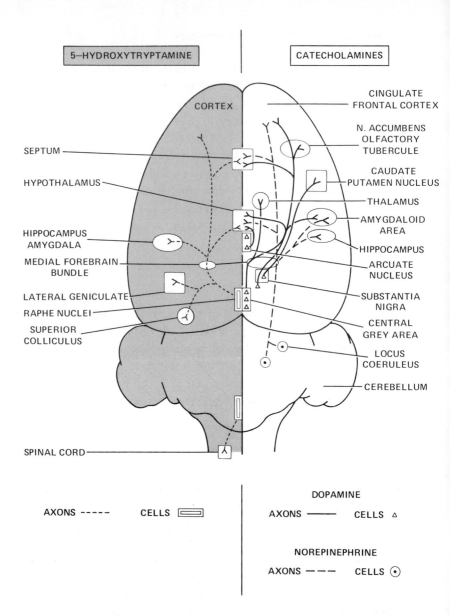

5–HYDROXYTRYPTAMINE | CATECHOLAMINES

CORTEX

CINGULATE
FRONTAL CORTEX

N. ACCUMBENS
OLFACTORY
TUBERCULE

SEPTUM

HYPOTHALAMUS

CAUDATE
PUTAMEN NUCLEUS

THALAMUS

AMYGDALOID
AREA

HIPPOCAMPUS
AMYGDALA

HIPPOCAMPUS

MEDIAL FOREBRAIN
BUNDLE

ARCUATE
NUCLEUS

LATERAL GENICULATE

RAPHE NUCLEI

SUBSTANTIA
NIGRA

SUPERIOR
COLLICULUS

CENTRAL
GREY AREA

LOCUS
COERULEUS

CEREBELLUM

SPINAL CORD

DOPAMINE

AXONS ----- CELLS ▭   AXONS ——— CELLS △

NOREPINEPHRINE

AXONS — — — CELLS ⊙

FIGURE 3-2. Schematic Representation of Pathways in the Rat Brain
Dopaminergic and noradrenergic pathways are also indicated for comparison. We wish to thank Dr. Stanley J. Watson for supplying this drawing, adapted from Ungerstedt (8) and Lindvall and Björklund (9).

of either 5-hydroxytryptophan or 5-hydroxytryptamine. Thus, feed-back inhibition, which plays such an important role for the catechol-amines (Chapter 2), does not seem to be a factor in this system.

Reuptake into Serotonergic Terminals

After its release into the synapse, 5-hydroxytryptamine is rapidly taken back into the presynaptic terminal ending by an active, energy-requiring process. It is not known whether there are physiological mechanisms for adjusting the activity of this system. However, inhibi-tion of this uptake mechanism is thought to be an important action of the tricyclic antidepressants (Chapter 11) and has been suggested as one of the effects of ethanol consumption (Chapter 20).

Neuronal Feedback

One aspect of serotonergic regulation in which significant progress has been made involves neuronal feedback loops. Aghajanian and his co-workers (11) have been particularly instrumental in helping to elaborate this mechanism. Direct application of 5-hydroxytryptamine to serotonergic cells in the raphé depresses their firing rate (7). This might provide a mechanism by which serotonergic cells can poten-tially inhibit their own firing by a feedback mechanism. Such a feed-back loop could provide the necessary balance to maintain the proper synthetic rate. This system has also been of major importance in elu-cidating the action of indoleamine hallucinogens (Chapter 22).

5-Hydroxytryptamine Receptors

Little is known about the receptor for 5-hydroxytryptamine or about the effects of receptor activation (11). 5-Hydroxytryptamine appears to be inhibitory both at receptors on the serotonergic cell bod-ies and at receptors in the terminal fields. However, these two recep-tors respond differently to LSD and other pharmacological agents, suggesting that variations in receptor configuration could be another mechanism by which the activity of the serotonergic system is modu-lated.

PHARMACOLOGICAL AGENTS

A brief list of substances which are known to interfere with the se-rotonergic system is presented in Table 3-1. These compounds are of

TABLE 3-1.

PHARMACOLOGICAL AGENTS WHICH INTERFERE WITH SEROTONERGIC ACTIVITY

SITE	ACTION	AGENT
Tryptophan Hydroxylase	Inhibition	p-Chlorophenylalanine
Monoamine Oxidase	Inhibition	Iproniazid, Clorgyline
Storage Vesicles	Inhibition	Reserpine, Tetrabenazine
Reuptake	Inhibition	Tricyclic Antidepressants, Tryptolines
Terminal	Destruction	5,6-Dihydroxytryptamine
Receptors	Antagonist	Cinanserin, Methysergide
Receptors	Agonist	LSD*

* See Chapter 22.

variable specificity. For example, reserpine acts with about equal potency on both serotonergic and catecholaminergic systems, while the tryptolines have little effect on reuptake mechanisms other than that for 5-hydroxytryptamine. However, in evaluating reports which depend upon the presumed activities of these compounds, it is important to remember that any pharmacological agent exerts a number of known and unknown effects, so that it is unwise to depend solely upon any single test. Efforts are still being made to improve the potency and selectivity of this pharmacological arsenal. For example, it would be particularly valuable to have a specific, short-acting inhibitor of tryptophan hydroxylase; p-chlorophenylalanine is maximally effective at forty-eight hours and also produces effects on the catecholamines.

ACETYLCHOLINE

HISTORY

While the history of 5-hydroxytryptamine has been intimately connected with psychopharmacology, that of acetylcholine has been closely associated with the development of the entire concept of chemical neurotransmission (Chapter 1). Acetylcholine is the neurotransmitter in a number of systems, including neuromuscular junctions, postganglionic parasympathetic fibers, and preganglionic fibers of both sympathetic and parasympathetic systems. Although acetylcholine is also probably a major transmitter in the central nervous system, much less is known about its function there. Even specific pathways remain to be identified. However, acetylcholine systems in the brain have been associated with arousal mechanisms, temperature regulation, and memory (12). In addition, there have been recent suggestions that these systems might play some role in schizophrenia and the affective disorders (Chapters 8 and 10).

SYNTHESIS

Choline, the precursor of acetylcholine, is probably not synthesized in the brain. However, it can be readily synthesized in the liver, from which it is transported to the brain either as free choline or as phosphatidyl choline (4). Choline is converted to acetylcholine by choline acetyl transferase (Fig. 3-3). The acetyl function is supplied as acetyl CoA, derived primarily from the metabolism of glucose or citrate. As with the serotonergic system, there are suggestions that the substrate

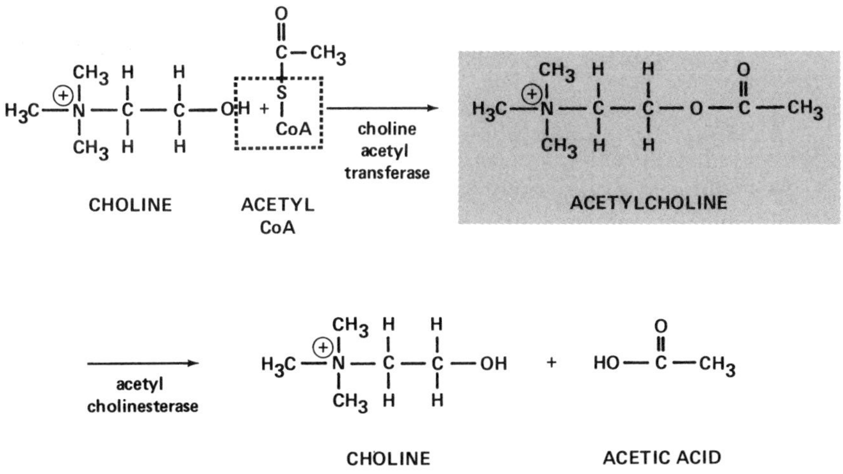

FIGURE 3-3. Synthetic and Metabolic Pathways for Acetylcholine

concentration may be rate-limiting. Thus, *in vitro* rates of synthesis increase with greater amounts of choline.

CATABOLISM

The inactivation of acetylcholine involves hydrolysis to choline and acetic acid (Fig. 3-3). Two classes of cholinesterases have been identified—a "true" cholinesterase, acetylcholinesterase, and a "pseudo" cholinesterase, butyrocholinesterase. As the names suggest, the former of these hydrolyzes acetylcholine faster than does the latter. Neuronal tissues generally contain acetylcholinesterase, while others contain the butyrocholinesterase. The elegant work which has been done in defining the active site of these enzymes is beyond the scope of this book but does make fascinating reading (13).

REGULATORY MECHANISMS

Despite the apparent simplicity of this system, or perhaps because of it, investigators have had little success in attempts to identify the means by which the cholinergic system is regulated. The cyclical nature of the metabolism makes it difficult to use tracers in following changes in the system activity. The recent introduction of choline derivatives which are labeled with the stable isotope deuterium have offered a means to circumvent this problem and may provide a powerful tool for future use (14).

Control of Synthesis

As mentioned earlier, there is some evidence that acetylcholine synthesis may be regulated by the availability of choline. Dietary increases in choline produce increases in brain acetylcholine, so that circulating concentrations of choline may be important in determining the synthetic rate (15). Others have stressed that the important factor may be the high-affinity uptake system for choline (14).

Reuptake into Cholinergic Terminals

Once it is released from the nerve terminal, acetylcholine is hydrolyzed almost immediately. Although there is no high-affinity reuptake system for acetylcholine, such a system does exist for choline (4,14). This system is able to recover 30–50 percent of the choline released by hydrolysis. In addition, it presumably supplies additional choline to the cell as needed for synthetic purposes. Interestingly, reuptake of choline is competitively inhibited by acetylcholine, creating the potential for a negative feedback loop (14). Thus, as more acetylcholine is released, less choline would be taken up, causing less acetylcholine to be synthesized for future release. The functional significance of this interaction is still unknown.

Acetylcholine Receptors

The isolation and characterization of the acetylcholine receptor has been an area of considerable progress in the past few years (16). Much of the success of this work rests upon two fortuitous circumstances: first, the electric tissues of the electric eel provide a tremendously rich source of the receptor; second, certain snake venoms, such as α-bungarotoxin, display a high affinity and specificity for acetylcholine receptors. These receptors have been highly purified, and investigators are now trying to reconstitute the receptor activity in artificial membranes. Studies are also under way to compare the electric eel receptors to receptors from mammalian tissues, including brain. Available evidence suggests that many of the essential features of the receptor have been conserved through the evolutionary process.

PHARMACOLOGICAL AGENTS

An important obstacle for studies of relationships between acetylcholine and behavior has been the lack of adequate pharmacological tools. To date, there are no known inhibitors which specifically block the uptake mechanism for choline. Specific inhibitors of the synthetic enzyme, choline acetyl transferase, have only recently been identified; their properties remain to be studied (14). There are, of course, a tremendous variety of cholinesterase inhibitors (13). However, many of these do not cross the blood-brain barrier and, therefore, are not centrally active. Similar statements can be made about receptor antagonists. Studies of central activity are further complicated by accompanying peripheral effects. Thus, the anticholinesterase physostigmine raises brain acetylcholine, but its peripheral effects also produce a variety of unpleasant and interfering side effects. Nevertheless, physostigmine has proven to be a valuable tool in human studies (Chapter 10).

γ-AMINOBUTYRIC ACID

History

The introduction of γ-aminobutyric acid (GABA) into the class of neuroregulators should be credited largely to the efforts of Eugene Roberts (17). Although GABA had long been recognized as a product of microbial and of plant metabolism, it was not demonstrated in mammalian systems until the early 1950's, when GABA was found to be present in very high concentrations only in the brain and spinal cord. In fact, brain concentrations of GABA are ten to fifteen times higher than those for the catecholamines or 5-hydroxytryptamine. The high concentration and marked localization of GABA naturally led to speculations that it might have some physiological role in the central nervous system. Elucidation of that role has not been a simple task. However, techniques are now available which promise to greatly expand our understanding of the function of GABA in the brain (18).

Synthesis

Like acetylcholine, GABA is synthesized in one step from its amino acid precursor (Fig. 3-4). Glutamic acid decarboxylase, the enzyme which converts glutamic acid to GABA, is present primarily in central nervous tissue. The enzyme has been purified to homogeneity, and antibodies to it are presently being used to identify GABA pathways in the brain (19). Enzymatic activity requires the co-enzyme pyridoxal phosphate and can be inhibited by various ions, including chloride and zinc (4,17).

Catabolism

The major metabolic pathway for GABA is indicated in Figure 3-4. The first step involves transamination to succinic semialdehyde, cata-

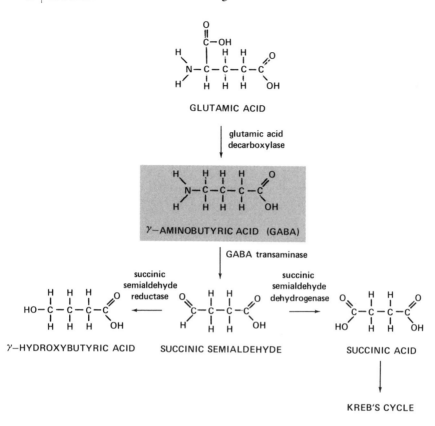

FIGURE 3-4. Synthetic and Metabolic Pathways for GABA

lyzed by GABA transaminase. In the transamination process, α-keto-glutarate acts as an amine acceptor and is converted to glutamic acid, the GABA precursor. The transaminase is widely distributed throughout the body. Even in the brain, it is present in higher concentrations than is glutamic acid decarboxylase, and it is a strong competitor for pyridoxal phosphate (4). *In vitro*, GABA transaminase catalyzes both the forward and the reverse reactions; however, the reverse reaction does not appear to occur under normal *in vivo* conditions.

Like 5-hydroxyindoleacetaldehyde, succinic semialdehyde may undergo further metabolism through either oxidation or reduction. The ratio. Under normal conditions, further oxidation occurs to yield suc-direction of the reaction is, again, determined by the NAD/NADH cinic acid, which then enters the Krebs cycle. Succinic semialdehyde dehydrogenase is highly specific for succinic semialdehyde. Its activity is so great that succinic semialdehyde is not normally detectable in neuronal tissue.

ROLE OF GABA

Interest in GABA as a neurotransmitter is so recent that we still have little specific information either about its role in the central nervous system or about the mechanisms which control its activity. GABA generally inhibits postsynaptic activity. Thus, GABA may be of major importance as an inhibitory system which "uncovers" effector systems as they are needed (17,18). For example, recent histochemical studies suggest that GABAergic systems have extensive connections on the dopaminergic neurons of the limbic system (19). It is possible that these synapses normally act to restrict the firing of the dopaminergic system.

GABA synapses have also been implicated in presynaptic inhibition (17). This effect was first discovered in spinal neurons but may also occur in the brain. Although the mechanism is not completely understood, it appears to involve a depolarization which makes the membrane refractory to the normal electrical signal. Presynaptic inhibition by GABA has already been implicated in the action of the benzodiazepines (Chapter 19).

PHARMACOLOGICAL AGENTS

Investigational tools for the GABA system are completely inadequate (4,17). No specific antagonists have been found for glutamic acid decarboxylase or for the GABA reuptake mechanism. Bicuculline and picrotoxin are good receptor antagonists, and muscimol has recently been shown to be a specific receptor agonist. Intensive studies of purified glutamic acid decarboxylase are being made in an attempt to identify a specific inhibitor.

OTHER NEUROREGULATORS

In the past few years, scientists have made tremendous advances in developing specific and sensitive techniques for measuring small amounts of a variety of substances. These have been supplemented with progress in theoretical and practical means of monitoring brain function (Chapter 1). These developments have resulted not only in the rapid expansion of our understanding of relatively well known neuroregulators but also in the recognition of a growing number of additional compounds which may act as neurotransmitters or neuroregulators. For example, one recent conference examined information about more than twenty-five substances which may have a neuroregulatory role in normal and abnormal brain function (20).

Naturally there is great interest in elaborating our understanding of familiar neurotransmitters such as dopamine, norepinephrine, 5-hydroxytryptamine, acetylcholine, and GABA, as well as of new candidates such as the enkephalins (Chapter 18). In addition, however, attention is being given to compounds which may be physiologically relevant only during pathological conditions; to compounds which may modulate the activity of neurotransmitters, rather than serve as transmitters themselves; and to substances which help to translate the activation of a synaptic receptor into biochemical events in the postsynaptic cell. Each of these areas has already impinged upon psychopharmacology.

The possibility that some psychiatric disorders might result from the formation of abnormal substances is of continuing interest. For example, a number of hallucinogenic N-methyltryptamine derivatives have been detected in both normals and schizophrenics, and investigators have still not determined whether that formation has any physiological or pathological significance (Chapter 8). Similarly, there are hypotheses that some of the effects of alcohol ingestion may result from the formation of aldehyde condensation products with catecholamines or indoleamines (Chapter 20).

Neuromodulation is a somewhat newer concept whose full implications remain to be explored. Neuromodulators are thought to "fine-tune" synaptic activity. For example, it is possible that such substances might act upon the reuptake mechanisms for neurotransmitters, prolonging the synaptic signal without altering the firing rate. Such substances might be present in only low concentrations and be metabolized very quickly, so that they would be difficult to detect under normal circumstances.

Finally, there is an intense interest in trying to uncover the processes of neuronal function which lie beyond the synaptic receptor. In the past few years, investigations of a group of substances called "cyclic nucleotides" have brought us much closer to an understanding of at least the next step. These substances are thought to act as "second messengers," translating the chemical signal into appropriate biochemical reactions. Already, investigators are beginning to seek possible abnormalities in these systems as a cause of psychiatric disturbances (Chapter 10). As our understanding improves, such studies will become increasingly sophisticated.

REFERENCES

1. Page, I. H. Serotonin (5-hydroxytryptamine). *Physiol. Rev.* *34*:563–588, 1954.
2. Barchas, J. and Usdin, E. *Serotonin and Behavior.* New York: Academic Press, 1973.
3. Tong, J. H. and Kaufman, S. Tryptophan hydroxylase. Purification and some properties of the enzyme from rabbit hindbrain. *J. Biol. Chem.* *250*:4152–4158, 1975.
4. Cooper, J. R., Bloom, F. E., and Roth, R. H. *The Biochemical Basis of Neuropharmacology,* 2nd ed. New York: Oxford University Press, 1974.
5. Hidaka, H., Nagatsu, T., and Yagi, K. Occurrence of a serotonin sulphotransferase in the brain. *J. Neurochem.* *16*:783–785, 1969.
6. Koslow, S. Bio-significance of N- and O-methylated indoles to psychiatric disorders. *In: Neuroregulators and Psychiatric Disorders.* E. Usdin, D. A. Hamburg, and J. D. Barchas, *eds.,* New York: Oxford University Press, 1977, pp. 210–219.
7. Edelman, A. M., Berger, P. A., and Renson, J. F. 5-Hydroxytryptamine: basic and clinical perspectives. *In: Neuroregulators and Psychiatric Disorders.* E. Usdin, D. A. Hamburg, and J. D. Barchas, *eds.,* New York: Oxford University Press, 1977, pp. 177–187.
8. Ungerstedt, U. Stereotaxic mapping of the monoamine pathways in the rat brain. *Acta Physiol. Scand., Suppl. 367*:1–48, 1971.
9. Lindvall, O. and Björklund, A. The glyoxylic acid fluorescence histochemical method: a detailed account of the methodology for the visualization of central catecholamine neurons. *Histochemistry 39*:97–127, 1974.
10. Wurtman, R. J. and Fernstrom, J. D. Control of brain monoamine synthesis by diet and plasma amino acids. *Am. J. Clin. Nutr. 28*:638–647, 1975.
11. Aghajanian, G. K., Haigler, H. J., and Bennett, J. L. Amine receptors in CNS. III. 5-Hydroxytryptamine in brain. *In: Handbook of Psychopharmacology.* L. L. Iversen, S. D. Iversen, and S. H. Snyder, *eds.,* New York: Plenum, 1975, pp. 63–96.
12. DeFeudis, F. V. *Central Cholinergic Systems and Behavior.* New York: Academic Press, 1974.
13. Goldstein, A., Aronow, L., and Kalman, S. M. *Principles of Drug Action: The Basis of Pharmacology,* 2nd ed. New York: John Wiley and Sons, 1974.
14. Jenden, D. J. Some recent developments in the biochemical pharmacology of cholinergic systems. *In: Neuroregulators and Psychiatric Disorders.* E. Usdin, D. A. Hamburg, and J. D. Barchas, *eds.,* New York: Oxford University Press, 1977, pp. 425–433.
15. Cohen, E. L. and Wurtman, R. J. Brain acetylcholine: increase after systemic choline administration. *Life Sci. 16*:1095–1102, 1975.
16. Karlin, A. The acetylcholine receptor: isolation and characterization. *In: The Nervous System. Vol. 1: The Basic Neurosciences.* R. O. Brady, *ed.,* New York: Raven Press, 1975, pp. 323–331.
17. Roberts, E. GABA in nervous system function—an overview. *In: The*

Nervous System. Vol. 1: The Basic Neurosciences. R. O. Brady, *ed.,* New York: Raven Press, 1975, pp. 541–552.
18. Roberts, E., Chase, T. N., and Tower, D. B., *eds. GABA in Nervous System Function.* New York: Raven Press, 1975.
19. Hökfelt, T., Ljungdahl, Å., Fuxe, K., Johansson, O., and Perez de la Mora, M. Some attempts to explore possible central GABAergic mechanisms with special reference to control of dopamine neurons. *In: Neuroregulators and Psychiatric Disorders.* E. Usdin, D. A. Hamburg, and J. D. Barchas, *eds.,* New York: Oxford University Press, 1977, pp. 358–372.
20. Usdin, E., Hamburg, D. A., and Barchas, J. D., *eds. Neuroregulators and Psychiatric Disorders.* New York: Oxford University Press, 1977.

4 | Neurophysiological Aspects of Brain Function

WALTON T. ROTH

INTRODUCTION

Neurophysiological studies stand somewhere along the spectrum from biochemical to behavioral analyses of brain function (1–3). As detailed in the two preceding chapters, information about neuroregulators offers a good basis for understanding the regulatory parameters of individual synapses. But how do these synaptic building blocks interact to form a functional neuronal circuit? Neurophysiology provides one means of examining that question.

This chapter contains brief descriptions of the major levels of analysis in neurophysiology, ranging from single cell recordings and iontophoresis, in which the electrical and chemical parameters of individual cells are measured, to recordings of the aggregate activity of large groups of neurons, so that more general influences can be assessed. There is no attempt to provide an exhaustive review of this complex and often controversial field. Rather, the chapter is designed to indicate the utility of each of these methods for increasing our understanding of normal and abnormal brain function.

SINGLE UNIT ACTIVITY

A spike potential from the firing of an individual neuron is called single unit activity. Such activity can be recorded from tiny electrodes, a few micra in diameter, which are implanted close to the neuron. Electrodes are placed stereotaxically according to atlases that give the coordinates of the neural structure to be investigated. At the end of the experiment, the animal is killed, so that the placement of the electrodes can be verified histologically. The influence of drugs on single unit activity can be observed after systemic administration of the drugs or after administration of the drugs via the electrode itself, which may be a micropipette filled with electrically conducting solutions. This latter method is called iontophoresis, since ions of the drug are driven into the brain by pulses of current of the appropriate polarity.

The effects of compounds on single unit activity provide information about their exact cellular location and mechanism of action. For example, the spontaneous discharge of Purkinje cells in the rat cerebellum is reduced shortly after an iontophoretic injection of norepinephrine (4). Since cyclic AMP produces a similar reduction and since inhibitors of cyclic AMP catabolism alter the effects of both norepinephrine and cyclic AMP, investigators have suggested that cyclic AMP mediates the effects of norepinephrine in those neurons. Stimulation of noradrenergic neurons in the locus coeruleus, which project to the Purkinje cells, produces the same inhibitory response as that obtained with direct applications of norepinephrine. This provides an interesting method for examining the effects of substances on the transmission of a signal through this system. For example, iontophoretic application of prostaglandin E_1 on the Purkinje cell prevents the inhibition which normally follows stimulation of the locus coeruleus (4).

A comparable, model system for dopaminergic neurons is that found in the substantia nigra and the caudate-putamen of the rat. When given systemically, substances which enhance dopamine release, such as amphetamine, inhibit neural firing in both of these locations. In contrast, substances which block dopaminergic activity increase firing. Interestingly, iontophoretic administration of amphetamine markedly inhibits dopaminergic neurons in the caudate-putamen but only minimally depresses those in the substantia nigra (5). Furthermore, if the possible pathways between these brain regions are lesioned, systemic amphetamine also fails to inhibit firing in the substantia nigra. These and other findings have led to suggestions of a feedback loop, whereby decreased firing of dopaminergic neurons in the caudate-putamen causes parallel decreases in the substantia nigra. Both negative (5) and positive (6) feedback loops have been postulated to account for these effects.

As a model for studying drug interactions with 5-hydroxytryptamine (serotonin), recordings have been made from single units in the midbrain raphé nuclei. Extremely small oral doses of lysergic acid diethylamide (LSD) completely but reversibly inhibit firing in these neurons (7). The clinically inactive LSD analogue, 2-bromo-LSD, has less than 1 percent of the activity of LSD in depressing raphé neurons, even though it is more effective than LSD in blocking serotonergic effects on smooth muscle. Iontophoretic application of LSD to these neurons also produces inhibition of firing, but that effect is not specific to serotonergic neurons. The use of this system in elucidating the effects of hallucinogens is described in Chapter 22.

MULTIPLE UNIT ACTIVITY

Using larger electrodes, one records continuously graded voltages instead of the all-or-none spikes that microelectrodes pick up. These result from spatial and temporal summation of electrical activity in many different neurons. These voltages fluctuate spontaneously, but they can also change in response to sensory stimulation (evoked potentials). Information from macroelectrodes is more difficult to relate to biochemical mechanisms than is that from microelectrodes; however, in some instances it is easier to relate to behavior. Three areas in which studies of multiple unit activity have been of particular interest to psychopharmacologists have been the reticular activating systems, the limbic system, and the cerebral cortex.

Reticular Activating System

In its simplest conception, the reticular activating system is a core of ventral neuronal tissue which extends from the spinal cord to the thalamus. The area receives input from the sensory pathways, which travel through its diffuse polysynaptic nets to produce widespread changes throughout the nervous system. Electrical stimulation of this core leads to behavioral and electroencephalographic (EEG) evidence of arousal and alertness. In psychological terms, the reticular activating system is related to the continuum of arousal from deep coma to hypervigilant agitation. Anxiety states and sleep disturbances are two common psychiatric symptoms that can be viewed as disturbances in the regulation of arousal. Disturbances of this sort are often very severe in schizophrenia and psychotic depression. Early studies on the site of drug effects on cortical arousal compared their effects on the intact brain, *cerveau isolé*, and *encéphale isolé* preparations (8). The *cerveau isolé* preparation is made by transecting the brainstem just posterior to the colliculi; this produces a perpetual state of sleep, since the ascending pathways of the reticular activating system are broken. The *encéphale isolé* preparation is created by transecting at the junction of the brain and spinal cord; thus, although sensory input from most of the body is excluded, the cranial nerves and the reticular activating system within the brainstem still permit cortical wakefulness. Table 4-1 shows how a comparison of these three preparations can permit inferences about where psychoactive drugs act. Amphetamine has an alerting, desynchronizing effect on the cortical EEG only while the pathway between the reticular activating system and the cortex is intact, suggesting that it acts on that system. In contrast, the actions of physostigmine and atropine are unaffected by sectioning, suggesting that these drugs act at higher centers. Since LSD and chlorpromazine have their maximum effects in the intact brain, their action on the reticular activating system probably depends on the integrity of somatic afferent stimulation.

The reticular activating system also has descending pathways which can modulate afferent input. These pathways are probably responsible for habituation to repeated stimuli. Thus, if the reticular activating system is stimulated just prior to a peripheral stimulus, the resulting evoked potentials are decreased, as if the system were acting as a filter (9). Chlorpromazine enhances this filtering effect from reticular stimulation, while phenobarbital antagonizes it. In agreement with this, chlorpromazine also accelerates habituation of the EEG arousal response to auditory stimuli.

LIMBIC SYSTEM

The limbic system is a loosely defined group of brain structures which includes the hippocampus, the septal area, the hypothalamus, and portions of the cerebral cortex and rhinencephalon. Rich interconnecting pathways between these structures give them a certain func-

TABLE 4-1.
EFFECTS OF DRUGS IN CONSCIOUS ANIMAL AND ACUTE PREPARATIONS*

| DRUG | CONSCIOUS ANIMAL | | ENCÉPHALE ISOLÉ | CERVEAU ISOLÉ |
	BEHAVIOR	ELECTRICAL ACTIVITY	ELECTRICAL ACTIVITY	ELECTRICAL ACTIVITY
Amphetamine	Excited	Fast, low amplitude	Fast, low amplitude	No effect
Physostigmine	Normal	Fast, low amplitude	Fast, low amplitude	Fast, low amplitude
Atropine	Normal or excited	Slow, high amplitude with spindles	Slow, high amplitude with spindles	Slow, high amplitude with spindles
LSD	Excited	Fast, low amplitude	No effect	No effect
Chlorpromazine	Drowsy and indifferent	Slow	Increased slow with spindles	No effect

* Adapted from Table 1 of Schallek *et al.* (10).

tional unity. The system appears to be involved in emotional and motivational behavior, in that lesions or stimulation within this system can lead to alterations in sexual, aggressive, and fear responses. Rats with electrodes implanted in certain areas of the limbic system will work to exhaustion pressing a lever that delivers electrical impulses to those electrodes; in contrast, if the electrodes are implanted in other areas of the system, the animals may actively avoid electrical stimulation. Since emotional and motivational behavior is often the target for psychoactive drugs, investigators have been particularly curious about drug action on the limbic system.

One method of assessing limbic system function utilizes electrodes in the septum, amygdala, and hippocampus of unanesthetized cats, so that these brain structures can be stimulated with a brief burst of impulses (10). If the EEG is then recorded from these same locations, an afterdischarge is observed. The EEG and behavioral effects of this procedure resemble those of a psychomotor seizure in man. Whereas chlorpromazine reduces the threshold for afterdischarge in the amygdala, phenobarbital, and chlordiazepoxide increase it. Phenobarbital alone raises the hippocampal threshold. An alternate way to study the anticonvulsant properties of the benzodiazepines and other drugs involves experimentally induced epileptogenic foci obtained by implanting aluminum oxide crystals in the intralaminar thalamic nuclei of kittens or in the hippocampus of adult cats (11).

EEG activity in different parts of the limbic system is differentially altered by various psychoactive compounds. In one study, spontaneous activity of the immobilized cat was measured at seven subcortical sites: the caudate, amygdala, hippocampus, septum, medial and lateral hypothalamus, and reticular formation (12). Chlordiazepoxide produced its greatest changes in the hippocampus, chlorpromazine had its greatest effects on the medial hypothalamus, and the target of pentobarbital was the reticular formation. Diazepam had little effect in this preparation.

CEREBRAL CORTEX

Spontaneous Activity

The electrical activity of the cortex can be measured either at the surface of the brain or from electrodes on the scalp, as is common in clinical EEG recording. The effects of spatial summation are much greater at the scalp than at the surface of the brain, and localization of neural activity is correspondingly worse. In spite of the fact that scalp recording prevents precise localization of cortical activity and is generally insensitive to subcortical activity, it offers the advantage of being nontraumatic, so that it can be used without danger in human subjects.

EEGs can be analyzed by breaking them into a sum of individual wave forms of varying amplitudes. For the resulting frequency spectrum of the spontaneous EEG in man, the component with the greatest amplitude, or power, is generally found around 10 cps (cycles/sec). The spectrum of spontaneous activity is arbitrarily divided into the following frequency bands: delta, 0.5–3.5 cps; theta, 3.5–7.5 cps; alpha, 7.5–13 cps; and beta, 13–40 cps. The exact distribution of these frequency bands and their relative importance vary both with the individual and with the state of consciousness. During sleep stages III and IV, theta and delta frequencies predominate (Chapter 14). Alpha activity is greatest when a subject is relaxed but not sleepy, and drowsiness or anxiety reduce alpha amplitude. Acute brain syndromes, such as delirium, are associated with a lower alpha frequency, regardless of the etiology of the delirium.

Different psychoactive drugs produce different profiles of change in the frequency spectrum of the human EEG, as summarized in Table 4-2 (13). There are four major patterns of alteration in spontaneous activity. Pattern I is characteristic of some of the antipsychotics, pattern II is found with barbiturates and other antianxiety drugs, such as the benzodiazepines; pattern III is associated with anticholinergic drugs, such as the tricyclic antidepressants; and pattern IV is produced by alcohol and two opiates.

This classification scheme appears to be useful for evaluating the psychoactive properties of new drugs (14). For example, fenfluramine was originally presumed to have stimulant properties; however, its EEG profile was more similar to amobarbital than to d-amphetamine. Subsequent clinical testing confirmed its sedative properties. Similarly, the EEG profile of doxepin was found to resemble imipramine and diazepam before the drug was shown to be both a sedative and an antidepressant.

The EEG profile can also serve as an index of the bioavailability of psychoactive drugs (14). Thus, when doxepin HCl and doxepin pamoate were compared in several doses, it was found that, at equal doses,

TABLE 4-2.
EEG PATTERNS OF PSYCHOACTIVE DRUGS*

CLASS	EEG PATTERN	BAND (cps)					DRUG
		DELTA (0–3.5)	THETA (3.5–7.5)	ALPHA (7.5–13)	BETA 1 (13–22)	BETA 2 (22–33)	
Ia	Slow	+	++	±	0	–	chlorpromazine, haloperidol, thioridazine
Ib	Slowing with increased alpha	+	++	++	0	±	trifluoperazine
IIa	Fast activity, increased amplitude	0	+	0	++	+	barbiturates, benzodiazepines
IIb	Fast activity, decreased amplitude	0	–	–	+	++	amphetamine, LSD, methylphenidate
IIIa	Fast and slow activity	++	+	–	+	++	atropine, Ditran
IIIb	Fast and slow activity increased seizure	+	++	–	+	+	imipramine, amitriptyline
IV	Alpha increase	–	+	+	0	0	ethanol, heroin, methadone

+ : increase   0 : no effect   – : decrease   ± : variable
* Adapted from Table 1 of Fink (13).

the two had equivalent effects at the onset; but the latter had a greater effect after two hours. A comparison of thiothixene capsules and liquid concentrate confirmed that the concentrate affected the brain more quickly. While measurement of drug plasma levels might have given similar results, the EEG effects are more pertinent to the drug action on the central nervous system. Furthermore, the blood-brain barrier and other factors of metabolism and distribution make hazardous the prediction of bioavailability from plasma levels alone.

Evoked Potentials

When a discrete stimulus is presented to man or other animals, neuronal activity is elicited at various locations in the central nervous system, with various time lags. When electrodes are placed appropriately within the brain tissue, the effects of each stimulus can be distinctly seen in the evoked potential or in the change of single unit firing; but when recordings are made from the scalp, spontaneous, multicellular activity overlaps and obscures individual evoked responses. A transitory suppression of alpha rhythm may initially follow stimuli, but the higher frequency components of the evoked cortical potential are buried in the "noise" of the ongoing EEG. This situation can be improved by making a time-point-by-time-point average of the response, using the stimulus as the starting point. In this way, the evoked response can be averaged over a number of repetitions of the same stimulus, thus identifying the activity which is "time-locked" to the stimulus. Spontaneous background activity which is not synchronized with the stimulus will eventually average to a mean close to zero, thus improving the signal-to-noise ratio of the underlying evoked potentials (2).

One series of experiments examined the acute effects of psychotropic drugs on somatosensory evoked potentials in normal volunteers (15). Average evoked potentials were elicited by repetitively stimulating the median nerve percutaneously at the wrist with brief painless shocks. Table 4-3 presents the profile of changes produced by various classes of compounds. There is some evidence that specific thalamocortical pathways mediate the earlier components, while collaterals to the reticular activating systems and diffuse thalamic projections to the cortex mediate the later components. Thus, a decrease in the amplitude of later components could be interpreted as a depressant effect on the reticular activating system. Whatever the validity of these neurophys-

TABLE 4-3.
SOMATOSENSORY EVOKED POTENTIAL DRUG PROFILES IN HUMAN
SUBJECTS

	EARLY PEAKS (0–40 msec)		LATE PEAKS (40–300 msec)	
	LATENCY	AMPLITUDE	LATENCY	AMPLITUDE
Antianxiety drugs	+	−	− −	−
Antipsychotic drugs	+	0	+ + +	−
Stimulants	− −	−	− −	+
Tricyclic antidepressants	− −	0	+	0

+, −, 0's indicate direction and approximate degree of drug-induced changes

iological interpretations, the profiles of evoked potential change can be used to predict the clinical effects of a drug in a manner similar to that of the power spectrum profiles. For example, two compounds with evoked potential profiles which were similar to the antianxiety profile have subsequently been shown to reduce anxiety (15).

Since changes in psychological variables such as attention affect evoked potentials (16), the impact of psychoactive drugs on psychological functioning can be quantified by measuring these potentials. In one experiment, human subjects performed a reaction time task in which a warning flash of light was followed by a tone, signaling that the subjects were to quickly press a telegraph key (17). Between the warning signal and the tone, a negative potential shift called the contingent negative variation (CNV) occurs in the scalp EEG. As with the evoked potentials to wrist shocks, computer averaging of a number of repetitions is necessary for reliable measurements. The amplitude of the negative shift is a function of the subjects' direction of attention and of their level of alertness. Amphetamine was found to have one of two subjective effects on these subjects: some became more alert, while others became drowsy. For the alert subjects, the negative shift increased in amplitude; for the drowsy subjects, however, the negative shift decreased in amplitude. Thus, the negative shift corresponded to the psychological effects of amphetamine, rather than to its mere presence in the body.

Psychological functions other than attention and alertness are also reflected in components of the evoked potential. For example, the subjective probability of a stimulus event is inversely related to the amplitude of a positive wave occurring at a mean latency of 300 msec. Unexpected events of the type that would produce an orienting response elicit these waves. There is a clear biological function for an "unexpected event" detector: potentially dangerous changes in the environment need immediate evaluation and response by the organism. Both marihuana and alcohol can decrease the amplitude of this wave without affecting other waves that reflect subjective stimulus intensity and attention (18).

CONCLUSIONS

Limitations to a neurophysiological understanding of drug action stem both from the state of neurophysiology and from the lack of empirical data about the effects of drugs on neurophysiological systems. Although neurophysiological analyses range from single neurons to scalp-recorded evoked potentials, only general facts are known about the relationships between these levels. When we advance to the behavioral level, our understanding of relationships is even more limited; for there are, at best, only a few hints about the neurophysiology of thinking, memory, or emotion. Similarly, we are still seeking the neurophysiological substrates of diseases such as schizophrenia and the affective disorders—or even of their symptomatic manifestations, such as looseness of association, delusions, or psychomotor retardation. Empirical data about drug effects on neurophysiological systems are quite spotty. An action common to phenobarbital and chlorpromazine may have some interest, but it will not go far in explaining the antipsychotic effects of the latter drug. More confidence in the relevance of a drug effect comes from finding a specific effect at a dose comparable to doses used clinically. Of course, different species may have different sensitivities to a drug—a fact that limits the generalizability of findings in rats, cats, and even chimpanzees to human beings.

In spite of these problems, it is likely that neurophysiological approaches to the study of psychoactive drugs will become increasingly important. For both ethical and practical reasons, the ultimate test of psychiatrically useful compounds—i.e., their effects on the mentally ill—must be preceded by tests in nonhuman species. A neurophysiological system which is sensitive for and specific to a class of psychoactive compounds would be very useful in the screening of new chemicals, particularly if it provided information about dose-response and time-action relationships. Neurophysiological measurements in humans also have a special place. There are many advantages to direct measures of the effects of drugs on the brain. Furthermore, whether or not a certain individual will respond to a given drug may become predictable, if the relevant individual differences can be assessed neurophysiologically.

As discussed in Chapter 1, all experimental findings must be considered in terms of the state of the organism. Variations in alertness, attention, and motivation have important neurophysiological consequences which can completely reverse drug effects. The mutual influences between "psychological" and "neurophysiological" variables should not be dismissed as troublesome artifacts (cf. Chapter 31). Instead, these influences should be regarded as manifestations of an intrinsic unity. Whenever posible, the methodologies of biochemistry, neurophysiology, and psychology should be applied together to elucidate mechanisms of drug action.

REFERENCES

1. Shagass, C. *Evoked Brain Potentials in Psychiatry*. New York: Plenum Press, 1972.
2. Thompson, R. F. *Foundations of Physiological Psychology*. New York: Harper & Row, 1967.
3. Bloom, F. E. Modern concepts in electrophysiology for psychiatry. *Psychopharmacol. Commun. 1*:579–585, 1975.
4. Bloom, F. E., Hoffer, B. J., and Siggins, G. R. Norepinephrine-mediated cerebellar synapses: a model system for neuropsychopharmacology. *Biol. Psychiatry 4*:157–177, 1972.
5. Bunney, B. S. and Aghajanian, G. K. *d*-Amphetamine-induced inhibition of central dopaminergic neurons: mediation by a striato-nigral feedback pathway. *Science 192*:391–393, 1976.
6. Groves, P. M., Wilson, C. J., Young, S. J., and Rebec, G. V. Self-inhibition by dopaminergic neurons. *Science 190*:522–529, 1975.
7. Aghajanian, G. K. LSD and CNS transmission. *Ann. Rev. Pharmacol. 12*:157–168, 1972.
8. Bradley, P. B. The central action of certain drugs in relation to the reticular formation of the brain. *In: Reticular Formation of the Brain*. H. H. Jasper, L. D. Proctor, R. S. Knighton, W. C. Noshay, and R. T. Costello, *eds.*, Boston: Little, Brown, 1958, pp. 123–149.
9. Killam, E. K. Pharmacology of the reticular formation. *In: Psychopharmacology: A Review of Progress 1957–1967*. D. H. Efron, *ed.*, U.S. Public Health Service Publication No. 1836, 1968, pp. 411–445.
10. Schallek, W., Zabransky, F., and Kuehn, A. Effects of benzodiazepines on central nervous system of cat. *Arch. Int. Pharmacodyn. Ther. 194*: 467–483, 1964.
11. Randall, L. O., Schallek, W. S., Sternbach, L. H., and Ning, R. Y. Chemistry and pharmacology of the 1,4-benzodiazepines. *In: Psychopharmacological Agents, Vol. III*. M. Gordon, *ed.*, New York: Academic Press, 1974, pp. 175–281.
12. Schallek, W. and Thomas, J. Effects of benzodiazepines on spontaneous electrical activity of subcortical areas in brain of cat. *Arch. Int. Pharmacodyn. Ther. 192*:321–337, 1971.
13. Fink, M. EEG classification of psychoactive compounds in man: a review and theory of behavioral associations. *In: Psychopharmacology: A Review of Progress 1957–1967*. D. H. Effron, *ed.*, U.S. Public Health Service Publication No. 1836, 1968, pp. 497–507.
14. Fink, M. EEG applications in psychopharmacology. *In: Psychopharmacological Agents, Vol. III*. M. Gordon, *ed.*, New York: Academic Press, 1974, pp. 159–174.
15. Saletu, B. Classification of psychotropic drugs based on human evoked potentials. *In: Psychotropic Drugs and the Human EEG*. T. M. Itil, *ed.*, Basel: S. Karger, 1974, pp. 258–285.
16. Callaway, E. Averaged evoked responses in psychiatry. *J. Nerv. Ment. Dis. 143*:80–94, 1966.
17. Tecce, J. J. and Cole, J. O. Amphetamine effects in man: Paradoxical

drowsiness and lowered electrical brain activity (CNV). *Science 185:* 451–453, 1974.

18. Roth, W. T., Tinklenberg, J. R., and Kopell, B. S. Ethanol and marihuana effects on event-related potentials in a memory retrieval paradigm. *Electroencephalogr. Clin. Neurophysiol.* 42:381–388, 1977.

5 | Effects of Drugs on Psychological Processes in Humans

BERT S. KOPELL

INTRODUCTION

This chapter will examine aspects of methods for studying drug effects in humans. Psychoactive medications operate through complex biochemical and physiological processes to achieve reparative and compensatory effects on the affective, psychomotor, and cognitive state of the patient. Traditionally, the clinical efficacy of psychoactive medications has been assessed by global rating scales and behavioral inventories. Although global measures can provide valuable clinical information, they are less useful as tools for determining specific effects of drugs on psychological processes such as the ability to focus attention, to register information in memory, and to retrieve it for later use.

If malfunction in the above capacities underlies certain psychiatric syndromes, the specific psychological effects of psychoactive medication can provide insights into how these drugs achieve their therapeutic effect. As an example, one popular hypothesis of schizophrenia postulates that it is a condition involving overarousal, resulting in excessive sensitivity to external stimulation (1). Theoretically, such a state could produce great anxiety. Thus, psychotic behaviors such as hallucinations, paranoia, and catatonia might represent defenses against the anxiety caused by an imperfect attentional system. Chlorpromazine minimizes psychotic symptoms (Chapter 9). By examining the effects of this drug on sensitivity to external stimuli, it may be possible not only to examine its behavioral effects but also to test the validity of the attentional theory of schizophrenia. Such behavioral studies need not be incompatible with the biochemical studies described in Chapter 9, which concentrate upon the neurochemical mechanisms by which the drug exerts its effects.

Psychological testing is becoming an increasingly important part of both clinical psychiatry and basic psychiatric research. And yet, results from experiments which are designed to investigate the psychological aspects of drug action are often marred by inadequate attention to definitions, quantification, reliability, validity, and baselines. Changes in drug administration, subject selection, and variable definition can prevent comparisons of studies by different investigators or even of different studies by the same investigators. Therefore, it is important to understand the general methodological considerations of any drug research (cf. 2,3).

Methodological problems are often particularly acute when psychological variables are being studied (Chapter 32). Frequently there is, at best, only a tenuous relationship between the test and what is being tested. In addition, individual differences can be so immense that the important effects are difficult to detect. These difficulties are complicated by the fact that psychological drug research has yet to develop a tradition of standardized, replicable techniques or to fully utilize recent advances in cognitive psychology. In light of the massive body of paradoxical and often incomprehensible data which presently exist in this field, it seems particularly appropriate to provide a brief survey of vital methodological considerations for psychological evaluation of drug effects in humans.

DRUG ADMINISTRATION

DOSE-RESPONSE CURVES

Drugs can differ in the concentrations at which medication has any effect at all (potency level), the extent to which an effect is intensified by graded increases in dose (slope), and the maximum effect obtainable (ceiling). Naturally, differences in potency level must be considered when comparing two drugs; however, more subtle differences in the slope and shape of the dose-response curve may be equally important. While dose-response curves for a wide range of physiological variables are documented, dose-response curves for performance on different psychological tests are often unknown. Most studies employ a single dose, usually one considered clinically "moderate"; only a few compare even a "high" and "low" dose.

Figure 5-1a illustrates hypothetical dose-response curves for three drugs of different potencies with regard to a single psychological or physiological variable. By selecting the correct dosage, one can obtain three different rank orders of potency. As shown in Figure 5-1b, the same drug can produce quite different dose-response curves for two different psychological variables. Thus, unless the full range of the dose-response curve is known, it is difficult to interpret the significance of a finding at any single point.

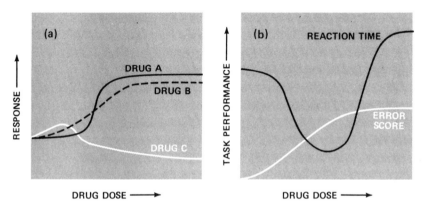

FIGURE 5-1. Dose-Response Curves
a. Three drugs of different potency. b. Two different behavioral measures.

TIME-ACTION CURVES

The time-action curve of a drug's effects constitutes a dose-response curve over time. Typically, studies of psychological drug effects employ a single testing period at the "peak" response time. This peak is generally deduced from physiological responses, and the assumption that the same time-action curve applies for psychological variables is seldom tested. As with dose-response curves, time-action curves are a source of variability which can affect comparisons between different drugs and between different studies of the same drug. Figure 5-2a il-

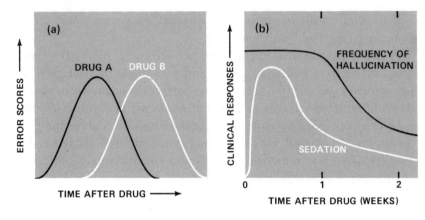

FIGURE 5-2. Time-Action Curves
a. Fast- and slow-acting drug. b. Two different clinical measures.

lustrates curves for a fast-acting drug (A) and a slow-acting drug (B). Inattention to time could produce a wide scattering of apparent relative potencies for these two drugs. Time-action curves can also uncover differential sensitivities of different variables to a given drug. For example, Figure 5-2b compares the time-action curve of two clinical effects of phenothiazines (see Chapter 9). Sedation can occur within an hour of drug administration; but after several days, patients develop tolerance to this effect. In contrast, it can take two weeks for an antipsychotic effect to develop, and this effect does not disappear with repeated administrations. Similarly, the cortical depressant action of the sedative hypnotic diazepam persists long after clinical and subjective signs of intoxication have passed (4).

CHRONIC VS. SINGLE-DOSE ADMINISTRATION

In clinical situations, psychoactive medication is administered over a period of time with a delay ranging from minutes to weeks or even months before therapeutic effects are seen. Unfortunately, studies of cognitive effects of chronically administered drugs are rare. The single-dose design is preferred, both because it is simpler to administer and because it is more appropriate for studies of normals. However, the acute and chronic effects of a drug may be quite different. The delayed antipsychotic action of the phenothiazines offers a clear example of the potential difficulties. Alternatively, many of the effects which are important initially may disappear with chronic administration, as tolerance develops or as the patient learns to compensate for the drug-induced change.

SUBJECT SELECTION

NORMALS VS. PATIENTS

Acute and chronic drug administration is only one aspect of the problems encountered in comparing the effects of psychoactive drugs on normal healthy subjects with those on patients exhibiting symptoms which the drug is believed to affect. Studies which employ healthy subjects do not need to accommodate for problems caused by distressed patients; they therefore tend to be more methodologically rigorous, with greater attention to the specification of dependent variables and the control of experimental setting. Such methodological rigor, however, may be achieved at the expense of clinical relevance. Additionally, studies may fail to control for important environmental effects such as hospital wards simply because it is easier and less expensive to use controls who are not housed in the hospital.

BASELINES

A crucial consideration in all drug research is the baseline from which changes occur. Patients are usually operating at different physical and psychological baselines than are persons defined as "healthy." Duffy (5) and Malmo (6) have hypothesized that the relationship between the degree of activation of an individual and his level of performance can be expressed as an inverted U (Fig. 5-3). Thus, for a time, increasing levels of arousal will improve performance. However, once a plateau is reached, continuing increases in arousal not only produce no increment in performance but actually result in a deterioration. Thus, drug effects must be evaluated not only in terms of direc-

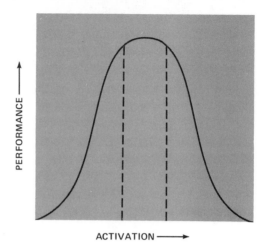

FIGURE 5-3. Inverted-U Relationship Between Activation and Performance

tion but also in terms of initial state. A particularly interesting application of this model is offered by the effects of chlorpromazine on arousal, as described later in this chapter.

INDIVIDUAL VARIATION

Individual differences within diagnostic categories of patients or among "normal" subject populations can mask important drug effects. Thus, the sedative hypnotic meprobamate is most likely to improve performance in subjects who score high on predrug levels of anxiety. Meprobamate's positive effect is best seen with tests involving experimentally induced anxiety (7). Among nonanxious populations or in unstressful experimental situations, the drug tends to have no effect, or even a negative one.

Although they have not yet been adopted universally, there are methodological techniques for coping with problems of individual variability (Chapter 32). These include use of a subject as his own control by administering placebo and drugs to the same subject on separate test days and comparing performance under different drug conditions, determination of predrug baseline levels of performance in order to compare drug-induced changes in performance, careful subject selection to minimize obvious sources of difference, and subdivision of subject population along relevant variables with separate analysis for subgroup data.

TEST SELECTION

Assuming a satisfactory solution to problems of drug administration and subject selection, the ultimate value of a study must lie in the selection of tests which not only provide reliable and valid measures of the psychological variable of interest but are also sensitive to the drug being studied. Even when standardized psychological tests are used, many prove stubbornly resistant to drug effects or, even worse, are affected inconsistently. A recent survey of one hundred studies of antianxiety agents divided the tests which had been used into "winners" and "losers" on the basis of their sensitivity to drug effects (8). Of the forty-three tests, ten were classified as highly sensitive, in that 50 percent or more of the relevant studies reported significant drug effects; ten more were of average sensitivity, with 25–44 percent of studies reporting significant drug effects. The remaining twenty-three tests were of either low or indeterminate sensitivity. Interestingly, the most popular tests were in the average or low sensitivity groups. This clearly illustrates the way in which certain tests are persistently included in drug protocols, even though they have regularly proved to be insensitive to drugs.

It is apparent that certain skills and functions are more drug sensitive than others. The capacity of humans to compensate for drug-induced impairments challenges the ingenuity of the investigator. Another important aspect of this phenomenon is the "placebo effect," which is discussed in Chapter 31. The complexity of events underlying performance on psychological tests makes it essential to use tests which can distinguish among different aspects of this performance. For example, a popular model of memory postulates the following stages (9,10):

- Selective attention to relevant stimuli
- Coding of relevant stimuli in a limited-capacity, short-term store
- Transfer of information from the short-term store to an unlimited, long-term store
- Retrieval of appropriate information when needed through recognition or recall.

Confounding this already complex sequence are the sensory processes involved in initial input of information and the motor processes involved in its final behavioral manifestation. In common test situations for this system, subjects are instructed to press a button as soon as they see a prearranged visual cue. A lengthened reaction time might indicate a change in cortical function, but it could also reflect impairment of the sensory organs or retardation of the motor response. It is not surprising, therefore, that many reaction-time paradigms yield inconsistent or paradoxical results. Cortical correlates of various behavioral parameters can also be monitored physiologically, through measures such as the evoked response (Chapter 4). These techniques are sensitive to certain hormones and socially abused drugs (11).

EFFECTS OF VARIOUS CLASSES OF DRUGS

ANTIPSYCHOTICS

The psychological effects of chlorpromazine and related phenothiazine drugs exhibit marked differences between schizophrenics and normals. For that reason, studies involving schizophrenics must be distinguished from those involving normals. An important focus of studies on the psychological effects of chlorpromazine has been a comparison of effects on the Digit Symbol Substitution Test and the Continuous Performance Test (1,12). The former test requires subjects to use a provided code to substitute as many symbols for digits as they can in ninety seconds. The task requires an intense cognitive or associative effort, but only for a short period of time; it is believed to involve cortical mechanisms. The latter test requires subjects to monitor a screen for a test stimulus, as different letters are presented briefly. The test lasts for ten minutes and requires little cognitive effort; but it does require sustained attention, since the display is constantly changing. It is believed to reflect skills mediated by the subcortical reticular activating system.

Chlorpromazine has little effect on cognitive associative tasks, but it does impair sustained attention. This latter effect appears to be most marked in normal subjects (1). The performance of schizophrenics on the Continuous Performance Test was relatively unchanged with acute administrations of chlorpromazine and improved during chronic administration, in parallel with clinical improvement (13). The inverted-U hypothesis can be employed to resolve this apparent paradox (Fig. 5-4). As mentioned in Chapter 4, chlorpromazine is thought to reduce arousal by acting on the reticular activating system. Normals operate on the upward slope of the curve, so that their performance suffers from a decrease in arousal. However, if schizophrenics operate on the downward slope of the curve, then a decrease in arousal actually improves their ability to perform the task (1).

An intriguing model, based on computer programming concepts, has been devised to explain the different responses of schizophrenics

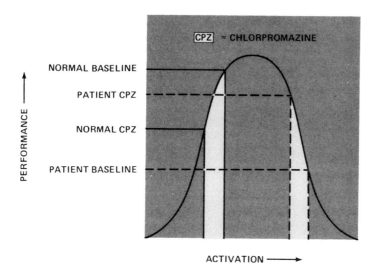

FIGURE 5-4. Inverted-U Model for Differential Effects of Chlorpromazine on Normals and Patients

and normals to chlorpromazine (14), although it has not been tested with empirical data. In this model, schizophrenics are hypothesized to be vulnerable to interference during the normal progression through "Test-Operate-Test-Exit" routines. This interference causes schizophrenics to jump prematurely to "Exit," thus disrupting their performance. According to the model, chlorpromazine causes delays in the "Test" phase, overcoming the tendency for premature "Exits." This delay is hypothesized to result from a reduction in the positive reinforcement of "Good, go on to the next step," which justifies proceeding to the next step. In contrast, normals do not "Exit" prematurely, so that a reduction in positive reinforcement causes delays which impair their performance.

Studies from a variety of sources, conducted under varying conditions, tend to support the clinical impression that chlorpromazine does not impair mental capacity. In fact, patients on chlorpromazine tend to show improvement in a variety of behavioral tasks paralleling clinical improvement (15). Normals receiving chlorpromazine also appear to experience no disruption of cognitive abilities, although the effects of the drug on psychomotor and attentive skills have been less clear-cut (16).

The importance of individual personality variables in drug response has been demonstrated in a study of the effects of chlorpromazine on two groups of normal subjects characterized by different psychological traits. The first group was physically vigorous, extroverted, and self-assertive, while the second was thought to be intellectual and introverted (17). While all subjects subjectively experienced sedating effects of 200 mg chlorpromazine and showed impairment on tasks requiring motor coordination and intellectual performance, subjects in the first group were more apprehensive, irritable, and unhappy about the drug's effects; those in the second group seemed to be tranquil and indifferent to their surroundings. Performance on learning nonsense syllables was impaired for subjects in the first group but improved for subjects in the second group.

Generally, the tranquilizing effect of chlorpromazine can be described as a reduction of stimulus significance. This reduction can account for the greater sensitivity seen with some tests. Since chlorpromazine causes outside events to become less salient or "attention grabbing," subjects are less inclined to maintain an attentive set. However, cognitive functions, which are not dependent on sustained attention, remain intact.

ANTIDEPRESSANTS

The effects of antidepressants on psychological processes of normals have not been investigated, and relatively little is known about their psychological effects on patients. To date, these drugs appear to have only slight effects on cognitive, perceptual, and psychomotor abilities. Recent studies have investigated their effects on tests believed to reflect different components of attention and of long- and short-term memory. The results have been contradictory (18,19). Depressed patients appear to have problems with memory. The extent to which memory improvement parallels clinical recovery and the role of antidepressant medication in these changes need to be investigated further.

ANTIANXIETY AGENTS

Studies of the psychological effects of the antianxiety agents are numerous, and the literature about their psychological effects is growing (4). Within this field, most investigators continue to adopt research designs which are inappropriate for understanding psychological effects of these drugs in the specific populations for whom they are most commonly prescribed, i.e., persons over forty-five years of age, women, and the anxious. Males, rather than females, and "normal" college students, rather than anxious patients, are the typical research subjects. In addition, testing is usually done after a single dose, rather than after chronic medication.

The results of separate studies can be drawn together to suggest that the benzodiazepine diazepam, the drug most frequently studied, has less of an effect on tasks requiring sustained attention than it does on tasks requiring associative cognitive effort. These characteristics resemble those of meprobamate and secobarbital and differ from those of chlorpromazine. The cortical depressant effects of diazepam persist long after other objective and subjective measures of intoxication have passed. The few studies of the psychological effects of antianxiety agents on patients have tended to employ idiosyncratic tests, so that it is still unclear whether there is a pattern of differential responsiveness between patients and normals.

Some studies have utilized the range of anxiety found in normal populations to examine the interaction between the trait of "anxiety" and the effects of an antianxiety agent. With meprobamate, improvement in performance is most likely to be found among subjects scoring high on predrug levels of anxiety and in tests involving experimentally induced anxiety (7). Among nonanxious populations or in unstressful experimental situations, meprobamate tends to have no effect or even a negative effect. Baseline conditions are obviously essential to predicting specific drug effects, and the inverted-U hypothesis again appears to be applicable.

In addition to its antianxiety effects, diazepam can produce amnesia, particularly when given intravenously. Many studies of the effects of diazepam on learning and memory have been inconclusive (4). More recent studies, employing sophisticated tests and designs, have documented significant memory impairment; in addition, they have identified the stage of memory processing which is affected (20). Recall from short-term memory is not altered, nor is retrieval of already learned material. Instead, diazepam inhibits the transfer of information from short- to long-term memory.

CONCLUSION

This chapter has explored some parameters for studying specific psychological effects of drugs. We have concentrated upon the use of behavioral tests as a measure of such psychological effects. However, it is quite apparent that drug actions are multifaceted, with behavior providing at best only an indirect measure of important effects. It is for this reason that clinical psychopharmacology is so inextricably linked to neurochemistry, neurophysiology, and behavioral biochemistry. As suggested in Chapter 1, multidisciplinary approaches are essential if we hope to uncover the connections between the effects of drugs on the brain and the ultimate expression of those effects as behavioral changes. For example, electroencephalographic (EEG) responses to stimuli involved in attention and reaction-time tests can be recorded from intact humans, providing information about the neuronal processes associated with a given behavior (Chapter 4). Since most psychoactive drugs are distinguished primarily by their effects on humans, sophisticated techniques for evaluating their influence upon the human brain ultimately must play a major role in elucidating their mechanisms of action.

REFERENCES

1. Kornetsky, C. and Mirsky, A. F.   On certain psychopharmacological and physiological differences between schizophrenics and normal persons. *Psychopharmacologia 8:*309–328, 1966.
2. Smith, R. G. and Baker, W. J.   Drug effects on learning and memory in man. *In: Drugs and the Brain.* P. Black, *ed.*, Baltimore: Johns Hopkins Press, 1969, pp. 261–276.
3. Fingl, E. and Woodbury, D. M.   General principles. *In: The Pharmacological Basis of Therapeutics,* 5th ed. L. S. Goodman and A. Gilman, *eds.*, New York: Macmillan Publishing Co., 1975, pp. 1–46.
4. Kleinknecht, R. A. and Donaldson, D.   A review of the effects of diazepam on cognitive and psychomotor performance. *J. Nerv. Ment. Dis. 161:*399–410, 1975.
5. Duffy, E.   The psychological significance of the concept of "arousal" or "activation." *Psychol. Rev. 64:*265–275, 1957.
6. Malmo, R. A.   Activation: a neuropsychological dimension. *Psychol. Rev. 66:*367–386, 1959.
7. Latz, A.   Cognitive test performance in normal adults under the influence of psychopharmacological agents: a brief review. *In: Psychopharmacology: A Review of Progress, 1957–1967.* D. Efron, *ed.*, Washington, D.C.: USPHS Bulletin #1836, 1968, pp. 83–90.
8. McNair, D. M.   Anti-anxiety drugs and human performance. *Arch. Gen. Psychiatry 29:*611–617, 1973.
9. Atkinson, R. and Shiffrin, R. M.   The control of short-term memory. *Sci. Am. 224:*82–90, 1971.
10. Anderson, J. R. and Bower, G. H.   Recognition and retrieval processes in free recall. *Psychol. Rev. 79:*97–123, 1972.
11. Kopell, B. S. and Rosenbloom, M. J.   Scalp-recorded potential correlates of psychological phenomena in man. *Adv. Psychol. Assess. 3:*433–476, 1975.
12. Mirsky, A. F. and Kornetsky, C.   On the dissimilar effects of drugs on the Digit Symbol Substitution and Continuous Performance Tests. *Psychopharmacologia 5:*161–177, 1964.
13. Orzack, M. H., Kornetsky, C., and Freeman, H.   The effects of daily administration of carphenazine on attention in the schizophrenic patient. *Psychopharmacologia 11:*31–38, 1967.
14. Callaway, E.   Schizophrenia and interference. *Arch. Gen. Psychiatry 22:*193–208, 1970.
15. Angle, H.   Role of chlorpromazine in maintaining timing behavior in chronic schizophrenics. *Psychopharmacologia 28:*185–194, 1973.
16. Uhr, L.   Objectively measured behavioral effects of psychoactive drugs. *In: Drugs and Behavior.* L. Uhr and L. L. Miller, *eds.*, New York: John Wiley & Sons, 1960, pp. 610–634.
17. Heninger, G., DiMascio, A., and Klerman, G. L.   Personality factors in variability of responses to phenothiazines. *Am. J. Psychiatry 121:*1091–1094, 1965.
18. Henry, G. M., Weingartner, H., and Murphy, D. L.   Influence of affective states and psychoactive drugs on verbal learning and memory. *Am. J. Psychiatry 130:*966–971, 1973.

19. Sternberg, D. E. and Jarvik, M. E. Memory function in depression: improvement with antidepressant medication. *Arch. Gen. Psychiatry* 33:219–224, 1976.
20. Ghoneim, M. M. and Mewaldt, S. P. Effects of diazepam and scopolamine on storage, retrieval, and organizational processes in memory. *Psychopharmacologia* 44:257–262, 1975.

6 | Sociopharmacology

PATRICIA R. BARCHAS and JACK D. BARCHAS

INTRODUCTION

Other chapters in this volume have discussed physiological actions of drugs, the use of drugs in treatment of some of the recognized psychiatric syndromes, and the effect of drugs upon certain psychological processes which seem to underlie some symptomatology. This chapter will discuss the relationship of drugs to the social situation, focusing upon small group situations. Our goal is to present some of the tools and approaches of sociopharmacology, an emerging discipline which has relevance to an understanding of some of the mechanisms through which drugs act and of some of the reasons that they are used by humans—intensely social organisms.

A connection between the social setting and pharmacological action is suggested by three lines of evidence: 1) social situations can markedly alter spontaneous physiological processes, 2) the social situation can govern an individual's interpretation of drug effects and can alter the effect of drugs, and 3) drug action feeds back into the social system itself.

The behaving individual is at a vortex of experience that he patterns according to his perceptions. Experience and perceptions are, to a great extent, formed by the social processes in which he acts. As the individual behaves, his physiology adjusts to his position in the environment. Through his behavior he may alter the environment for himself and others, producing a continuous flow of interrelationships between physiology, behavior, and social structure. Social life is inextricably bound to biological life, each influencing and setting the stage for the other. We are just beginning to understand how to inquire into that interaction. There is strong evidence attesting to the powerful impact of social environments, relations, and structures upon physiology—and, as an intervening variable, upon drug effects. There is yet to be developed a typology of social situations by drug or by disease.

There are larger societal processes in which psychoactive drugs play an important role. These include legal and illegal distribution of drugs, drug-related crime, inducement of individuals into a drug culture, the economics associated with drug use, and deviant and nondeviant behaviors. Although these are critically important areas, they will not be considered in this chapter.

PHYSIOLOGICAL RESPONSE TO SOCIAL SITUATIONS

Physiological sociology is concerned with those areas in which an explanation of changes in biology is aided by reference to the individual's relation to the social system (1). In physiological sociology the relation of prime interest is between internal physiological processes and external social events. Perceptions and emotions are mediating variables which are related to and important in physiological sociology but which are determined, in part, by sociological events. Social situations alter physiology in the same kinds of ways that pharmacological agents do. We do not know if mood, cognitions, and feeling tones are modified in exactly the same way, although we do know that both social and pharmacological events may change affect and behavior.

Physiological processes related to social structure can be most effectively investigated using small group social processes such as the establishment and maintenance of status, conformity, and normative behavior. These processes are as basic to social interaction as the metabolism of glucose is to biochemistry.

To date, studies have concentrated primarily upon the endocrine correlates of hierarchical processes (2). Thus, adrenal cortical function is known to vary with dominance in a variety of species. In ongoing groups of monkeys, dominance was found to correlate roughly with androgen levels, although aggression, a particularly complex behavior, was not so related (3). In rodents, adrenal medullary function and social interaction were studied using interconnected cages—a technique that leads to confrontations and severe social stimulation. Catecholamine-synthesizing enzymes were decreased in the dominant animals in groupings exposed to the situation for prolonged periods (4).

More recently, the relationship between social status processes and catecholamine secretion has been studied in humans (5). Individuals of equal external status, as determined by education, age, race, and sex, were allowed to interact for one hour. The status differential that was established between the individuals through interaction was assessed by observers and by questionnaires to the subjects. There was no relationship between acquired status and the concentration of catecholamines in urines taken before the interaction. However, there was a pattern of association between acquired status and the urinary catecholamines sampled after interaction: individuals with higher acquired status had higher epinephrine secretion and lower norepinephrine secretion.

A means of studying the relationship of social processes to endocrine and other physiological processes is suggested from investigations of free fatty acids and social behavioral states. Free fatty acid levels are believed to correlate highly with sympathetic activation, of which adrenal-medullary activity would be an important component. There are demonstrated correlations between free fatty acid levels and behavioral measures of conformity and leadership (6). The meaning of the social situation to the individual was found to intervene between the physiological and behavioral response. This suggests that the meaning of a situation may dictate what the individual reacts to as arousing stimuli.

Neurochemical measures may also be altered by social behavior, as suggested in rodent studies. Few variables have been investigated, but studies have shown changes in brain catecholamine utilization in relation to housing conditions and to behaviors, including aggression (7).

While we have focused on data which relate endocrine and neurochemical function to social processes, there is also evidence that neurophysiological processes may be altered by social structural manipulation. These studies have used contingent negative variation (CNV), a slow brain wave which occurs prior to a response to a stimulus about which the subject has been warned. The CNV may well be altered in certain psychiatric states (Chapter 4). The CNV may reflect various internal events, including motivation, expectation, preparedness for action, and attention. Using attention to link sociological findings with the CNV physiological events, it has been demonstrated that individuals who are manipulated into a high status relative to another exhibit heightened CNVs (1). Thus there is empirical evidence that position in a social structure alters brain events in a patterned way, mediated by psychological variables.

EFFECTS OF SOCIAL SITUATION ON ACTIONS
OF PHARMACOLOGICAL AGENTS

Physicians are becoming increasingly aware of the potential contribution of social setting to the effectiveness of pharmacological agents. A seminal study was conducted by Schachter and Singer (8). Subjects received either adrenaline or a placebo under varying conditions of information about what to expect. In the adrenaline/no information condition, subjects used the social cues provided by the experimental setting to give meaning to their aroused condition. Both interpretation of feeling and behavior were affected.

The clinical relevance of such concerns is illustrated by a study with phenothiazines in which it was shown that schizophrenics treated with the drugs exhibited differential improvement rates, depending upon the environmental characteristics of their wards (9). That is, milieu modified the effect of the drug. Thus, there is evidence—for one drug, for one severe symptomatology—that aspects of the social situation alter the effect of treatment agents.

Moos and his group (10) have stimulated the application of studies of the environment to psychiatry. They have proposed that social situations affect physiologies through changes in perception. They provide evidence that environments, such as psychiatric wards, classrooms, and work groups, tend to have characteristic profiles, according to perceptions of persons in them. The dimensions upon which perceptions of environments cluster are: relationship, examples of which are involvement, affiliation, peer cohesion, staff support, and expressiveness; personal development, which consists of autonomy or independence and responsibility; and system maintenance and change, which include order and organization, clarity, and control. Work pressure and innovation or change are found in some environments. The social environment, as it is perceived by individuals, exerts influences on the individual within that environment. These investigators stress that the environment does not act directly upon the individual but through perception of the social environment as mediated by personality variables, roles and status relationships, and behavior.

Individuals who interact closely with each other come to show a similarity on certain physiological indices. For example, the secretion of 17-hydroxycorticoids in same-sex groups in different studies has been shown to cluster (11); in females, covariation of menstrual cycles occurs among friends and roommates in a college dormitory but not among randomly selected pairs. Other studies using galvanic skin response suggest that positive or negative involvement promotes physiological covariation but that neutrality does not (12).

EFFECTS OF PHARMACOLOGICAL AGENTS ON THE SOCIAL SITUATION

Social behaviors are the building blocks of social structure. Although social structure is tolerant of some behavioral variants, severe, critical, or prolonged alterations of behavior will pull the structure itself out of shape. We see this behaviorally in damaged communication patterns in families, though there are as yet no biological referents for these altered social structures. Drugs can modify individual behavior and, through the behaviors, affect social structures and the processes which maintain them. The structures themselves influence behavior and feelings of individuals, as they markedly influence who does what with whom.

Alteration of central neurotransmitters has been found to produce major effects upon social behavior. Studies would suggest that certain forms of social behaviors may be mediated by catecholamine-containing neurons and are altered by drugs which affect catecholamine mechanisms. For example, in nonhuman primates, administration of drugs which decrease brain catecholamines decreases social initiation and may result in decreased dominance. Such animals may be more peripheral to their social group and exhibit both decreased threat behavior and decreased affiliative behavior in the form of social grooming (13). The findings that central catecholamine systems are profoundly involved in primate social behaviors raises questions as to the role of central catecholamines in human social behaviors. The processes that have been studied—status, affiliation, and dominance—are related to basic social processes that have previously been shown to be similar in non-human and human primates.

Limited studies have been conducted of the effects of normally used psychopharmacological agents on social processes. There are marked changes in communication patterns after alcohol in dyadic, mixed-sex groups (14). Alcohol—in the form of a couple of glasses of wine—also alters the processes by which groups of previously unacquainted individuals interact to create a social structure (1). Interestingly, the structure that is created when group members are under the influence of alcohol tends not to carry over to the situation in which the same members are not under the influence of alcohol. Ordinarily, created structures do tend to carry over. This raises the interesting question of whether agents which have been found to have state-dependent (dissociative) effects on human memory for cognitive tasks also have such effects on social learning. Alcohol and marihuana, as well as stimulants and barbiturates, have been demonstrated to have state-dependent learning effects in humans. For example, doses of marihuana which are equivalent to a moderate "social high" can produce state-dependent effects on cognitive tasks (15). It is as if relationships learned under some pharmacological states may be difficult to retrieve in nonpharmacological states, thus creating gaps in the social fabric. This may also have important implications in clinical situations in terms of the effects of drugs used in treatment (cf. Chapter 1).

FUTURE DIRECTIONS

As sociopharmacology links particular structural patterns to physiological responses, it may be able to delineate effects by drug and dose, by type of social structure, and by disease. As this is done, the field will undoubtedly come to be concerned with issues of time and timing of exposure to certain social structures. Thus, developmental aspects will be explored, as will conditions under which physiological responses are and are not mutable. From such investigation should come knowledge which will permit the physician to design intervention strategies that will optimize conditions for a patient's development and growth.

At this stage, it seems reasonable to assume that physiological and sociological processes are intimately related. Sociological processes set in motion events that influence physiological mechanisms. Drugs also alter internal states. Drugs and social context each modify the effect of the other upon the individual—physiologically, emotionally, and cognitively. In the simplest scheme, we assume that sociological events affect the body chemistry and that, in turn, the chemical change affects the probability of future sociological events. Psychopharmacological agents logically should influence social processes. An understanding of resulting changes in social processes so altered is likely to provide important information about one level of the mechanism of action of such drugs.

REFERENCES

1. Barchas, P. Physiological sociology: interface of sociological and biological processes. *Ann. Rev. Sociology 2:*299–333, 1976.
2. Barchas, P. and Barchas, J. Physiological sociology: endocrine correlates of status behavior. *In: American Handbook of Psychiatry.* Vol. 6. D. Hamburg and H. K. H. Brodie, *eds.,* New York: Basic Books, 1975, pp. 623–640.
3. Rose, R. M., Gordon, T. P., and Bernstein, I. S. Plasma testosterone levels in the male rhesus: influences of sexual and social stimuli. *Science 178:*643–645, 1972.
4. Henry, J. P., Ely, D. L., and Stephans, P. M. Changes in catecholamine-controlling enzymes in response to psychosocial activation of the defense and alarm reactions. *In: Physiology, Emotions, and Psychosomatic Illness.* New York: CIBA Foundation, 1972, pp. 225–251.
5. Barchas, P. R. and Barchas, J. D. Social behavior and adrenal medullary function in relation to psychiatric disorders. *In: Neuroregulators and Psychiatric Disorders.* E. Usdin, D. Hamburg, and J. Barchas, *eds.,* New York: Oxford University Press, 1977, pp. 95–102.
6. Back, K. W. and Bogdonoff, M. D. Plasma lipid responses to leadership, conformity, and deviation. *In: Psychobiological Approaches to Social Behavior.* P. H. Leiderman and D. Shapiro, *eds.,* Stanford: Stanford University Press, 1964, pp. 24–42.
7. Stolk, J. M., Conner, R., and Barchas, J. D. Social environment and brain biogenic amine metabolism. *J. Comp. Physiol. Psychol. 87:*203–207, 1974.
8. Schachter, S. and Singer, J. E. Cognitive, social and physiological determinants of emotional state. *Psychol. Rev. 69:*379–399, 1962.
9. Kellam, S., Goldberg, S., Schooler, N., Berman, A., and Schmelzer, J. Ward atmosphere and outcome of treatment of acute schizophrenia. *J. Psychol. Res. 5:*145–163, 1967.
10. Kiritz, S. and Moos, R. H. Physiological effects of social environment. *Psychosom. Med. 36:*96–114, 1974.
11. Mason, J. and Brady, J. The sensitivity of psychoendocrine systems to social and physical environment. *In: Psychobiological Approaches to Social Behavior.* P. H. Leiderman and D. Shapiro, *eds.,* Stanford: Stanford University Press, 1964, pp. 4–23.
12. Kaplan, H. B., Burch, N. R., and Bloom, S. W. Physiological covariation and sociometric relationships in small peer groups. *In: Psychobiological Approaches to Social Behavior.* P. H. Leiderman and D. Shapiro, *eds.,* Stanford: Stanford University Press, 1964, pp. 92–109.
13. Redmond, D. E., Maas, J. W., Kling, A., Graham, C. W., and Dekirmenjian, H. Social behavior of monkeys selectively depleted of monoamines. *Science 174:*428–431, 1971.
14. Smith, R. C., Parker, E. S., and Noble, E. P. Alcohol's effect on some formal aspects of verbal social communication. *Arch. Gen. Psychiatry 32:*1394–1398, 1975.
15. Stillman, R. C., Weingartner, H., Wyatt, R. J., Gillin, J. C., and Eich, J. State-dependent (dissociative) effects of marihuana on human memory. *Arch. Gen. Psychiatry 31:*81–85, 1974.

II | Theory and Practice of Psychopharmacology

Part II describes the diagnosis and pharmacological treatment of severe psychiatric disorders and reviews the biochemical hypotheses of their etiologies. The affective disorders and schizophrenia are major public health problems which require a significant proportion of hospital beds and physician effort. Substantial progress has been made in defining biochemical mechanisms which might be involved in these psychiatric illnesses and in suggesting mechanisms by which psychopharmacological agents exert their effects. The greatest concern of many physicians is the effective diagnosis and the immediate and long-term treatment of ill patients, using available agents. We have provided detailed descriptions of the appropriate uses and of the side effects of the major psychopharmacological medications. We have also attempted to highlight areas of continuing research into the etiology and treatment of these states.

For some psychiatric illnesses, such as anxiety states, insomnia, and aggression, little is known about the underlying biochemistry. The overwhelming importance of psychological and sociological factors in these disorders is clear. However, the powerful effects of drugs such as the antianxiety agents are equally undeniable and suggest important relationships between behavioral and biochemical processes. As yet, we lack even a vocabulary to describe such interactions. Hopefully, one will emerge as we continue to study this important area, so that we can begin to effectively deal with the complex issues which arise.

7 | Emergency Treatment

BURR EICHELMAN

INTRODUCTION

Early in training, a psychiatrist frequently serves as admitting physician for an active inpatient service. Beyond making the decision to hospitalize a patient and constructing a differential diagnosis, he will be pressured to "do something"—to "stop the crazy behavior" and reduce the dysphoria and panic of a patient or the staff anxiety level of the ward or emergency room. This chapter raises some warnings and suggests some guidelines for fulfilling that role. The general emphasis is on pharmacological interventions which can be initiated in a well-staffed emergency room or during the first twenty-four to forty-eight hours of hospital admission. This chapter is intended only as a brief introduction to the management of psychiatric emergencies. More detailed discussions of pharmacological treatments for psychiatric disorders are presented in subsequent chapters of this volume.

GENERAL PRINCIPLES

Four principles can facilitate the initial treatment of a psychiatric patient.

WHEN IN DOUBT, OBSERVE

A correct diagnosis is extremely helpful in selecting an appropriate pharmacological treatment. Hasty pharmacological intervention may contribute to the problem rather than alleviate it. For example, suppose a patient reports that he took an overdose of amphetamines when, in fact, he took amitriptyline. In this case, treatment with chlorproma-

91

zine (Thorazine), which could be appropriate for amphetamine toxicity, would compound the sedation that follows amitriptyline ingestion.

CONSIDER BEHAVIORAL INTERVENTIONS PRIOR TO PHARMACOLOGICAL ONES

The night light for the agitated patient with an organic brain syndrome, the structured "talk-down" of a patient on a bad trip, or the use of physical restraints for the undiagnosed violent patient may be wise investments during the initial hours of treatment and evaluation.

WHEN THE DIAGNOSIS IS IN DOUBT BUT MEDICATION IS NECESSARY, GIVE THE MOST BENIGN

For example, if the differential diagnosis includes acute schizophrenic episode and psychosis from "street drug" administration, a benzodiazepine may provide adequate symptomatic treatment for a more prolonged period of observation and history-gathering, until the weight of evidence strongly favors one diagnosis over the other. If an antipsychotic agent were given, its anticholinergic effects might contribute to possible toxic psychosis.

USE A DRUG'S SIDE EFFECTS FOR ADDITIONAL CLINICAL EFFICACY

For instance, agitated patients can benefit from the sedating effects of antipsychotics or antidepressants.

ACUTE PSYCHOTIC STATES OF UNKNOWN ETIOLOGY

Hyponatremia, bromide intoxication, encephalitis, scopolamine poisoning, hallucinogen ingestion, pheochromocytoma, thyroid dysfunction, and many other problems—each can present as a schizophreni-form psychosis. Thus, careful history-taking and diagnosis are crucial. The patient and accompanying friends should be questioned about over-the-counter medications, industrial occupations, and medical diseases. In addition, the physician should ask whether the .psychotic symptoms are new, whether they have been experienced by another family member, and whether there are other nonbehavioral symptoms, such as vomiting, headache, or fever, which might be important to the diagnosis.

The history should be supplemented with a thorough physical examination and adequate laboratory screening. Depending on the institution, this may be carried out by the psychiatrist or by an internal medicine consultant. Patients with syphilis or carcinomas do appear on psychiatric units. These diseases, along with others such as tuberculosis, can be diagnosed on admission after routine screening.

The medical examination at the time of admission also can alert the physician to contraindications for and possible complications with certain medications. If contraindications are absolute, the medication can be avoided. In addition, a report of difficulty with urination or of glaucoma-like eye pain can alert the physician to possible exacerbation of both conditions by the anticholinergic effects of phenothiazines.

In general, if the etiology of a psychotic state remains undetermined after a thorough initial evaluation, the patient should be managed with vigorous behavioral interventions supplemented by benzodiazepines, while additional studies are undertaken and further behavioral observation continues.

AMPHETAMINE PSYCHOSIS

Psychosis precipitated *solely* by amphetamines can be efficiently treated with phenothiazines, such as chlorpromazine, in doses comparable to those discussed below for schizophrenia. If the patient might also have taken an hallucinogen with anticholinergic properties, chlorpromazine is contraindicated and a benzodiazepine should be used. The treatment of adverse reactions to amphetamines and related compounds is discussed in detail in Chapter 24.

SCHIZOPHRENIA

Many different types of antipsychotic medications are available to the physician for treating acute schizophrenia. Early in his career, the psychiatrist should gain experience with at least one drug from each of the major drug classes (Chapter 9). For a newly admitted schizophrenic patient, the choice among the antipsychotic medication classes depends mainly on whether sedative action is needed to control agitation, anxiety, or disruptive behavior. In general, the low-potency agents have greater sedative activity. Therefore, agitated schizophrenic patients can be treated with chlorpromazine, 50–100 mg orally four times a day. This can be supplemented with additional oral doses of 50–100 mg as often as every four hours, as needed. Since chlorpromazine can produce hypotension, intramuscular injections of the drug should be limited to 50 mg every four hours. The physician should be aware that intramuscular chlorpromazine is painful. If hypotension develops, it can usually be treated by having the patient lie down. If pharmacological intervention becomes necessary, a drug with α-adrenergic and no β-adrenergic activity, such as norepinephrine, should be used. Norepinephrine, 4 mg in 500 ml of solution, can be given intravenously by continuous infusion. Isoproterenol and epinephrine, which have β-adrenergic activity, can exacerbate the hypotension.

The high-potency antipsychotic haloperidol (Haldol) can also be used for the agitated or disruptive patient, even though haloperidol is less sedating than chlorpromazine in the usual therapeutic range. Severely agitated, violent, or excited patients often respond well to haloperidol, 10 mg orally or 5 mg intramuscularly, given every four hours. Some physicians have suggested that, for patients in severe catatonic excitement, haloperidol can even be given in these doses as often as every thirty minutes. If medication must be given prior to transporting a patient who is unmanageable by restraints alone, haloperidol has advantages over chlorpromazine, since there is less risk of hypotension in transit.

For patients who do not require sedation, an antipsychotic with less sedative activity, such as fluphenazine (Prolixin) can be used. Fluphenazine can be initiated at 2.5–5.0 mg, two times a day, and increased to 20 mg, two times a day. It can also be given in depot injections as the enanthate or decanoate, for sustained release. However, such long-term, irreversible treatment generally is premature during the initial period of hospitalization; rather, it should be used only after careful, long-term planning with the patient prior to discharge. Often, suspicious or paranoid patients will tolerate fluphenazine better than chlorpromazine, since there is less sedation and patient vigilance is less impeded. Similarly, patients experiencing an initial schizophrenic psychosis often accept this drug more readily than they do the more sedating antipsychotics. A detailed discussion of the use of antipsychotic medications and of their side effects is provided in Chapter 9.

The prophylactic use of antiparkinsonian agents in patients treated with antipsychotics is controversial. Unquestionably, they help to prevent some of the disturbing side effects of antipsychotics. An acute dystonic reaction in a patient who is psychotic or who is emerging from a psychosis can be a frightening experience and may cause the patient to refuse further treatment. Consequently, it may be appropriate to use antiparkinsonian agents prophylactically in young, acutely psychotic patients being treated with high-potency antipsychotics such as haloperidol. To avoid extrapyramidal reactions, one can use benztropine mesylate (Cogentin), 1-2 mg orally, one to two times a day. For the acute treatment, intramuscular injections of 50 mg of diphenhydramine (Benadryl), of 500 mg of caffein sodium benzoate, or of 2 mg of benztropine mesylate, can be given. However, antiparkinsonian drugs also have anticholinergic activity, which may increase the risk of anticholinergic reactions with antipsychotics (Chapter 24). If the anticholinergic activity results in urinary retention, bethanecol chloride (Urecholine), 10–30 mg orally, three or four times a day, can be helpful. As the psychosis resolves, the antiparkinsonian medication should be discontinued as soon as possible. Sample admission orders for a newly admitted patient with acute schizophrenia are presented in Table 7-1.

MANIA

Initially, manic episodes can be treated with antipsychotic agents such as chlorpromazine, 100 mg orally, four times a day, or haloperi-

TABLE 7-1.

SAMPLE ADMITTING ORDERS FOR AN ACUTE SCHIZOPHRENIC PATIENT

---

1. Admit to ward no. 7, tentative dx.: acute schizophrenia
2. Vital signs: pulse, respir., temp, BP bid
3. Regular diet
4. Mark chart allergic to . . .
5. CBC, UA, SMA 6 and 12 in a.m.
6. Haloperidol 5 mg po bid
7. Haloperidol 5 mg im or 10 mg po, 4 hr prn agitated or assaultive behavior
8. Benztropine mesylate 1 mg po bid
9. Benzotropine mesylate 2 mg, im or po, q 6 hr, prn extrapyramidal reaction
10. Restrict to unit
11. Seclude and restrain prn.; then call physician; order expires in 24 hr

---

dol, 5 mg orally, two times a day. As needed, these can be augmented every four hours with chlorpromazine, 100 mg orally or 50 mg intramuscularly, or haloperidol, 10 mg orally or 5 mg intramuscularly. On subsequent days, the total antipsychotic medication should be adjusted to prevent disruptive behavior without undue sedation. Soon after treatment is begun, the patient should be evaluated for lithium therapy, as detailed in Chapter 12. Within seven to ten days, lithium alone will probably be sufficient to prevent disruptive behavior, and other medications can be reduced and eventually discontinued.

DEPRESSION

Only severe depressions, depressions with psychosis, or depressions with suicidal risk should be treated immediately with antidepressant medications. Patients with psychotic or severely agitated depressions can be given antipsychotics; others who require immediate treatment should be started on tricyclic antidepressants (tricyclics). Less severely depressed patients should first be evaluated for the characterological and situational aspects of the depression. In these patients, benzodiazepines may be used to promote sleep or to reduce agitation. A detailed discussion of the pharmacological treatment of depression is presented in Chapter 11.

Physicians should remember that the tricyclics are not as safe as the antipsychotics and benzodiazepines. Thus, when prescribing tricyclics, they should evaluate the patient's potential for overdosing, restrict the number of pills given in each prescription, and seek the assistance of the patient's friends who could supervise the administration of this potentially lethal medication.

ACUTE ANXIETY

Benzodiazepines such as diazepam (Valium), 5–10 mg, can be given as needed as often as every four hours for management of acute anxiety. Some kinetic studies of benzodiazepines suggest that they need not be given this frequently. However, patients often report that frequent administration is more helpful. This effect may be due to an as yet unrecognized metabolic aspect of the drugs. Alternatively, the resulting increase in staff-patient interactions may provide additional therapeutic effects through a placebo response (Chapter 31). Flurazepam (Dalmane) can be given for sleep in doses of 15–30 mg at bedtime. This dose can be repeated an hour later, if the patient requests additional medication. If a patient has a history of taking meprobamate (Miltown), if he forcefully requests this drug, and if an antianxiety agent is indicated, he may be given the analogue tybamate (Tybatran), 250–500 mg three to four times a day, as indicated. Tybamate is metabolized more rapidly than meprobamate and discontinuance of it is not accompanied by the severe withdrawal symptoms which are often seen with meprobamate. A detailed discussion of the treatment of anxiety is found in Chapter 13.

ADVERSE REACTIONS TO ADDICTIVE DRUGS AND ALCOHOL

Sedative-hypnotics, narcotic analgesics, and alcohol are three classes of addictive drugs whose use can lead to emergency room visits. The abuser of addictive drugs presents with an overdose, a withdrawal syndrome, or a medical illness which may be related to his drug abuse. Overdoses of sedative-hypnotics and alcohol require immediate evaluation of cardiopulmonary function. Resuscitation and assisted ventilation, blood pressure support, and admission to an intensive care unit may all be necessary. Overdoses of narcotic analgesics are treated in the same way, except that a specific opiate antagonist can be administered after resuscitation has begun. Naloxone (Narcan), 0.4 mg, can be given intravenously. This dose can be repeated every three minutes, two to three times, if necessary. Since naloxone is a pure opiate antagonist, it will not worsen mixed overdoses and can even be used when a patient presents with coma from unknown causes. Management of overdose syndromes of addictive drugs of abuse is described in Chapter 23.

Withdrawal reactions from addictive drugs are treated by substituting a cross-tolerant medication, followed by gradually decreasing the dose. Opiate withdrawal syndromes can be treated with oral methadone. The amount used in the first twenty-four hours can be individualized, but for many daily opiate users, 10–20 mg of methadone twice daily is sufficient. Once the twenty-four-hour dose is determined, it can be reduced by 10–20 percent of the original dose each day, until the patient is free of opiates after five to ten days. Sedative-hypnotic withdrawal is a potentially fatal syndrome and should be treated rapidly. Phenobarbital is cross-tolerant to sedative-hypnotics and can be used to prevent or diminish the serious abstinence syndrome. Again, the amount used in the first twenty-four hours can be individualized. In some cases, this amount can be approximated by using a simple test of tolerance described in Chapter 23. When the twenty-four-hour requirement of phenobarbital is established, this amount can be reduced by 10 percent each day for ten days. Phenobarbital should be given in three to four divided doses.

Chlordiazepoxide (Librium) is often used to manage impending delirium tremens or alcohol hallucinosis (Chapter 23). When possible, it should be given orally, since absorption from intramuscular injection sites is unreliable. For mild withdrawal syndromes, chlordiazepoxide, 25 mg, can be given every four hours; more severe cases may require as much as 100 mg every two hours. The physician or a well-trained nurse should evaluate the patient every two to four hours, to ensure adequate therapy without oversedation. Seizures can be treated acutely with intravenous diazepam (Valium) at an infusion rate of 5 mg per minute, until the seizure stops or until 20–30 mg of drug has been given. Phenothiazines are contraindicated in alcohol withdrawal, since they can lower the seizure threshold. Withdrawing alcoholics who have poor nutritional status should also receive intramuscular injections of multivitamins and of 100 mg of thiamine.

Emergency rooms increasingly encounter the "polydrug abusers," who may be intoxicated simultaneously with alcohol, barbiturates, and other drugs of abuse. The treatment of this complex problem is discussed in Chapter 24. The physician must carefully evaluate all the drugs involved before initiating a systematic campaign to remove specific components of the abused drugs in an appropriate order.

"BAD TRIPS"

Patients presenting with "bad trips" are most often simply "talked down" in the emergency room. If they need acute ancillary medication, diazepam, 10–30 mg, can be given orally or intramuscularly. Phenothiazines should not be used, since they may add to anticholinergic effects which are present in many street drugs and may mask a coexisting schizophrenia. The treatment of the nonaddictive drug abuser is discussed in Chapter 24.

ORGANIC BRAIN SYNDROME

Etiology is important in deciding on appropriate medication for organic brain syndrome. If it is induced by toxins, drug overdose, infection, or metabolic imbalance, the direct cause should be treated. However, in cases of organic brain syndrome which are secondary to senile dementia or arteriosclerotic vascular disease, small doses of antipsychotic agents such as haloperidol, 2 mg, one to two times a day, or antihistamines such as diphenhydramine, 50 mg, four times a day, can be helpful (Chapter 28).

8 | Biogenic Amine Hypotheses of Schizophrenia

JACK D. BARCHAS, GLEN R. ELLIOTT,

and PHILIP A. BERGER

INTRODUCTION

In the last twenty years, studies of biochemical and pharmacological correlates to schizophrenia have yielded an impressive body of data. And yet, not only are the etiology and pathogenesis of schizophrenia still unknown, but even the mechanisms by which some pharmacological agents are able to ameliorate schizophrenic symptoms remain obscure. Although there have been numerous variants, two hypotheses have dominated the search for a biological substrate of schizophrenia: one suggests that schizophrenic symptoms arise from the endogenous production or abnormal accumulation of a methylated psychotogen, while the other postulates that schizophrenia results from a functional hyperactivity of one or more cerebral dopaminergic systems.

THE TRANSMETHYLATION HYPOTHESIS OF SCHIZOPHRENIA

Osmond and Smythies (1) were the first to suggest that the aberrant formation of methylated amines might play an etiological role in schizophrenia. They noted that mescaline, a powerful hallucinogen (Fig. 8-1), is an O-methylated derivative of the catecholamines and that the synthesis of epinephrine requires an N-methylating enzyme. They therefore proposed that this or another enzyme might incorrectly O-methylate catecholamines to yield a "mescaline-like" substance such as dimethoxyphenylethylamine (DMPEA) (Fig. 8-1). With the subsequent discovery of the indoleamine 5-hydroxytrypta-

mine (serotonin) in mammalian brains and the identification of methylated indoleamines such as N,N-dimethyltryptamine (DMT) psilocin, psilocybin, and D-lysergic acid diethylamide (LSD) (see Fig. 8-1)
as powerful hallucinogens in man, the original methylation hypothesis
of Osmond and Smythies was expanded to what has been called the
"transmethylation" hypothesis of schizophrenia, which postulates that
schizophrenia arises from the abnormal accumulation of a psychoto-

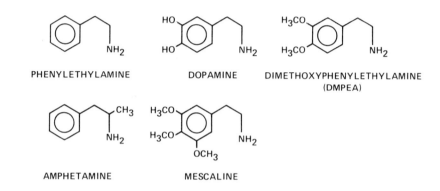

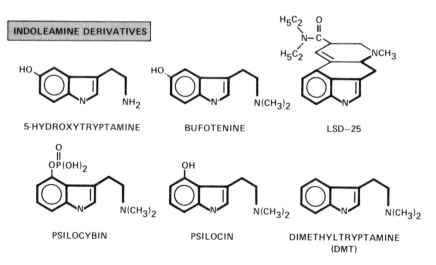

FIGURE 8-1. Compounds Relevant to Hypotheses of Schizophrenia

genic N- or O-methylated biogenic amine derivative (2). (For a good compendium of the hallucinogenic properties of methylated biogenic amines, see 3.)

Investigations of the transmethylation hypothesis may be conveniently divided into three types: 1) efforts to detect methylated derivatives of biogenic amines in biological fluids, 2) pharmacological interventions aimed at altering the turnover of such methylated derivaitves, and 3) attempts to identify and characterize enzymes which might be involved in the synthesis of these compounds.

Excretion of Methylated Amines

Dimethoxyphenylethylamine (DMPEA). As mentioned earlier, dimethoxyphenylethylamine was proposed as a possible endogenous psychotogen. In 1962, a compound which was characterized as dimethoxyphenylethylamine was found in urine samples from 15 of 19 schizophrenics and none of 14 controls (4). It became known as the "pink spot," because of its color on staining. Despite the promise of the original report, a large number of subsequent studies have failed to establish not only whether this compound plays any role in schizophrenia but even whether it is an abnormal constituent of urine (5).

Methylated Indoleamines. With the discovery that methylated indoleamines are powerful hallucinogens (Chapter 22), a search was made for these compounds in urines of schizophrenics. Although bufotenine and N,N-dimethyltryptamine (DMT)—the N,N-dimethylated derivatives of 5-hydroxytryptamine and tryptamine, respectively (Fig. 8-1)—have been detected in urine and plasma samples from both schizophrenics and normal controls, no consistent differences between schizophrenics and controls have emerged (5). It is important to emphasize, however, that failure to identify a methylated amine which is uniquely associated with schizophrenia cannot eliminate the possible existence of such a compound. First, the list of reasonable candidates is enormous and has in no way been studied exhaustively. Second, appropriate controls for the effects of diet, drug treatment, hospitalization, and other factors is both crucial and extremely difficult. Third, methylated amines may be a normal constituent of biological systems, so that changes in accumulation, excretion, or receptor mechanisms may be far more important than are absolute concentrations. Finally, it is conceivable that the important changes are occurring in specific cerebral nuclei, so that sampling at distant sites such as plasma or even cerebrospinal fluid may provide no information about the important phenomena.

ATTEMPTS TO ALTER THE PRODUCTION OF THE PROPOSED PSYCHOTOGEN

A second strategy for evaluating the transmethylation hypothesis has centered about attempts to alter schizophrenic symptoms by "loading" with amino acids which might act as precursors for the psychotogen. This approach was stimulated by a report that, in the presence of a monoamine oxidase (MAO) inhibitor, large oral doses of methionine produced an increase in psychotic symptoms of schizophrenics (6). It was suggested that methionine might increase the psychotic symptoms by supplying methyl groups, thus enhancing transmethylation reactions. Since this first study, at least fifteen other reports have appeared about the effects of methionine loading in schizophrenia, as summarized in a recent review (7). Despite a wide variety of study populations, drug regimens, and experimental designs, there is unanimous agreement that methionine produces a deterioration in mental status. What remains unclear is whether this deterioration represents a true increase in schizophrenic symptoms or an additional toxic psychosis. Some have argued that methionine does not produce new symptoms but, instead, increases pre-existing schizophrenic symptoms; others have suggested that methionine loading probably induces a superimposed intoxication. Furthermore, even if schizophrenia were specifically exacerbated by methionine, the effect need not result from an increase in methylation. Although animal studies have shown that methionine loading does lead to increased concentrations of the methyl donor S-adenosylmethionine (SAM) in brain and liver, there are undoubtedly other direct and indirect effects of this compound (8). Thus, while the methionine-loading studies are suggestive, they neither confirm nor disprove the transmethylation hypothesis.

If, as suggested by the methionine-loading studies, an increase in methylating activity exacerbates schizophrenic symptoms, then blockade of methylation reactions might ameliorate the disorder. Nicotinamide therapy for schizophrenics was, in part, based on the *in vitro* ability of this substance to serve as an acceptor of methyl groups. Although this treatment is still favored by some physicians, controlled studies have failed to show significant improvement in schizophrenics receiving nicotinamide (5). Similar "megavitamin" therapies have been attempted with a variety of other vitamins for many reasons. While there may be some instances in which individuals with specific vitamin deficiencies improve, double-blind trials of these treatments have not demonstrated their efficacy. Similarly, efforts to decrease methylations with a low methionine diet have failed to produce significant improvement in schizophrenic symptoms (9).

Like the studies of methylated amines, efforts to alter psychotogen production have failed to establish whether methylation reactions are involved in schizophrenia. Again, there are mitigating circumstances for this failure. Just as the excretion studies may be confounded by processes which are unrelated to the disease, so too are the loading studies unable to differentiate between specific actions on the systems of interest and other direct and indirect effects produced by large doses of the drugs. In addition, relevant effects of the agents may be impossible to characterize precisely, since it can be extremely difficult to distinguish between increases in specific psychotic symptomatology and the addition of an overlying organic psychosis. Furthermore, day-to-day fluctuations in individual symptomatology may either be mistaken for or mask the effects of the drug.

Attempts to Identify N-Methylating Enzymes

A third approach to investigating the transmethylation hypothesis has entailed identification of enzymes which might produce methylated biogenic amines. In 1961, Axelrod (10) described an enzyme which could transfer a methyl group from S-adenosylmethionine (SAM) to a variety of indoleamine substrates, producing potentially psychotogenic compounds (Fig. 8-2A). Although Axelrod originally isolated this SAM enzyme from rabbit lung, it has subsequently been detected in several other organs and species, including man (11). A recent study examined the activity of the SAM enzyme in preparations of red blood cells, plasma, and platelets from controls, chronic schizophrenics, and psychotic depressives (12). No differences were found in either red-blood-cell or plasma activities; but platelet preparations from schizophrenics and psychotic depressives did have significantly higher activities than did those of normal controls, although the variability was high and the difference was partially produced by a dialyzable factor in the nonpsychotic group. Studies of the SAM enzyme in preparations of autopsied brain parts from chronic schizophrenics and normal controls have also failed to reveal marked differences between chronic schizophrenics and controls (13).

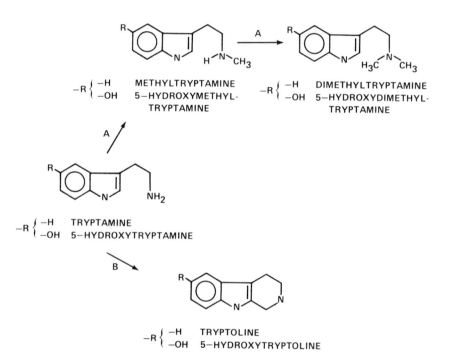

FIGURE 8-2. *In Vitro* Enzymatic Reactions Using SAM or 5-MTHF as Cofactors and Tryptamines as Substrates

A. N-Methylation occurs in some *in vitro* tissue preparations of the SAM-dependent enzymatic system and can proceed in two steps. Methylation has not been demonstrated for a 5-MTHF-dependent enzymatic system.

B. Tryptolines are the major, perhaps sole, products for *in vitro* preparations of the 5-MTHF-dependent enzymatic system. This reaction may also be a significant component of some SAM-dependent enzymatic preparations.

Both the blood and the brain-parts studies are greatly complicated by uncertainty about product identification. Although the products of this SAM-dependent reaction have been absolutely identified as methylated tryptamines in some systems, there is evidence suggesting that a competing reaction, illustrated in Figure 8-2B, can also occur (14). This latter reaction may well be strictly an *in vitro* artifact, but the resulting products are sufficiently similar to methylated tryptamines to interfere with many of the assays used to measure "methylating" activity. Thus, differences in actual methylating activity might be masked by this competing reaction.

New interest in N-methyltransferase enzymes was spurred by reports of enzymatic activity in preparations from rat brain, which appeared to use 5-methyltetrahydrofolic acid (5-MTHF) as a methyl donor (15). Other investigators were unable to detect any N-methylation with this enzymatic system (16). They found that tryptamines yielded products which consistently failed to match the thin-layer chromatographic properties of any of the possible N- or O-methylated derivatives. Instead, the reaction was shown to involve a one-carbon-unit transfer from 5-MTHF to the tryptamine substrate, followed by an intramolecular cyclization to form a tryptoline (Fig. 8-2B). This has now been shown to be the major, probably the sole, reaction in the enzymatic preparations using 5-MTHF (17). Although it is possible that tryptoline formation might occur under special circumstances, it now seems certain that this system is not involved in methylation reactions (16).

To date, studies of N-methylating enzymes have failed to show the relevance of such enzymes to schizophrenia. However, the SAM-dependent enzyme, currently the only one known to N-methylate indoleamines, remains to be fully characterized. In addition, other enzymes with this capability may yet be discovered. Even if the correct enzyme were isolated, it is possible that enzymatic activity would be present in both normals and schizophrenics, while modulators or activating mechanisms might differ between these groups. Thus, a tremendous amount of work remains to be done before the relevance of methylating enzymes in schizophrenics can be determined. In addition to the extension of available *in vitro* techniques, the work may also require the development of specific pharmacological agents for *in vivo* manipulation of the formation and metabolism of methylated amines (13).

SUMMARY

More than two decades after the introduction of the transmethylation hypothesis, no conclusions can be drawn about its relevance to or
involvement in schizophrenia. Numerous methylated biogenic amines
remain as viable candidates for the endogenous psychotogen, yet none
has been shown to occur exclusively in schizophrenics or even to exist
in relatively high concentrations in schizophrenics. As Kety (2) observed nearly ten years ago, however, the transmethylation hypothesis
transcends considerations of any individual substance: for each substance which is eliminated, several new ones are introduced. While this
resilience keeps the hypothesis viable, it can prevent a precise focus
for new research. This, perhaps, explains the intense interest in methylating enzymes, since they represent a clearly defined aspect of a complex and often unwieldy hypothesis.

THE DOPAMINE HYPOTHESIS OF SCHIZOPHRENIA

ACTIONS OF ANTIPSYCHOTIC MEDICATIONS ON CENTRAL DOPAMINE

The second major hypothesis of schizophrenia arises from the suggestion that schizophrenic symptoms result from abnormal cerebral
dopaminergic activity. This suggestion is based on several types of
evidence, the most important of which is the growing conviction that
antipsychotic agents act by decreasing central dopaminergic transmission. Although investigators have yet to establish exactly how these
drugs exert their effects, most attention has focused on their actions
on postsynaptic sites, where they could block effective transmission
of a neuronal impulse. This exciting area has continued to depend on
interesting and innovative advances in technology.

Several years ago, Greengard suggested that a dopamine-sensitive
adenylate cyclase might mediate the postsynaptic actions of dopamine
(18) and that this enzyme activity might correlate with postsynaptic
effects of dopamine (cf. Chapter 2). It was of great interest, therefore,
that the ability of several phenothiazine antipsychotics to inhibit this

cyclase correlates well with their clinical potency, while related compounds which lack antipsychotic activity are also far less potent inhibitors of the cyclase (19). The correlation was marred, however, by the fact that the butyrophenones are less active against the dopamine-sensitive adenylate cyclase than would be predicted from their clinical potencies. This might suggest either that the butyrophenones are not exerting their normal actions in these *in vitro* preparations or that their primary effect involves some other mechanism, such as a presynaptic action (20).

Another approach to studying the postsynaptic actions of dopamine has been developed more recently by Seeman and co-workers (21) and by Snyder and his associates (22). Both groups label brain dopamine "receptors" by binding radiolabeled dopamine or dopamine antagonists to synaptic membranes in brain homogenates. The relative potency of phenothiazines against this dopamine receptor binding closely parallels both their clinical potency and their ability to inhibit dopamine-sensitive adenylate cyclase (21,22). Again, however, the butyrophenones are not as active as would be predicted by their clinical potency. Interestingly, potency of the antipsychotics against binding of the antagonist haloperidol exhibits a rather different pattern, since the correlation between clinical efficacy and the inhibition of haloperidol binding is good for both phenothiazines and butyrophenones (21,22). These data have been interpreted as evidence that dopamine and haloperidol bind to discrete "agonist" and "antagonist" states of the dopamine receptor, leading to suggestions that antagonist binding is more directly relevant to clinical efficacy (22).

In addition to these *in vitro* studies, there is also good *in vivo* evidence from both human and animal studies to suggest that antipsychotic agents can affect dopamine neurotransmission. For example, the response of striatal neurons to the direct application of dopamine is blocked by chlorpromazine (23). Furthermore, antipsychotics increase dopamine turnover in the brain, which may reflect increased dopamine neuronal activity in response to postsynaptic receptor blockade (24). They also block amphetamine- and apomorphine-induced stereotypic behaviors, which appear to be mediated by central dopaminergic pathways (25). In addition, these drugs produce Parkinson-like motor effects in humans—motor abnormalities which are thought to reflect, in part, a decrease in central dopaminergic activity.

PHARMACOLOGICAL MANIPULATION OF CENTRAL DOPAMINE

Other pharmacological agents also have clinical effects which lend support to the dopamine hypothesis of schizophrenia. The synthetic and metabolic pathways of dopamine are detailed in Chapter 2 (Fig. 8-3). α-Methyl-*p*-tyrosine (AMPT), which inhibits catecholamine synthesis, reportedly potentiates the antipsychotic action of phenothiazines (26). Similarly, reserpine, which depletes monoamines and thus reduces dopamine activity, also has antipsychotic properties. In contrast, L-dihydroxyphenylalanine (L-DOPA), the immediate precursor

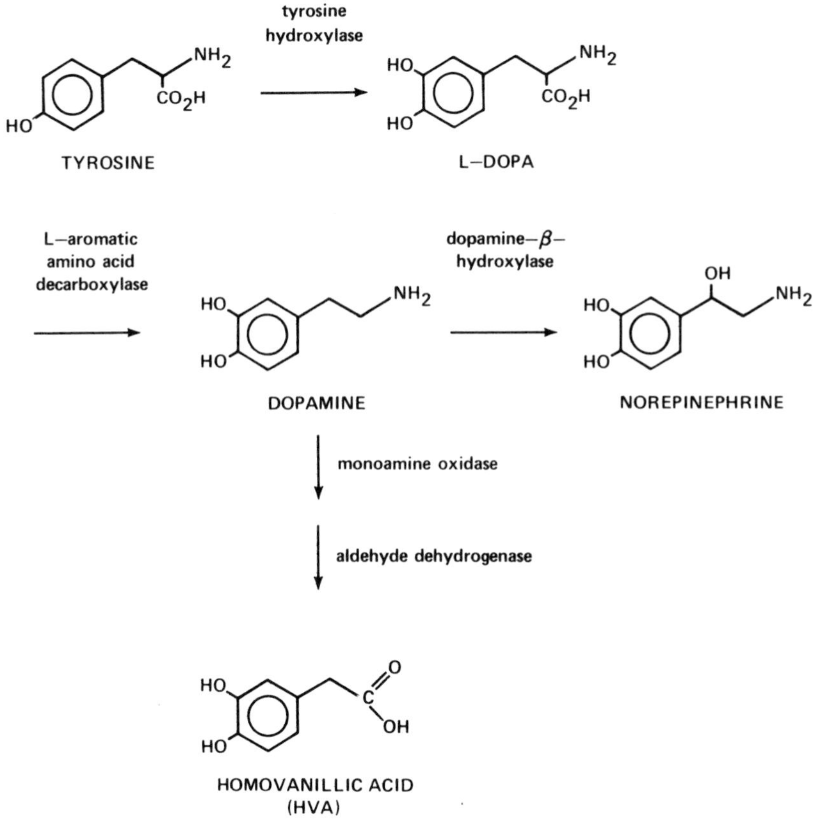

FIGURE 8-3. Dopamine Metabolic Pathway

of dopamine, apparently induces psychosis in some patients with Parkinson's disease (27) and increases symptomatology in schizophrenics (28). Unfortunately, all of these studies are confounded with the possible effects these treatments may have on other central and peripheral systems.

The pharmacological and behavioral effects of amphetamines in man and in animals are particularly important for arguments that dopamine has a role in schizophrenia. Amphetamine psychosis was first reported in 1938 (29). It is particularly striking because it closely resembles—and is often mistaken for—acute paranoid schizophrenia (Chapter 24). Although the psychosis usually follows chronic amphetamine use, it has resulted from a single, large dose. Amphetamine psychosis differs from most toxic psychoses because with the former, patients remain oriented and retain a good memory of the psychotic episode (30). Although patients with amphetamine psychosis rarely have the formal thought disorder or blunted affect of chronic schizophrenics, many of them have been diagnosed as acute paranoid schizophrenics, suggesting a considerable overlap in the clinical picture. In addition, amphetamines have been reported to worsen schizophrenic symptoms (31).

The neurochemical basis of amphetamine psychosis is not known; but, as described in Chapter 21, catecholamines have been implicated. Whether the primary actions involve dopamine or norepinephrine is less certain, but many investigators have concluded that most of the important actions are mediated through dopaminergic systems.

The direct evidence that dopamine is involved in amphetamine action is varied and inconclusive. One important argument relies upon a possible pharmacological difference between the d- and l-stereoisomers of amphetamine (31). From *in vitro* studies on uptake into striatal synaptosomes, the two forms appeared to be nearly equipotent for dopaminergic synaptosomes, while d-amphetamine had a much greater affinity for noradrenergic synaptosomes. This, combined with clinical reports that d- and l-amphetamine are approximately equipotent in inducing psychosis or worsening schizophrenic symptoms, led to the suggestion that dopamine is involved in both amphetamine psychosis and schizophrenia—an hypothesis which remains unconfirmed. It is unclear how well the synaptosomal affinity of amphetamines correlates with their pharmacological actions. Furthermore, investigators have failed to confirm the reported asymmetry between the amphetamine stereoisomers (13). These inconsistencies by no means rule out important interactions between dopamine and amphetamines. The recent demonstration of a good correlation between the abilities of antipsychotics to inhibit haloperidol binding and block amphetamine- and apomorphine-induced behavioral syndromes (32) certainly implicates dopaminergic systems, although parallel effects on norepinephrine and upon other neuronal transmitters and modulators remain to be examined.

BIOCHEMICAL AND METABOLIC STUDIES ON THE DOPAMINE HYPOTHESIS

Although pharmacological studies strongly suggest that antipsychotics work through a central dopaminergic system, the evidence that schizophrenia is caused by a defect in that system is far weaker. Investigators have employed a variety of direct and indirect approaches for detecting a defect in cerebral activity. Two reasonably direct attempts to monitor dopaminergic activity have been measurement of the dopamine metabolite homovanillic acid (HVA) in cerebrospinal fluid and examination of catecholamine-related enzymes in autopsied brains.

Measurement of Homovanillic Acid in Cerebrospinal Fluid. To date, no differences have been found for homovanillic acid in the spinal fluid of schizophrenics and controls (33). It is possible that turnover is more relevant than absolute levels; however, in the only available study of turnover, no differences between normals and unmedicated, acute schizophrenics were detected (34).

Since antipsychotic medications increase dopamine turnover in animals, they might also be expected to increase homovanillic acid levels in humans. This could be an important indication, in humans, that they are acting through dopaminergic systems. Indeed, some schizophrenic patients on antipsychotic medication have recently been shown to have elevated cerebrospinal concentrations of homovanillic acid (35). It will be important to examine possible relationships between increases in homovanillic acid and clinical response to antipsychotic medication.

Measurement of Cathecholamine Enzymes. If schizophrenics suffer from a central defect in the dopaminergic system, one might hope to detect it in autopsied brain. The few studies which are available to date have failed to reveal such a defect. Recently, both synthetic and degradative enzymes in the catecholamine pathway (Fig. 8-3) were examined in samples of several regions of brain from schizophrenics and controls (36). Although the mean values for schizophrenics were generally 10 to 20 percent lower than those of controls for all enzymes and all parts, there was a substantial overlap between the groups and none of the differences reached statistical significance. In contrast, one group has reported that dopamine-β-hydroxylase, the enzyme which converts dopamine to norepinephrine, is 30–50 percent less active in schizophrenics than in controls, with almost no overlap (37). This is consistent with their suggestion that schizophrenia might result from a defect in a noradrenergic reward system. Unfortunately, other enzymes in the pathway were not examined in this latter study.

The possible sources of the discrepancies between these two studies are numerous. Parameters such as subject selection and experimental details may not be directly comparable. More important, the defect, if present, might require an active process which deteriorates at variable rates after death. Furthermore, enzyme activity might be only a poor indicator of a defect in some other part of the system, such as the receptor. Alternatively, the catecholamine system may not be of central importance in schizophrenia, so that changes which may occur are correlated with some other parameter, such as degree of compensation. Although each of these possibilities is potentially important, we still know far too little about the schizophrenic state to be able to assess their impact upon the above studies.

SUMMARY

Dopaminergic systems are central to most recent explanations of psychotic disorders, and the dopamine hypothesis has generated tremendously exciting and important research. Still, direct confirmation that dopamine is involved in schizophrenia continues to elude investigators. We have emphasized that the dopamine hypothesis draws heavily upon the fact that all known antipsychotic agents inhibit dopaminergic activity. An analogy might be made to the effects of acupuncture on pain. Although it is obviously of great interest to establish the mechanisms by which acupuncture is able to block pain, it would not be surprising if those studies did little to reveal the central mechanisms by which pain impulses are recognized in the brain. Instead, acupuncture might work by blocking the normal transmission of those impulses to the central nervous system. Might not dopamine play a similar role in schizophrenia? The analogy certainly has strong parallels to suggestions that antipsychotics may be active primarily by affecting dopamine-mediated attentional mechanisms (38). For example, although amphetamines exacerbate the psychotic state of active schizophrenics, they rarely precipitate a psychotic episode during remission (31). If dopamine were involved in a compensatory system, manipulation of dopaminergic activity might be effective only when an underlying defect is expressed. It would also fit well with suggestions that the basic defect in schizophrenia involves GABAergic systems and that antipsychotics work by preventing an overloading stream of dopaminergic impulses to that defective system (39). Thus, as we extend our knowledge of cerebral function in schizophrenics, it will be important not only to examine dopaminergic systems but also to obtain additional information about other neuroregulators.

OTHER BIOGENIC AMINE HYPOTHESES OF SCHIZOPHRENIA

There are two other interesting hypotheses which should be mentioned in a review of biogenic amines and schizophrenia: the phenylethylamine hypothesis and the balance hypothesis. Both are relatively recent suggestions and have only begun to receive the attention necessary for a careful evaluation. However, they do suggest other intriguing alternatives for research on schizophrenia.

PHENYLETHYLAMINE HYPOTHESIS

Good, recent summaries of the phenylethylamine hypothesis are available (40,41). Phenylethylamine contains the ring and sidechain of the catecholamines, differing from amphetamine only by a methyl group (Fig. 8-1). It appears to be formed endogenously, where it is rapidly metabolized to phenylacetic acid by monoamine oxidase

(MAO). It readily passes the blood-brain barrier and appears to have both peripheral and central activity. It can produce amphetamine-like hyperactivity and stereotypy which is blocked by antipsychotics.

As discussed in the next section of this chapter, there is some evidence that MAO activity is decreased in schizophrenics. Since this is the major metabolic pathway for phenylethylamine, such a decrease might result in an abnormal accumulation of the amine. In addition, schizophrenics might also be heterozygotes for phenylketonuria, which would increase the production of phenylethylamine (40). A combination of the two abnormalities might be expected to greatly increase the circulating concentrations of the amine. These suggestions are interesting, but further studies are needed. The recent development of sensitive and specific assays for both phenylethylamine and phenylacetic acid (41) should permit acute and longitudinal studies of these substances in cerebrospinal fluid, plasma, and urine of schizophrenics and controls, to see what association they have with the onset and course of the disease process, if any.

BALANCE HYPOTHESES

One important aspect of our increasing insight into cerebral function has been the discovery that many neuroregulators seem to work in parallel with or in opposition to one another. An outstanding example of this co-operativity between neuronal systems has come from the work on Parkinson's disease, in which there appears to be a balance between dopaminergic and cholinergic systems. Interestingly, a similar "balance hypothesis" of these two systems has been suggested for schizophrenia. We have already reviewed the evidence for a dopaminergic overactivity in schizophrenia. In addition, it has been suggested that the effects of inhibiting dopaminergic transmission might be enhanced by increasing central cholinergic activity (42). This same strategy is also reported to reverse the exacerbation of an active psychosis by methylphenidate (42). These data have led to the suggestion that schizophrenia may result from a relative predominance of dopaminergic over cholinergic activity (42,43). It is important to note that, to date, there is no evidence that manipulation of the cholinergic system alone produces an effect on schizophrenia, suggesting either that dopamine is more directly involved or that dopaminergic activity is being altered more effectively. Other balance hypotheses can be formulated involving serotonergic and dopaminergic pathways.

MONOAMINE OXIDASE IN SCHIZOPHRENIA

For the past several years, there has been considerable interest in and controversy about the possible relevance of monoamine oxidase (MAO) activity to the schizophrenic process. MAO is a major metabolic enzyme in the degradation of many monoamines, including 5-hydroxytryptamine, dopamine, and norepinephrine; as such, it may help to regulate their intracellular storage. The possible relevance of MAO activity to psychiatric disorders was first suggested by the antidepressant activity of a wide variety of MAO inhibitors (Chapter 10).

MAO is a mitochondrial constituent of many human tissues, including synaptosomes. The enzyme appears to exist in multiple forms, characterized by different substrate and inhibitor specificities. The relative abundance of these isoenzymes varies with both organ and species, and the exact role of each in physiological and pathological states promises to be an exciting area for future research (44).

Most studies of MAO activity in schizophrenia have utilized blood platelets as a ready source of the enzyme. The first study reported a marked reduction in the platelet MAO activities of some chronic schizophrenics (45); this has been followed by a number of conflicting reports (46). Several groups have found low platelet MAO activity in schizophrenics, and some have evidence suggesting that it might be a genetic marker for vulnerability to schizophrenia. Others either have been unable to find such a decrease in activity or have found it only for some enzyme substrates. In addition, preliminary investigations of MAO activity in postmortem brains of schizophrenics and controls have, to date, failed to find any significant differences between the groups (13). Possible explanations for these inconsistent results are many. For example, low MAO activity might be found only in certain subgroups of schizophrenics, as suggested by the recent report that only schizophrenics with auditory hallucinations had abnormally low platelet MAO activity (47). In addition, such a decrease might not be specific for schizophrenia, since some bipolar depressed patients are also reported to have reduced platelet MAO activity (48). In future studies, it will be crucial to control experimental conditions such as diet, medications, and circulating hormones, all of which may have profound influences upon platelet MAO activity. Various MAO substrates should also be used in assessing the enzyme activity, to detect possible alternations in the active site of the enzyme (49).

Even if low platelet MAO activity is found to characterize some subgroup of schizophrenic patients, direct relevance to the pathogenesis·of schizophrenia is unclear. Reduced activity is consistent with every hypothesis of schizophrenia which invokes a relative abundance of a biogenic amine. Dopamine, methylated tryptamines, phenylethylamine—all are metabolized by MAO. Thus, even if MAO activity is altered in schizophrenics, it will be necessary to determine the changes which this defect actually induces in biogenic amine metabolism.

CONCLUSION

Where, then, are we? Unquestionably, the transmethylation and the dopamine hypotheses of schizophrenia have led to many imaginative studies of the biochemistry of schizophrenia. And yet, they have not provided a complete elucidation either of etiological factors predisposing toward schizophrenia or of central mechanisms which mediate the psychotic state. Thus, the strong data suggesting that dopamine is involved in the successful treatment of schizophrenia are not matched by direct evidence that schizophrenics have a defect in dopaminergic systems. The elucidation of this complex disease process will require progress in lines of research ranging from basic biochemical to clinical. Many of the recent technological advances in these areas are reviewed in Part I.

Ultimately the various biochemical hypotheses of schizophrenia must be related to behavioral concepts of the disorder. Stress is known to markedly alter the functioning of individuals with a schizophrenic diathesis and also to alter neuroregulator function (see Chapters 1 and 2). A variety of behaviors and psychological processes, including family interaction styles, have been related to the development of psychotic reactions. A challenge for the future will be to demonstrate the means by which such psychological mechanisms interact with the biochemical ones (Chapter 6). Genetic factors set biochemical limits for the operation of neuroregulator systems. These systems, in turn, are altered by behavior. In susceptible individuals, such changes could lead to relative excess or deficiency for a given transmitter or to the activation or suppression of an enzymatic or receptor system. A pattern of such change could lead to the common symptom we identify as schizophrenia. Thus, "schizophrenia" may be a spectrum of illnesses, some highly controlled by genetic processes and others more determined by behavioral events.

We already have an array of effective medications for schizophrenia, but this is not sufficient. Although there are many antipsychotics from which to choose, they all seem to work by similar, if unknown, mechanisms. None is without potentially serious side effects, and none offers a cure for the disease. Furthermore, even with these medications, many schizophrenics continue to have a poor clinical course. On one level, then, continued research is potentially of value for the rational development of even more specific and less hazardous drugs with which to treat schizophrenia. On another level, schizophrenia provides us with a working model of a brain which is not quite right. If we can find out what goes wrong—if we can identify the altered pathways and the necessary functions they are unable to subserve—then we may have gained immensely important insight into how the normal brain is able to perform its incomprehensibly complex tasks.

REFERENCES

1. Osmond, H. and Smythies, J. Schizophrenia: a new approach. *J. Ment. Sci. 98:*309–315, 1952.
2. Kety, S. S. Summary. The hypothetical relationships between amines and mental illness: a critical synthesis. *In: Amines and Schizophrenia.* H. E. Himwich, S. S. Kety, and J. R. Smythies, *eds.*, Oxford: Pergamon Press, 1967, pp. 271–277.
3. Usdin, E. and Efron, D., *eds. Psychotropic Drugs and Related Compounds.* 2nd Ed., DHEW Publ. No. 72–9074. Washington, D.C., U.S. Govt. Printing Office, 1972.
4. Friedhoff, A. J. and Van Winkle, E. The characteristics of an amine found in the urine of schizophrenic patients. *J. Nerv. Ment. Dis. 135:*550–555, 1962.
5. Wyatt, R. J., Termini, B. A., and Davis, J. Biochemical and sleep studies of schizophrenia: a review of the literature—1960–1970. *Schizophrenia Bull. 4:*10–66, 1971.
6. Pollin, W., Cardon, P. V., and Kety, S. S. Effects of amino acid feeding in schizophrenic patients treated with iproniazid. *Science 133:* 104–105. 1961.
7. Cohen, S. M., Nichols, A., Wyatt, R., and Pollin, W. The administration of methionine to chronic schizophrenic patients: a review of ten studies. *Biol. Psychiatry 8:*209–225, 1974.
8. Baldessarini, R. J. Biological transmethylation involving S-adenosylmethionine: development of assay methods and implications for neuropsychiatry. *Int. J. Neurobiol. 18:*41–67, 1975.
9. Pscheidt, G. R., Berlet, H. H., Spaide, J., and Himwich, H. E. Variations of urinary creatinine and its correlation to secretion of indole metabolites in mental patients. *Clin. Chim. Acta 13:*229–334, 1961.
10. Axelrod, J. Enzymatic formation of psychotomimetic metabolites from normally occurring metabolites. *Science 124:*343–344, 1961.
11. Koslow, S. Bio-significance of N- and O-methylated indoles to psychiatric disorders. *In: Neuroregulators and Psychiatric Disorders.* E. Usdin, D. A. Hamburg, and J. D. Barchas, *eds.*, New York: Oxford University Press, 1977, pp. 210–219.
12. Wyatt, R. J., Saavedra, J. M., and Axelrod, J. A dimethyltryptamine forming enzyme in human blood. *Am. J. Psychiatry. 130:*754–760, 1973.
13. Barchas, J. D., Elliott, G. R., and Berger, P. A. Biogenic amine hypotheses of schizophrenia. *In: Second Rochester International Conference on Schizophrenia.* R. Cromwell and L. Wynne, *eds.*, New York: Wiley, in press.
14. Rosengarten, H. and Friedhoff, A. J. A review of recent studies of the biosynthesis and excretion of hallucinogens formed by methylation of neurotransmitters or related substances. *Schizophrenia Bull. 2:* 90–105, 1976.
15. Laduron, P. N-methylation of dopamine to epinine in brain tissue using N-methyltetrahydrofolic acid as a methyl donor. *Nature New Biol. 238:*212–213, 1972.
16. Elliott, G. R. and Holman, R. B. Tryptolines as potential modulators of serotonergic function. *In: Neuroregulators and Psychiatric Dis-*

orders. E. Usdin, D. A. Hamburg, and J. D. Barchas, eds., New York: Oxford University Press, 1977, pp. 220–228.

17. Taylor, R. T. and Hanna, M. L. 5-Methyltetrahydrofolate aromatic alkylamine N-methyltransferase: an artefact of 5,10-methylenetetrahydrofolate reductase activity. Life Sci. 17:111–112, 1975.

18. Kebabian, J. W., Petzold, G. L., and Greengard, P. Dopamine-sensitive adenylate cyclase in caudate nucleus of rat brain, and its similarity to the "dopamine receptor." Proc. Nat. Acad. Sci. U.S.A. 69:2145–2149, 1972.

19. Iversen, L. L. Dopamine receptors in the brain. Science 188:1084–1090, 1975.

20. Seeman, P. and Lee, T. Antipsychotic drugs: direct correlation between clinical and presynaptic action on dopamine neurons. In: Antipsychotic Drugs: Pharmacodynamics and Pharmacokinetics. G. Sedval, ed., New York: Pergamon Press, in press.

21. Seeman, P., Lee, T., Chau-Wong, M., and Wong, K. Antipsychotic drug doses and neuroleptic/dopamine receptors. Nature 261:717–718, 1976.

22. Snyder, S. H. The dopamine hypothesis of schizophrenia: focus on the dopamine receptor. Am. J. Psychiatry 133:197–202, 1976.

23. Bunney, B. S., Walters, J. R., Roth, R. H., and Aghajanian, G. K. Dopaminergic neurons: effect of anti-psychotic drugs and amphetamines on single cell activity. J. Pharmacol. Exp. Ther. 185:560–571, 1973.

24. Carlsson, A. and Lindqvist, M. Effect of chlorpromazine or haloperidol on formation of 3-methoxytryptamine and normetanephrine in mouse brain. Acta Pharmacol. Toxicol. 30:140–144, 1963.

25. Randrup, A. and Munkvad, I. Pharmacology and physiology of stereotyped behavior. J. Psychiatr. Res. 11:1–10, 1974.

26. Carlsson, A. Antipsychotic drugs and catecholamine synapses. J. Psychiatr. Res. 11:57–64, 1974.

27. Goodwin, F. K. and Murphy, D. L. Biological factors in the affective disorders and schizophrenia. In: Psychopharmacological Agents. M. Gordon, ed., New York: Academic Press, 1974, pp. 19–37.

28. Angrist, B., Sathananthan, G., Wilk, S., and Gershon, S. Amphetamine psychosis: behavioral and biochemical aspects. J. Psychiatr. Res. 11: 13–23, 1974.

29. Young, D., and Scoville, W. B. Paranoid psychosis in narcolepsy and the possible danger of benzadrine treatment. Med. Clin. N. Am. 22: 637–646, 1938.

30. Ellinwood, E. H., Jr. Amphetamine psychosis: individuals, settings, and sequences. In: Current Concepts on Amphetamine Abuse. E. H. Ellinwood and S. Cohen, eds., Bethesda: National Institutes of Mental Health, 1970, pp. 143–159.

31. Snyder, S. H. Amphetamine psychosis: a "model" schizophrenia mediated by catecholamines. Am. J. Psychiatry. 130:61–67, 1973.

32. Creese, I., Burt, D. R., and Snyder, S. H. Dopamine receptor binding predicts clinical and pharmacological potencies of antischizophrenic drugs. Science 192:481–483, 1976.

33. Rimon, R., Roos, B.-E., Räkköläinen, V., and Yrjö, A. The content of 5-hydroxyindoleacetic acid and homovanillic acid in the cerebrospinal fluid of patients with acute schizophrenia. J. Psychom. Res. 15: 375–378, 1971.

34. Fink, E. B., Post, R. M., Carpenter, W. T., and Goodwin, F. K. CSF

metabolites in acute schizophrenia. *New Res. Abst.*, APA Annual Meeting, May 1974, p. 24.

35. Sedvall, G., Fyrö, B., Nyback, H., Wiesel, F. A., and Wode-Helgodt, B. Mass fragmentometric determination of HVA in lumbar cerebrospinal fluid of schizophrenic patients during treatment with antipsychotic drugs. *J. Psychiatr. Res.* 11:75–80, 1974.

36. Barchas, J. D., Berger, P. A., Elliott, G. R., Erdelyi, E., and Wyatt, R. J. Studies of enzymes involved in biogenic amine metabolism in schizophrenia. *In: Biochemistry and Function of Monoamine Enzymes.* E. Usdin and N. Weiner, eds., New York: Marcel Dekker, in press.

37. Wise, C. D., Baden, M. M., and Stein, L. Post-mortem measurements of enzymes in human brain: evidence of a central noradrenergic deficit in schizophrenia. *In: Catecholamines and Schizophrenia.* S. W. Matthysse and S. S. Kety, eds., Oxford: Pergamon Press, 1974, pp. 185–198.

38. Matthysse, S. A theory of the relation between dopamine and attention. *J. Psychiatr. Res.*, in press.

39. Roberts, E. The GABA system and schizophrenia. *In: Neuroregulators and Psychiatric Disorders*, E. Usdin, D. A. Hamburg, and J. D. Barchas, eds., New York: Oxford Press, 1977 pp.347–357.

40. Wyatt, R. J., Gillin, J. C., Stoff, D. M., Moja, E. A., and Tinklenberg, J. R. β-Phenylethylamine (PEA) and the neuropsychiatric disturbances. *In: Neuroregulators and Psychiatric Disorders.* E. Usdin, D. A. Hamburg, and J. D. Barchas, eds., New York: Oxford Press, 1977, pp. 31–45.

41. Sandler, M. and Reynolds, G. P. Does phenylethylamine cause schizophrenia? *Lancet 1*:70–71, 1976.

42. Davis, J. M., Janowsky, D., and Casper, R. C. Acetylcholine and mental disease. *In: Neuroregulators and Psychiatric Disorders.* E. Usdin, D. A. Hamburg, and J. D. Barchas, eds., New York: Oxford Press, 1977, pp. 434–441.

43. Davis, K. L., Hollister, L. E., Berger, P. A., and Barchas, J. D. Cholinergic imbalance hypotheses of psychoses and movement disorders: strategies for evaluation. *Psychopharmacol. Comm.* 1:533–543, 1975.

44. Sandler, M. and Youdim, B. H. Multiple forms of monoamine oxidase: functional significance. *Pharmacol. Rev.* 24:331–348, 1972.

45. Murphy, D. and Wyatt, R. J. Reduced monoamine oxidase activity in blood platelets from schizophrenic patients. *Nature 238*:225–226, 1972.

46. Berger, P. A. and Barchas, J. D. Monoamine oxidase inhibitors. *In: Psychotherapeutic Drugs.* E. Usdin and I. Forrest, eds., New York: Marcel Dekker, 1977.

47. Schildkraut, J. J., Herzog, J. M., Orsulak, P. J., Edelman, S. E., Shein, H. M., and Frazier, S. H. Reduced platelet monoamine oxidase activity in a subgroup of schizophrenic patients. *Am. J. Psychiatry 133*: 438–439, 1976.

48. Murphy, D. L. and Weiss, R. Reduced monoamine oxidase activity in blood platelets from bipolar depressed patients. *Am. J. Psychiatry 128*: 1351–1357, 1972.

49. Zeller, E. A., Bashes, B., Davis, J. M., and Thorner, M. Molecular aberration in platelet monoamine oxidase in schizophrenia. *Lancet 1*:1385, 1975.

9 | Antipsychotic Medications and the Treatment of Schizophrenia

LEO E. HOLLISTER

INTRODUCTION

Schizophrenia may best be viewed as a disorder of the brain which is manifested primarily by a disturbance in logical sequencing, producing abnormal thinking, behavior, and affect. A genetic predisposition is probably a necessary condition for developing the disorder. The phenotypical expression may be contingent upon the degree of genetic load, the level of intelligence, the presence of unfavorable developmental influences before or after birth, and various life experiences of the affected individual, including both psychological and physiological stresses. The proximate cause of the brain disorder is uncertain. As described in Chapter 8, it could be a disturbance in neurochemical transmission or an abnormality of brain circuitry, since disruptions of either biochemical or neurophysiological functions of the brain might lead to aberrations in perception and in information processing. Clinical manifestations of such a complex disorder might be expected to be highly variable in relation to age of onset, natural history, and clinical manifestations. Many of the latter could be epiphenomena of the primary disorder. One could hypothesize that there is only one schizophrenia and only one necessary condition for it, with many of its expressions depending upon modifying factors (1).

For pharmacological treatment, an operational definition of types of schizophrenias suggests that three different syndromes occur (2):

- *Schizophrenic syndrome* in young adults, with insidious onset and appearance at 15–35 years of age.
- *Schizophreniform psychosis* with acute onset and obviously related to alcohol, drugs, brain damage, or serious emotional trauma.
- *Paranoid psychosis* in middle life, with onset from 35–64 years

121

of age, precipitated by systemic illness, organic brain disease, alcohol or drug abuse, social isolation, or cultural dislocation.

The above formulation of a combination of biological and environmental determinants of schizophrenia is consistent with experience gained from treating patients with schizophrenia. Few would disagree that chemotherapy is the basic treatment. Yet additional success in treatment may result from other interventions including those designed to reduce psychosocial stress, such as training the person for an appropriate role in life and providing family support.

Evidence derived from three major sources—consanguinity, twin, and adoptive studies—strongly suggests that genetic factors play a role in the development of schizophrenia, although the magnitude of the contribution remains to be clarified (3). The role of family as a provoking factor is less easily settled, for the family constellation of a schizophrenic may be confounded both by the same genetic influences affecting the patient and by the adaptational stresses of having a schizophrenic family member. Family influences are more easily evident in the content of specific symptoms of the patient (4).

HISTORY

Extracts from *Rauwolfia serpentina*, a climbing shrub found in India, may have been the first effective agents for treating schizophrenia (5). The use of these agents for snake bites, hypertension, insomnia, and insanity are described in ancient Hindu *ayurvedic* writings. In 1703, the French botanist Plumier named the plant for Rauwolf, an Ausburg botanist who probably never knew the plant existed, and for its snakelike appearance. In 1931, Sen and Bose published a medical paper claiming that *Rauwolfia* was useful for severely disturbed patients. In the next twenty years, scattered reports by several individuals, including Siddiqui, Chopra, Gutpa, Chakravarti, Kahali, Arnold, Wilkins, and Judson, confirmed these observations.

An active principle of *Rauwolfia serpentina*, the alkaloid reserpine (Fig. 9-1), was isolated by Müller, Schlittler, and Bein in 1952. The drug was first used to treat hypertension, but Kline soon reported antipsychotic activity. It is interesting that the discovery of the antipsychotic activity of reserpine was made at about the same time as was the antipsychotic activity of the chemically dissimilar phenothiazines. Today, reserpine is rarely used in the treatment of schizophrenia. However, its place in the history of pharmacology is assured by two other pharmacological properties. First, the occasional appearance of depressive symptoms during reserpine treatment is a keystone of the biogenic amine hypothesis of depression (Chapter 10). Second, the depleting action of reserpine on biogenic amines has made it an invaluable pharmacological tool for the investigation of biogenic amine neurotransmitters (Chapters 2 and 3).

The history of the first major class of antipsychotics began in 1883, when phenothiazine was first synthesized by Bernthsen in the course of the chemical investigation of two dyes, Lauth's violet and methylene blue. However, phenothiazines were not introduced into human pharmacological studies until the 1940's, when they were first investigated as possible antihelmintic agents and later as antihistamines. The French surgeon Laborit used the phenothiazine promethazine (Fig. 9-1), in combination with several other pharmacological agents, to potentiate and facilitate surgical anesthesia. Laborit was seeking an agent which was similar to promethazine but had greater central activity. He was not alone. The pharmaceutical company Rhône-Poulenc wanted to develop a phenothiazine amine with a strong central action; this led Charpentier to synthesize a variety of new phenothiazine derivatives, including chlorpromazine (see Fig. 9-2) in 1950. Chlorpromazine was tried by Laborit, who felt it might have some use in psychiatry. However, it was Sigwald and Bouttier, in late 1951, and Delay and Deniker, in early 1952, who first reported chlorpromazine's antipsychotic activity. Between 1953 and 1954 chlorpromazine, known in Europe as Largactil (large activity) was tested in England, Switzerland, and Canada and finally, in 1954, in the United States (6).

The story of the butyrophenones reflects a more rational development for a drug than is usual in biological psychiatry (5). In 1953, Janssen returned from military service as a physician to the small pharmaceutical company founded by his father. Since the company had no patents and no research, Janssen decided to synthesize and test new, reasonably inexpensive chemicals. The oldest member of his research group was twenty-seven. Today, Janssen admits that if they had not been so naive and inexperienced, they might not have continued. The

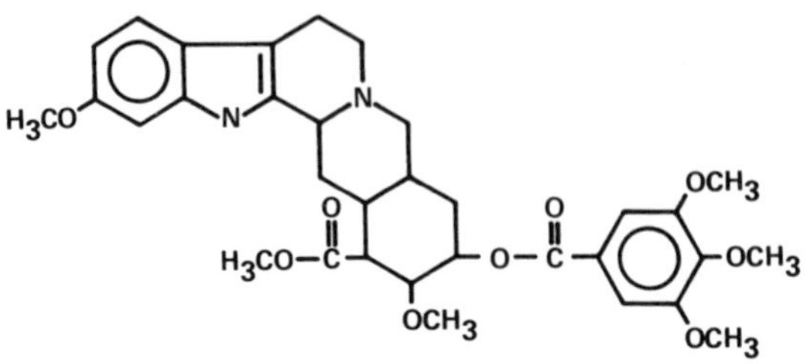

RESERPINE

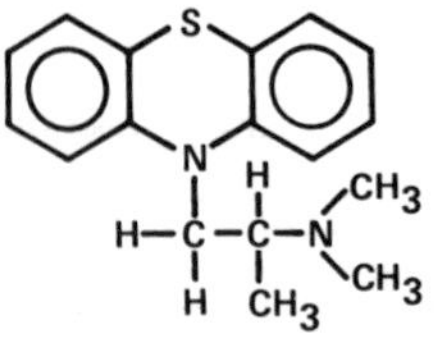

PROMETHAZINE

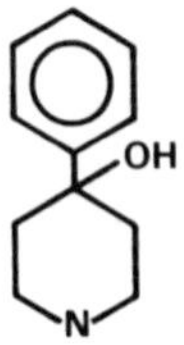

4—PHENYL—4—PIPERIDINOL

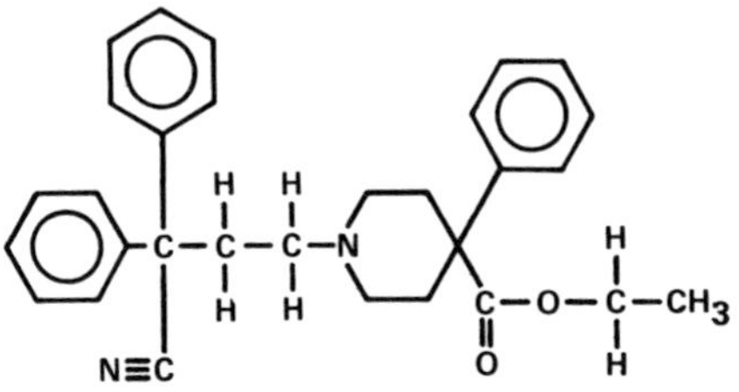

DIPHENOXYLATE
(LOMOTIL^R)

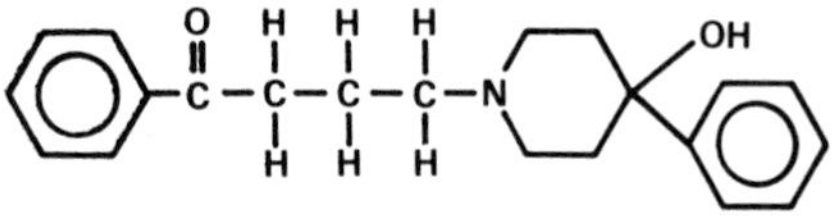

4—PHENYL—
4—PIPERIDINOLBUTYROPHENONE

FIGURE 9-1. Compounds of Historical Importance in the Development of Antipsychotics

group developed the strategy of taking a pharmacologically active chemical and modifying it, emphasizing modifications which could be done cheaply, with easy reactions and inexpensive starting materials. In one case they started with the 4-phenyl-4-piperidinol (Fig. 9-1) related to meperidine. They obtained both the antidiarrheal agent diphenoxylate (Lomotil) (Fig. 9-1) and a propiophenone with good analgesic activity. They modified this latter drug to increase potency and got a butyrophenone derivative. When they injected this last compound into mice, they detected not only morphine-like but also chlorpromazine-like activity, including sedation, calmness, and muscle rigidity. This was a surprise. Since there are obvious problems with a compound having both opiate and neuroleptic activity, they again modified it, this time to increase neuroleptic activity and reduce morphine-like activity. Soon, they developed 4-phenyl-4-piperidinolbutyrophenone (Fig. 9-1), which had only neuroleptic activity. This was further modified to produce haloperidol (Fig. 9-4), a compound which is many times more potent than chlorpromazine and has fewer autonomic effects. Haloperidol was first used at the Psychiatric Clinic of Liege University by Divry, Bobon, Collard, Pinchard and Nols, and successful trials were first reported in 1958. Haloperidol, the first of many active butyrophenones, was in common use in Europe by 1960.

PHARMACOLOGICAL PROPERTIES OF ANTIPSYCHOTICS

Almost two hundred drugs proposed somewhere in the world as antipsychotics have been given generic names. Bestowing a generic name suggests the possibility that the compound might come to the market, so many more compounds probably have shown antipsychotic properties but have not been pursued for reasons of toxicity. For a long while, only three chemical classes of drugs were available in the United States, but this number has recently grown.

STRUCTURE-ACTIVITY RELATIONSHIPS

Phenothiazine derivatives are both the most numerous and still the most widely used of antipsychotic drugs. Three chemical subfamilies can be distinguished, based on differences in the sidechain (Fig. 9-2). The aliphatic series and the piperidine series of compounds are generally regarded as low-potency compounds. All effective antipsychotic phenothiazines have some substituent at the 2-position. Some theories suggest that the structure-activity relationships involve creation of a three-dimensional configuration in which the nitrogen atom in the sidechain bears the same spatial relationship to the aromatic ring as ni-

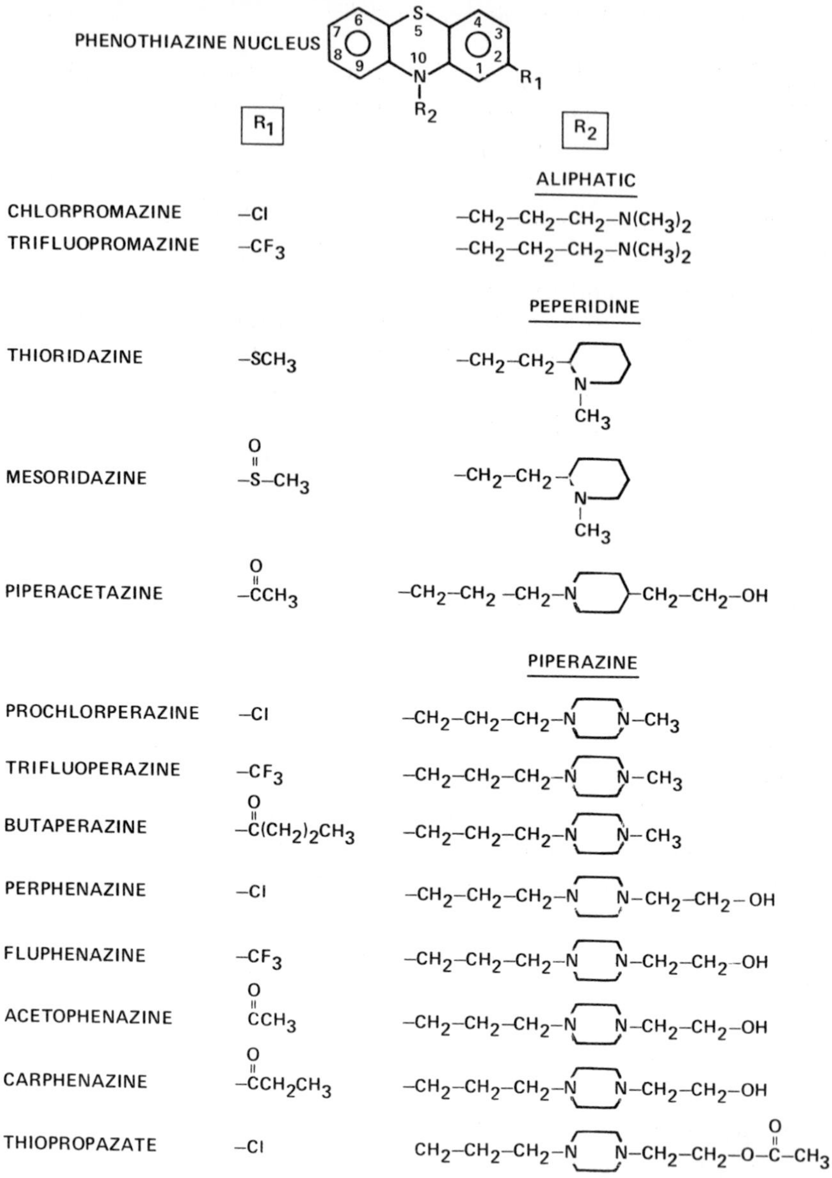

PHENOTHIAZINE NUCLEUS

	R_1	R_2

ALIPHATIC

	R_1	R_2
CHLORPROMAZINE	$-Cl$	$-CH_2-CH_2-CH_2-N(CH_3)_2$
TRIFLUOPROMAZINE	$-CF_3$	$-CH_2-CH_2-CH_2-N(CH_3)_2$

PEPERIDINE

THIORIDAZINE	$-SCH_3$	$-CH_2-CH_2-$ (piperidine, $N-CH_3$)
MESORIDAZINE	$\overset{O}{\overset{\|}{-S}}-CH_3$	$-CH_2-CH_2-$ (piperidine, $N-CH_3$)
PIPERACETAZINE	$\overset{O}{\overset{\|}{-C}}CH_3$	$-CH_2-CH_2-CH_2-N$ (piperidine) $-CH_2-CH_2-OH$

PIPERAZINE

PROCHLORPERAZINE	$-Cl$	$-CH_2-CH_2-CH_2-N$ (piperazine) $N-CH_3$
TRIFLUOPERAZINE	$-CF_3$	$-CH_2-CH_2-CH_2-N$ (piperazine) $N-CH_3$
BUTAPERAZINE	$\overset{O}{\overset{\|}{-C}}(CH_2)_2CH_3$	$-CH_2-CH_2-CH_2-N$ (piperazine) $N-CH_3$
PERPHENAZINE	$-Cl$	$-CH_2-CH_2-CH_2-N$ (piperazine) $N-CH_2-CH_2-OH$
FLUPHENAZINE	$-CF_3$	$-CH_2-CH_2-CH_2-N$ (piperazine) $N-CH_2-CH_2-OH$
ACETOPHENAZINE	$\overset{O}{\overset{\|}{C}}CH_3$	$-CH_2-CH_2-CH_2-N$ (piperazine) $N-CH_2-CH_2-OH$
CARPHENAZINE	$\overset{O}{\overset{\|}{-C}}CH_2CH_3$	$-CH_2-CH_2-CH_2-N$ (piperazine) $N-CH_2-CH_2-OH$
THIOPROPAZATE	$-Cl$	$CH_2-CH_2-CH_2-N$ (piperazine) $N-CH_2-CH_2-O-\overset{O}{\overset{\|}{C}}-CH_3$

FIGURE 9-2. Structural Relationships of Phenothiazines

trogen in the sidechain bears to the ring in dopamine. It is also possible that nuclear substituents increase lipid solubility of the molecule. Three variants of the piperazine sidechain, along with variations in the ring substituent, create a rather large group of piperazinylphenothiazines. These compounds are known as high-potency drugs. Piperacetazine is an example of a drug which is technically a piperidine, but whose structural geometry resembles that of the piperazines; accordingly, it has more properties in common with the latter group.

The modification in the ring of the thioxanthenes tend to make for a generally less potent group of compounds than for the phenothi-

PHENOTHIAZINE DERIVATIVES

PHENOTHIAZINE NUCLEUS

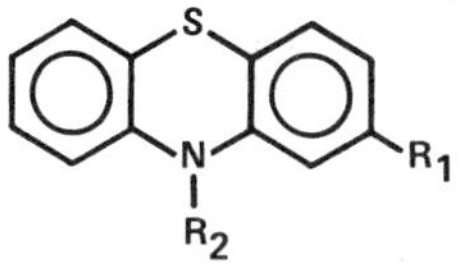

CHLORPROMAZINE

R_1 = $-Cl$ R_2 = $-CH_2-CH_2-CH_2-N(CH_3)_2$

THIOXANTHENE DERIVATIVES

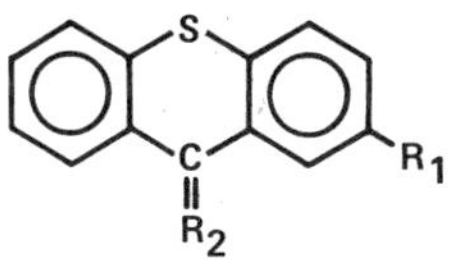

	R_1	R_2
CHLORPROTHIXENE	$-Cl$	$-CH-CH_2-CH_2-N(CH_3)_2$
THIOTHIXENE	$-SO_2N(CH_3)_2$	$-CH-CH_2-CH_2-N$⟩N$-CH_3$

FIGURE 9-3. Thioxanthene Compared with Phenothiazines

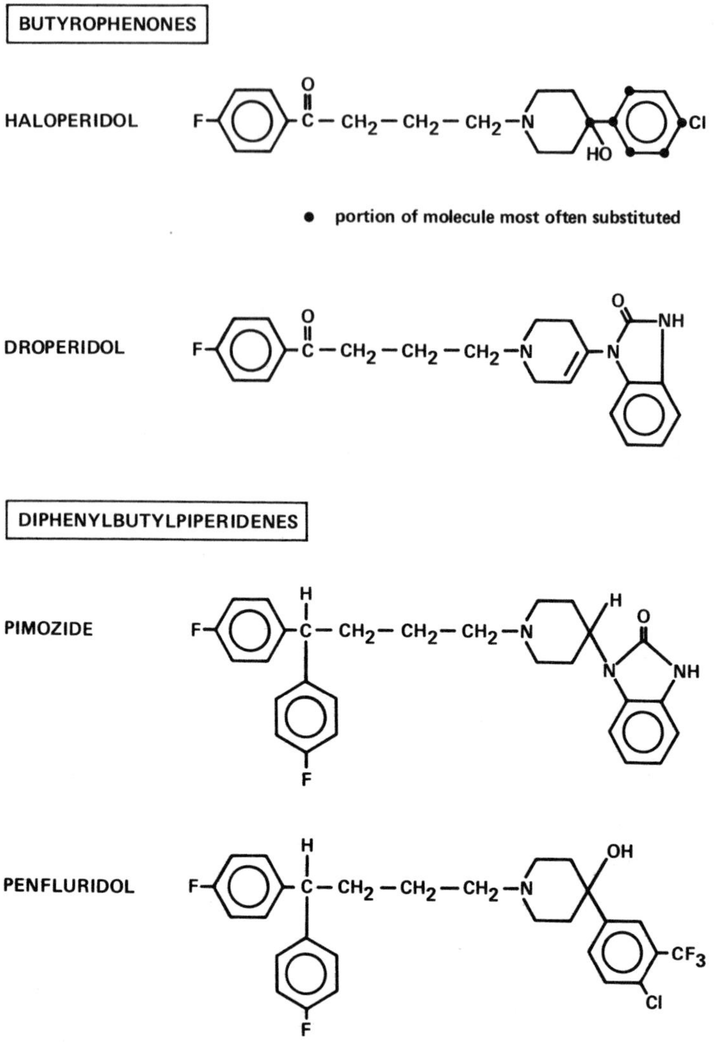

BUTYROPHENONES

HALOPERIDOL

● portion of molecule most often substituted

DROPERIDOL

DIPHENYLBUTYLPIPERIDENES

PIMOZIDE

PENFLURIDOL

FIGURE 9-4. Structural Relationship Between Butyrophenones and Diphenylbutylpiperidines

azines (Fig. 9-3). Such seems to be the case for chlorprothixene, the thioxanthene homolog of chlorpromazine. The slight loss of potency from the ring structure can be compensated for by the choice of ring substituents and sidechains. The dimethylsulfonamide ring substituent and piperazine sidechain of thiothixene make it a fairly potent drug. Still, it is less potent than its phenothiazine homolog, thioproperazine.

Potency should never be confused with efficacy, which is roughly the same overall among all these drugs. The separation of antipsychotic effects from other pharmacological actions of these drugs, such as sedation or α-adrenergic blockade, may reduce certain side effects, like the autonomic ones, while increasing others, such as extrapyramidal motor reactions. The French phrase for such a drug is *neuroleptique incisif*, the English equivalent being "a more specific antipsychotic drug."

Although many butyrophenone structures are possible, only two are currently marketed in the United States (Fig. 9-4). Virtually all the structural variations involve portions of the phenylpiperidine moiety, sometimes entailing formation of a single piperazine ring—or two piperidine rings or other ring conformations as in droperidol—but never disturbing the position of the nitrogen in the piperidine ring. The chemical resemblance between the diphenylbutylpiperidines and butyrophenones is easily visualized. Pimozide, penfluridol, and fluspirilene are the most advanced of this series. The latter two are of great interest because of their exceedingly long action following oral doses. Pimozide may soon reach the American market. It is reputed to be less sedative than other drugs and especially valuable for "resocialization" of chronic schizophrenics.

Several other chemical classes have antipsychotic activity. In America, reserpine is used almost exclusively for treating hypertension; however, a benzoquinolizine derivative, benzquinamide, is marketed in the United States as an antiemetic drug. Tetrabenazine is used elsewhere as an antipsychotic. Oxypertine is used elsewhere as an antianxiety and antidepressant drug as well as an antipsychotic. Molindone and loxapine are new entries into the American market. Although they are effective antipsychotic drugs, it remains to be seen whether they have any special advantage over previous drugs, other than the increasingly dubious one of representing a different chemical structure. Metiapine and clozapine are still under investigation. The latter drug is of great interest in that it appears to be an effective antipsychotic without producing extrapyramidal motor reactions.

METABOLISM

Both the phenothiazines and the butyrophenones are well absorbed from the gastrointestinal tract and slowly excreted in urine and feces.

Phenothiazine metabolites have been detected in body fluids months after their discontinuation. A tremendous amount of research has been done on the metabolic fate of chlorpromazine, which may form as many as 168 metabolites (7). Although a large number of derivatives have been detected, the primary metabolic pathway involves hydroxylation at carbons 3 and 7 (Fig. 9-2). Some metabolites, such as 7-hydroxychlorpromazine retain pharmacological activity. The hydroxy derivatives are then conjugated with glucuronic acid, and these conjugates are excreted in urine. Sulfoxide metabolites also account for a significant portion of the degradation products. The phenothiazines may increase the activity of the liver enzymes which are responsible for their metabolism, but this effect is not as marked as it is for the barbiturates (Chapter 19).

BIOLOGICAL EFFECTS

All antipsychotic drugs share two novel pharmacological actions which were unknown prior to their advent: the ability to ameliorate the symptoms of schizophrenia and the ability to evoke in many patients extrapyramidal syndromes of various types, including one that strongly mimics naturally occurring Parkinson's disease. For a long while, it was uncertain why these two unusual and seemingly unrelated effects should be linked. Now it appears that both are mediated through the same biochemical mechanism of decreased transmission in dopaminergic pathways of the brain. The antipsychotics are also called "neuroleptics" and are believed to act at four anatomical sites.

- at the reticular activating system of the midbrain, where sensory input is monitored;
- at the amygdala and hippocampus, structures in the limbic system that provide the emotional coloring attached to incoming signals;
- at the hypothalamus, which governs the peripheral responses to meaningful sensory information through both of the pituitary-endocrine system and the autonomic nervous system; and,
- at the globus pallidus and corpus striatum, where extrapyramidal syndromes are elicited, perhaps coincidentally.

Thus, these drugs affect the function of three major integrating systems of the brain—the reticular activating system, the limbic system, and the hypothalamus. One might speculate that they could reduce extraneous or distracting sensory information, reduce the affective charge of all sensations, and reduce the somatic responses to them.

All antipsychotics are sedative, which led to the erroneous term "tranquilizer." Although some have clinical reputation as "activating" drugs, they are by no means stimulants. Rather, this reputation is based upon the observation that treatment increases motor activity in some patients, particularly with those drugs which have a smaller sedative-to-antipsychotic ratio. Most antipsychotics are α-adrenergic blocking drugs. Some, such as chlorpromazine and thioridazine are especially so. With the conspicuous exception of thioridazine, all are antiemetic drugs, which provides an additional clinical use. This latter coincidental pharmacological action led to the paradox that for many years the animal pharmacological test which correlated most highly with antipsychotic activity was the prevention of apomorphine-induced emesis in dogs.

INDICATIONS FOR ANTIPSYCHOTIC DRUGS

SCHIZOPHRENIA

Antipsychotic drugs are the basic treatment of schizophrenia. The extensive literature of evaluative trials has demonstrated the value of antipsychotic drugs in all forms of schizophrenia, at all ages, at all stages of illness, and in all parts of the world. Unfortunately, they are not effective in all patients, at least to any meaningful degree.

Given that drugs are a primary treatment, does this necessarily mean that they should be given indiscriminately to all patients? Some schizophrenic patients have rather good premorbid adjustments and their psychosis has relatively clear precipitants. Such patients have been termed as having "reactive" schizophrenia or, in European literature, schizophreniform psychoses. Although they may present explosively, the course is often self-limiting, and a relatively full remission can be obtained. Many have responded to treatment without drugs. Drugs may be useful during the acute episode but are probably not required for maintenance after resolution of the acute psychosis. Another group of patients for whom drug therapy might be questioned are those with exceedingly chronic schizophrenia and long-term hospitalization. Frequently, such patients show only meaningless improvement from drug therapy, which is more often given for the benefit of the hospital staff than for that of the patient. The appropriateness of drug treatment for such patients has been questioned, especially because of the possible appearance of tardive dyskinesia.

This latter complication should promote a conservative use of these drugs. Unfortunately, the current trend is in the opposite direction. Even patients with acute schizophrenia, where drugs are most clearly indicated, may be overtreated in the zeal to reduce hospital stay or even to avoid hospitalization. Not all chronically psychotic patients require large doses of these drugs or prolonged, uninterrupted treatment. As has been cogently argued, the risks for some may outweigh the benefits (8).

SCHIZOAFFECTIVE DISORDERS

The preponderance of evidence suggests that antipsychotic drugs are the preferred treatment (9). Some patients respond to lithium alone and some respond better to combined treatment (10).

MANIA

Acute manic states associated with manic-depressive disorder often require antipsychotic drugs for effective management. Lithium is the primary treatment; but, because of its slow onset of action, concurrent use of an antipsychotic may be required for a period of several days (Chapter 12). Nonmanic excited states from a variety of causes may be managed with droperidol (Inapsine), a drug marketed mainly as an antiemetic. It is not proven that this butyrophenone is more effective than haloperidol or conventional sedatives.

Depression

Most studies comparing antipsychotic drugs with tricyclic antidepressants (tricyclics) in heterogeneous groups of depressed patients have failed to show much difference in response. Use of antipsychotics for treating depressed patients remains controversial, however. Arguments against their use can be made. First, they may make truly endogenous depressions worse. Second, they are not necessarily more effective than placebo, antianxiety drugs, or the sedative tricyclics in the mixed anxiety-depression syndrome so often associated with reactive depressions. Finally, the risk of tardive dyskinesias may be too great under these conditions. Some patients undoubtedly are helped more by these drugs than by any other type, but antipsychotic drugs are not a preferred treatment (Chapter 11).

Gilles de la Tourette Syndrome

This rare disorder responds to antipsychotic drugs. Haloperidol, the only drug adequately studied, is preferred, although benefit may not be unique to this drug. The unpredictable barking, tic, and outbursts of foul language these patients suffer are socially disabling and drug treatment is clearly warranted.

Psychoses Associated with Old Age

Although best results in true organic brain syndromes of senile or arteriosclerotic brain disease have been obtained from antipsychotics, the goals of treatment are limited (Chapter 28).

Acute Brain Syndromes

Acute brain syndromes due to withdrawal from alcohol or other drugs are best treated by replacing the abused drug with one that is pharmacologically equivalent (Chapter 23). Such is clearly not the case with antipsychotic drugs. In addition, they lower seizure thresholds and are therefore contraindicated. Acute disorders associated with hallucinogenic drugs are usually self-limiting and respond as well or better to antianxiety drugs or conventional sedatives (Chapter 24). Antipsychotic drugs may produce more disabling effects in these otherwise normal persons than the disorder being treated. When a schizophrenic-like psychosis is precipitated by hallucinogenic drugs, then antipsychotic drugs may be indicated; but this situation is usually not evident for several days. On the other hand, acute brain syndromes associated with being placed in recovery rooms, coronary care units, or other strange medical surroundings seem to respond better to potent antipsychotics, such as haloperidol, than to conventional sedatives, which often aggravate the delirium.

MINOR EMOTIONAL DISORDERS

Neuroses or psychophysiological disorders associated with anxiety respond preferentially to antianxiety drugs (Chapter 13). The latter are considerably safer than antipsychotics. Instances of tardive dyskinesia have occurred when even quite small doses of antipsychotic drugs have been used for such disorders (11).

CHOICE OF DRUG

Ten years of promising leads have failed to provide a completely rational system for choosing among antipsychotic drugs for individual patients on the basis of presenting symptoms and signs of schizophrenia (12). The target-symptom approach to drug evaluation remains valid, but to use it as a basis for choosing drugs is an error. Antipsychotic drugs do not treat specific symptoms: they treat an illness. The belief that drug X may be good for symptom A, drug Y for symptom B, and drug Z for symptom C has led to the most incredible polypharmacy. Suppose one were to have a patient who presented with the following symptoms: fever, chills, chest pain, cough, rusty sputum. Now suppose you were to treat his fever with aspirin, his chills with intravenous calcium, his chest pain and cough with codeine, and his expectoration with potassium iodide. You would properly be denounced as a quack! The patient's illness is lobar pneumonia, and the treatment is an appropriate antibiotic, with which the individual symptoms and signs will subside at varying rates. We should now apply the illness model to schizophrenia.

One is left, then, with a bewildering array of drugs from which to choose for an empirical trial in a given patient. Such a situation is analogous to the case of the numerous corticosteroids, antihistaminics, diuretics, and digitalis preparations which confront the clinician. The usual dictum has been to learn to use a few drugs well rather than all poorly. The differences between the proper and improper use of a drug will probably exceed any actual difference between drugs. One of the most rational ways to narrow the choice of antipsychotics would be to master one of each of the three types of phenothiazines and one of each of the remaining chemical classes of drugs. A possible selection, based on drugs currently available in the United States, is shown in Table 9-1.

A basic assumption in making these choices is that differences within a chemical class are less important than differences among them, allowing the choice of only a single drug for each. The assumption is also made that the puzzling differences between the responses of individual patients to different drugs are largely due to differences in the

TABLE 9-1.
RATIONAL CHOICE OF ANTIPSYCHOTIC DRUGS

Criteria: Example of chemical class
            Different pharmacological profile

Phenothiazines
        Aliphatic—chlorpromazine
        Piperidine—mesoridazine
        Piperazine—fluphenazine

Thioxanthenes—thiothixene

Butyrophenones—haloperidol

Dibenzoxazepines—loxapine

Indolics—molindone

Major guide: Patient's prior response

patient's metabolic handling of the drug, making chemical distinctions important.

A simplistic decision process for choosing a drug for an individual patient is based on his initial motor state. A highly agitated, combative patient might best be treated with a sedative-type antipsychotic such as chlorpromazine or thioridazine, while the withdrawn, slowed-down patient with primary thinking disturbance may be better suited for treatment with the more potent, more specific antipsychotics such as fluphenazine, thiothixene, or haloperidol. Overriding all other considerations is the patient's past history of response to a drug, if that information is available.

PRACTICAL ASPECTS OF PHARMACOLOGICAL TREATMENT

Doses

Few drugs have such great therapeutic margins and such a wide range of therapeutic doses as the antipsychotics. Dose ranges shown in Table 9-2 are only rough guides, somewhat reflecting current practice of using higher doses. It remains to be seen whether this trend is justified. The old idea of a "digitalizing" dose has been revived for antipsychotic drugs, following a plan of rapid increments of dose to 50–100 mg of fluphenazine (13). It is now known, of course, that digitalis produces a graded, not an all-or-none, effect. Since the same principle almost certainly applies to antipsychotics, one might question the advisability of potentially overtreating many patients for the somewhat dubious gain of shortening hospitalization for a few. We tend to hurry too much in treating schizophrenics, where it generally does not much matter, and too little in treating depressives, where it does.

Enthusiasm for using mega-doses of highly potent drugs, such as 1200 mg of fluphenazine or haloperidol, has waned, since the number of patients salvaged has been few and the potential dangers still uncertain. While no patient should be considered a drug failure without an intensive course of therapy, high doses should not become a routine for all patients. With the exception of thioridazine, where a maximal daily dose of 800 mg is recommended to avoid retinal pigmentary

TABLE 9-2.

DOSAGE RELATIONSHIP AMONG ANTIPSYCHOTICS

| NAMES | | | RANGE OF TOTAL DAILY DOSE | |
GENERIC	REPRESENTATIVE BRAND	RELATIVE POTENCY	OUTPATIENT (MG/DAY)	INPATIENT (MG/DAY)
Phenothiazines				
Aliphatic				
Chlorpromazine	Thorazine	100	50–400	200–1600
Piperidine				
Thioridazine	Mellaril	100	50–400	200–800
Mesoridazine	Serentil	50	25–200	100–400
Piperacetazine	Quide	10	10–40	20–160
Piperazine				
Carphenazine	Proketazine	25	50–150	75–400
Acetophenazine	Tindal	20	40–80	60–100
Prochlorperazine	Compazine	15	20–60	60–200
Perphenazine	Trilafon	10	8–24	12–64
Butaperazine	Repoise	10	10–30	10–100
Trifluoperazine	Stelazine	5	4–10	10–60
Fluphenazine	Prolixin	2	1–5	2–60
Thioxanthene				
Thiothixene	Navane	5	6–30	10–120
Butyrophenones				
Haloperidol	Haldol	2	2–6	4–100
Dibenzoxazepines				
Loxapine	Loxitane	10	15–60	40–160
Indolics				
Molindone	Moban	10	15–60	40–225

changes, no specific maximal doses have been set for any antipsychotic. The possibility of monitoring doses of antipsychotics by measuring plasma levels of the drugs seem to be quite remote at the moment, because of multiple metabolites. The clinician may surmise that an inadequate dose has been delivered in the absence either of an improved mental state or of an extrapyramidal reaction. These are the two unique pharmacological actions which bear somewhat upon each other. If neither outcome is evident, then more drug is needed. However, neither outcome necessarily indicates that the optimal dose has been attained. Exploration of the upper limits of effective dose should be based on other considerations. Obviously, routine use of an antiparkinson drug at the onset of treatment may rob the clinician of one of these two clinical criteria for assessing the adequacy of dose.

One of the more common errors of drug prescribing found in a large mental hospital is that of excessively low doses of drug. One should not be so afraid of doing harm that one does no good. Other errors commonly encountered are excessive use of antiparkinson medication and polypharmacy, including the use of antidepressants for schizophrenics (14). Nothing will substitute for careful thought if drugs are to be used well; treatment should never become routine.

DOSAGE SCHEDULES

At the beginning of treatment, divided doses are usually given. These minimize the initial impact of many of the unwanted pharmacological effects such as sedation and adrenergic blocking activity and allow better titration of dose. Unfortunately, this eminently sensible practice in initiating treatment is seldom changed, and patients may stay on divided doses for years. Since these drugs are intrinsically long acting, no pharmacokinetic basis for divided doses obtains. Once a patient reaches a satisfactory daily maintenance dose, it is feasible to reduce the frequency. Many clinicians aim for a single daily dose to be given just before retiring. Even when they use divided doses, they tend to give the major dose of the day at this time. Two advantages accrue. First, the patient sleeps when he should, rather than during the day because of oversedation. Second, he is less likely to suffer disabling extrapyramidal symptoms, if the major impact of the drug occurs while he is sleeping. For reasons which still are not clear, manifestations of Parkinson's disease are ameliorated by sleep.

The technique for reducing doses may vary. Some prefer to eliminate the morning dose first, consolidating it with one given later in the day and then progressively doing the same to noon and afternoon dose. If very large amounts of drug are required for maintenance treatment, one may still prefer to divide the total daily dose, giving perhaps one-third in the late afternoon and the remainder before bedtime. In most cases, however, the goal of a single daily maintenance dose can be attained, provided that the total daily maintenance dose is not too high. Many drugs are now available in larger, single-dose units to meet the growing acceptance of the single daily dose.

Maintenance Treatment

Antipsychotic drugs may be discontinued after brief periods of treatment of acute brain syndromes, some manic episodes, and some acute schizophrenic disturbances. Acute responses of patients newly treated with drugs are variable, ranging from days to weeks. Most clinicians would feel that failure of acute or newly admitted schizophrenics to improve after six to eight weeks of adequate treatment with a drug would be reason to try another. Newly treated chronic patients might require three to six months of treatment before a change of medication would be warranted. Improvement tends to be more rapid earlier than later on.

As a rule, schizophrenic patients are placed on maintenance doses which should be as low as suitable for retaining therapeutic gains. Dosage should be reduced gradually to avoid a sudden recrudescence of symptoms. The minimal dose at which the patient functions best is preferred to an arbitrarily imposed maintenance dose such as one-third or one-fourth of the peak dose. Reduction of doses for maintenance treatment is of considerable importance. Many instances of so-called post-schizophrenic depression may well result from overtreatment with antipsychotic drugs. As one becomes more "normal," these drugs become more noxious. One might even postulate biochemical reasons why an excess of drug might evoke depression.

Patients tolerate reductions in the maintenance doses of drug very well. No differences were found over a four-month period between patients who stayed on their usual maintenance doses and patients who skipped their treatment on two or three days of the week (15). "Drug holidays" are another way in which the total drug exposure of patients may be reduced. Such an approach is completely empirical, as it is impossible to predict in advance who will tolerate a drug holiday of any substantial period of time, although many patients will. Unless someone is around to watch the patient carefully for signs of relapse, so that treatment may be restarted immediately, this approach is neither feasible nor fair to the patient. Nor has it been shown that this approach has any compelling advantages over trying assiduously to find the least possible maintenance dose.

Many patients take their own drug holidays, either by discontinuing the drug altogether or by taking less than prescribed. In one study, thirty-nine of eighty-five chronic schizophrenic patients took less drug than prescribed when followed over a two-year period; the major reason proposed for discontinuation was the unpleasant effect of a subtle akathisia (16). Actually, this rate of noncompliance is not much different from that of patients taking antihypertensive drugs or those on prophylactic regimens of antitubercular drugs.

Assuming that one has found the minimal maintenance dose, the patient should be cautioned to continue medication, even though he feels well, and should be reassured about fears of becoming addicted. He should be cautioned about possible drowsiness and interference with skilled movements and warned against the concomitant use of alcoholic beverages. The patient's family should have the same instructions. Information should be provided to the family physician and pharmacist. An uninterrupted supply of medication should be assured. The ever-increasing number of patients discharged from hospitals on antipsychotic drugs poses a special challenge to follow-up clinics. One should make efforts to keep patients on drugs. In one study, only 15 percent of chronic schizophrenics were considered to be suitable for trial without drugs, and less than 1 percent were able to stay off drugs completely; the average time from discontinuation of drug to relapse was 4.5 months (17).

Long-acting depot preparations have been a boon to maintenance therapy, especially when patients are unreliable about taking medication. Several studies have suggested a decreased rate of relapse among patients so maintained, as contrasted with those taking daily oral medication, with marked reductions in readmission rates to hospitals and days spent in the hospital (18). Other results have been less spectacular (19).

CONCOMITANT NONDRUG THERAPY

Antipsychotic drugs are the foundation for an effective total treatment program of psychosis. Many patients with short-term psychoses are subsequently able to function normally. However, few patients who have been hospitalized for any appreciable period as schizophrenics ever function in a completely "normal" way thereafter. Accordingly, realistic efforts must be made to help such patients so that they can live in the community despite their handicap. Various types of therapy, including supportive psychotherapy and occupational therapies, can be very important and helpful. Recently, new approaches using behavioral modification techniques have become popular. It remains to be seen whether these approaches add substantially to the effects of drug therapy. Following hospital discharge, an emphasis on real-life adjustment should be constantly provided, just as might be appropriate in any other temporarily or permanently handicapped person.

The problem of maintaining patients on appropriate medication is a serious and continuing one. Close social casework follow-up may help to remedy this problem. When combined with vocational rehabilitation counseling, the relapse rate of patients was still further lowered (20).

TOXICITY AND SIDE EFFECTS

The adverse reactions to antipsychotic medications can be conveniently categorized into extensions of known pharmacological actions, hypersensitivity reactions, and idiopathic reactions. Despite the variety of antipsychotics which are available, the spectrum of major pharmacological actions is reasonably constant throughout the entire group (21,22).

Overdose

Antipsychotics have a wide therapeutic margin in adults, so that most fatalities with these drugs have occurred in children. Clinically, overdose presents as drowsiness, leading rapidly to coma. Other manifestations can include hypotension, seizures, hypothermia, extrapyramidal reactions, and cardiac arrhythmias. The hypotension results from α-adrenergic blockade and may be difficult to treat. Since phenothiazines are detoxified in the liver, coma may be prolonged in patients with hepatic insufficiency.

Central Nervous System Effects

Oversedation is a common side effect of antipsychotic medications, particularly when compounded by the addition of other sedatives. The low-potency phenothiazines are more sedative than are the high-potency ones.

Acute blockade of the dopaminergic striatonigral pathway probably leads to the extrapyramidal side effects of the antipsychotics. These are usually manifested as: a syndrome resembling Parkinson's disease; a syndrome of uncontrollable restlessness, known as akathisia; and acute dystonic syndromes. The parkinsonian symptoms can include muscular rigidity, "pill-rolling" tremor, altered posture, immobility or akinesia, immobile facies, and shuffling gait. Akathisia is manifested by constant pacing and "fidgeting"; by finger, hand, and foot movements; and by a powerful subjective sense of restlessness. It is often mistaken for psychotic agitation. Acute dystonic reactions often involve spasms of neck muscles (torticollis), occasionally include spasms of the spine and extremities (opisthotonus), and can mimic the oculogyric crises associated with Parkinson's disease, in which spasms of the eye muscles predominate. They tend to be more common in children and young adults and generally appear soon after medication is initiated. Tardive dyskinesia, another important central adverse effect of antipsychotic medication, is discussed in the final section of this chapter.

Autonomic Side Effects

An acute hypotensive crisis can be a troublesome side effect of anti-psychotic medication. Hypotension is more commonly seen in patients receiving parenteral phenothiazines but can occur when oral pheno-thiazines are given to elderly or debilitated patients.

Anticholinergic side effects can also be a problem. These effects include dry mouth, blurred vision, tachycardia, and constipation. Rarely, antipsychotics may exacerbate or precipitate narrow-angle glaucoma, urinary retention, or paralytic ileus.

Cardiac Effects

Thioridazine commonly produces prolonged ventricular repolariza-tion, with lengthened Q-T intervals and prominent U waves in the electrocardiogram (ECG). Other antipsychotics also produce these changes, although less frequently. This effect may be the result of a potassium shift to the intracellular compartment (23). The significance of this reversible cardiac side effect is not clear, and its relationship to the sudden deaths which are occasionally associated with phenothia-zines will require further study.

Metabolic and Endocrine Effects

Prolactin levels appear to be increased by antipsychotics (cf. Chapter 8). This is the probable cause of the milk production (galactorrhea) which sometimes is seen in women. Amenorrhea is also an occasional side effect. Men frequently complain of sexual disturbances, with loss of libido. Another disturbing metabolic concomitant of antipsychotic medication is weight gain, often to a remarkable degree. Hyperpyrexia can also be troublesome and usually occurs during prolonged hot spells in hospitals without air conditioning.

Allergic or Toxic Effects

Phenothiazines probably have a direct toxic effect on the myeloid elements of the bone marrow, since a decrease in white blood cell production occurs in many patients treated with these agents. Fortunately, this rarely progresses into agranulocytosis. Patients who initially present with low white cell counts or have concurrent medical illnesses may be at greater risk for agranulocytosis, as are those receiving low-potency antipsychotics. Agranulocytosis occurs most commonly during the first six weeks of treatment. However, since the patient may have a normal white count just prior to the onset of the agranulocytosis, frequent monitoring of the white count has been abandoned by most clinicians. Still, an initial leukocyte count is useful to help identify patients who are at risk.

The frequency of cholestatic jaundice produced by antipsychotics seems to be declining. The syndrome has many characteristics of an allergic reaction, occurring soon after the drug is started and being accompanied by fever, eosinophilia, and rashes. Many of the cases of clinically manifest cholestatic jaundice were associated with chlorpromazine.

Miscellaneous Adverse Effects

Thioridazine stands alone among the antipsychotics in producing a pigmentary retinopathy which can cause irreversible loss of visual acuity. This severe reaction appears to occur only at doses above 800 mg per day. Chlorpromazine sometimes produces pigment deposits in the skin and in the cornea or lens of the eye; it may also induce photosensitivity. Finally, the antipsychotics may produce seizures in some patients, particularly in those with a history of epilepsy.

Management of Adverse Reactions

Overdose with the antipsychotics is primarily treated symptomatically. Intravenous fluids and volume expanders should be used to combat hypotension; if these are insufficient, norepinephrine can be administered. The hypotension results from an α-adrenergic blockade; therefore, epinephrine should *not* be used, since its β-adrenergic stimulating effects may decrease blood pressure further. Control of extrapyramidal reactions is described below. Hypothermia may necessitate the use of warm blankets and baths. In light of the cardiac effects of these drugs, an overdose patient should be monitored by ECG. Once the patient is stable, increased removal of phenothiazines can be effected with lavage and forced diuresis; dialysis is of little value.

Oversedation can be minimized by dividing the doses in early stages of treatment, by avoiding other sedative medications, and by using the less sedating, higher potency antipsychotics. Extrapyramidal side effects can be managed by reducing the dosage and by administering antiparkinsonian agents such as trihexyphenidyl (Artane), 2–10 mg/day; benztropine mesylate (Cogentin), 4–6 mg/day; procyclidine hydrochloride (Kemadrin), 10–20 mg/day; or biperiden (Akineton), 2–8 mg/day. These anticholinergic agents should not be used in every patient, since the parkinsonian side effects do not always appear and since the combined anticholinergic effects can also lead to adverse reactions. Akathisia may be alleviated by a reduction in dosage, by diphenhydramine (Benadryl), or by the antiparkinsonian agents. Acute dystonic reactions will also respond to intramuscular diphenhydramine, 50 mg, to intravenous caffeine sodium benzoate, 500 mg, or to intramuscular antiparkinsonian agents. When a patient has had a severe extrapyramidal reaction, it may be best to continue the antiparkinsonian medications for six to eight weeks; however, they need not be continued indefinitely.

Autonomic side effects can also be troublesome. Because of hypotension, patients should probably lie flat for at least half an hour after the injection of antipsychotics, and blood pressures should be measured before and several times after drug administration. This is particularly important for patients at risk for hypotension. Occasionally, more vigorous treatment for hypotension is necessary, as described earlier. The anticholinergic side effects of antipsychotics rarely necessitate treatment other than dosage reduction. Local application of cholinomimetic drugs to the eye has been recommended for severe cases of blurred vision. The treatment of the anticholinergic crisis is described in Chapter 24.

Cardiac side effects may be more common for the low-potency antipsychotics, particularly thioridazine. Patients who have a history of cardiac arrhythmias or who develop abnormal electrocardiograms should probably be switched to a high potency antipsychotic, and the electrocardiogram should be checked frequently.

The galactorrhea, gynecomastia, and loss of libido seen with antipsychotics is troublesome but not dangerous. Hyperpyrexia, however, requires vigorous treatment with sponge or alcohol baths and the transfer to a cooler environment.

Agranulocytosis is a potentially fatal complication. It is usually first manifested by a sore throat and fever. The antipsychotic medication should be discontinued and infection should be combated in consultation with other specialists, using reverse isolation, antibiotics, and supportive measures. Cholestatic jaundice is increasingly uncommon, and the jaundice will usually decrease rapidly when the antipsychotic medication is discontinued. The retinal changes produced by thioridazine suggest that doses of this medication should not exceed 800 mg per day. The photosensitivity and skin and eye pigmentation caused by chlorpromazine probably should lead to use of other antipsychotics as a first choice for treating schizophrenics.

TARDIVE DYSKINESIA

Tardive dyskinesia has been of increasing concern, the frequency of occurrence almost depending on how closely one looks for the complication. In one survey, tardive dyskinesia was diagnosed in 36 percent of chronic mental hospital patients (24). The reaction is not restricted to old patients or to patients under long treatment, since it can develop within weeks. The fact that it may occur in nonpsychotic patients treated with antipsychotic drugs is warning enough against using these drugs for trivial indications (11).

Under the auspices of the American College of Neuropsychopharmacology and the Food and Drug Administration, a brief review of all neurologic syndromes induced by antipsychotic drugs has been presented (25). The essential feature of tardive dyskinesia is repetitive involuntary movements of a choreoathetoid type involving the mouth, lips, tongue, trunk, and extremities. The basic mechanism proposed for this syndrome is the development of dopaminergic hypersensitivity in the striatonigral system, with a relative reduction in cholinergic function (26,27). Such a formulation explains several clinical phenomena:

- Most, if not all, cases of tardive dyskinesia are preceded by the Parkinson syndrome, and occasionally one sees mixed syndromes.
- Anticholinergic drugs are not only ineffective but often unmask a latent dyskinesia.
- Augmenting doses of antipsychotic drugs, either by using more of the same or by adding another, often ameliorates the picture, at least temporarily.
- Sudden withdrawal from an antipsychotic drug may exacerbate a latent syndrome.
- L-DOPA administration, which increases dopaminergic activity, makes the syndrome worse; and physostigmine, which increases cholinergic activity, may briefly ameliorate it.

The pathogenesis of this disorder is not clearly understood. The initial perturbation produced by antipsychotic drugs is the postsynaptic block of dopamine receptors, which is thought to produce both of the novel pharmacological actions of these drugs. In the striatonigral dopamine system, the following sequences may occur with continued treatment. Continued block of postsynaptic receptors activates a feedback loop, presumably a dendritic connection from the postsynaptic to the presynaptic neuron (Chapter 2). An attempt is made to overcome the postsynaptic block by increased synthesis of dopamine and possibly by increased storage of the transmitter and increased receptor formation. As a result, dopaminergic transmission may be restored to normal, leading to loss of extrapyramidal motor reactions, or actually increased beyond normal, resulting in the appearance of earliest signs of tardive dyskinesia. If treatment is still continued, it has been postulated that alteration may occur to the neuronal membrane, producing a phenomenon of denervation supersensitivity, in which the receptors now are much more sensitive to the action of dopamine. At this point, the tardive dyskinesia may become quite severe and long-lasting, if not irreversible. Thus, from an initial situation of too little dopaminergic transmission one has progressed to a relative excess of activity. Therefore, this syndrome is completely opposite to that of drug-induced extrapyramidal reactions and requires totally opposite approaches to treatment.

A number of proposals for managing tardive dyskinesia have been made (28). Although Huntington's chorea was treated with antipsychotic drugs in the 1950's, the past is always waiting to be rediscovered. It is obvious that one might overcome the compensatory mechanism by increasing the antipsychotic medication. It should be apparent that this expedient solution is not without dangers, for one might be increasing one's bets in a losing game. Other tactics depend upon decreasing dopaminergic activity (Chapter 2). Blocking the synthesis of dopamine with the tyrosine hydroxylase inhibitor α-methyl-p-tyrosine seems logical but has not been very successful. Reserpine and tetrabenazine have been used to decrease the storage of transmitter in the synaptic vesicles, and results have been mixed. Methyldopa has been given to act as a precursor for a false transmitter, methyldopamine, which would displace dopamine and reduce its effects, again without much apparent benefit. Reducing the dose of drug seems the most natural thing to do, but if this is done precipitously, the motor disturbances may get temporarily worse. Lithium carbonate, if beneficial, might be so from two actions: first, by increasing the intraneuronal turnover of dopamine and, second, by decreasing receptor sensitivity. Diazepam is sometimes useful, possibly by reducing the intensity of the compensatory feedback loop through increasing cyclic AMP levels or inhibiting dopaminergic activity by a mechanism involving γ-aminobutyric acid (GABA) (Chapter 19). Recent reports of the use of deanol (2-dimethylaminoethanol), a possible choline precursor, for treating L-DOPA-induced dyskinesias, Huntington's chorea, and tardive dyskinesia have not yet been confirmed (29). This approach would work on the other side of the equation, attempting to increase cholinergic transmission.

SUMMARY

Drug treatment of schizophrenia has been the most successful approach to date for this devastating illness. It is far from ideal, as most schizophrenic patients show improvement, but relatively few recover. Current progress in developing new drugs provides hope for better ones. Even more important, the spur to biomedical research into the nature of schizophrenia, which the era of drug treatment provided, will lead to a much better understanding of the pathogenesis of the disorder. When we better understand the causes, our approach to treatment should become even more rational.

REFERENCES

1. Pollin, W.   The pathogenesis of schizophrenia: possible relationships between genetic, biochemical and experiential factors. *Arch. Gen. Psychiatry* 27:29–37, 1972.
2. Forrest, A. D. and Hay, A. J.   The schizophrenias: operational definitions. *Br. J. Med. Psychol.* 46:337–346, 1973.
3. Cancro, R.   The causes of the schizophrenias. *Ann. Intern. Med.* 77: 647–648, 1972.
4. Lidz, T.   The nature and origins of schizophrenic disorders. *Ann. Intern. Med.* 77:639–645, 1972.
5. Ayd, F. J. and Blackwell, B. *(eds.). Discoveries in Biological Psychiatry.* Philadelphia: Lippincott Co., 1970.
6. Swazey, J. P.   *Chlorpromazine in Psychiatry: A Study of Therapeutic Innovation.* Cambridge: MIT Press, 1974.
7. Byck, R.   Drugs and the treatment of psychiatric disorders. *In: The Pharmacological Basis of Therapeutics,* 5th ed. L. S. Goodman and A. Gilman, *eds.,* New York: Macmillan Co., 1975, pp. 152–200.
8. Baldessarini, R. J. and Lipinski, J. F.   Risks *vs* benefits of antipsychotic drugs. *N. Eng. J. Med.* 289:427–428, 1973.
9. Prien, R. F., Klett, J., and Caffey, E. M.   Lithium carbonate and imipramine in prevention of affective episodes. *Arch. Gen. Psychiatry* 29: 420–425, 1973.
10. Dinsmore, P. R. and Ryback, R.   Lithium in schizo-affective disorders. *Dis. Nerv. Syst.* 33:771–776, 1972.
11. Klawans, H. L., Bergen, D., Bruyn, G. W., and Paulson, G. W.   Neuroleptic-induced tardive dyskinesias in nonpsychotic patients. *Arch. Neurol.* 30:338–339, 1974.
12. Hollister, L. E., Overall, J. E., Kimbell, I., and Pokorny, A.   Specific indications for different classes of phenothiazines. *Arch. Gen. Psychiatry* 30:94–99, 1974.
13. Donlon, P. T. and Tupin, J. P.   Rapid "digitalization" of decompensated schizophrenic patients with antipsychotic agents. *Am. J. Psychiatry* 131:310–312, 1974.
14. Laska, E., Varga, E., Wanderling, J., Simpson, G., Logemann, G. W., and Shah, B. K.   Patterns of psychotropic drug use for schizophrenia. *Dis. Nerv. Syst.* 34:294–305, 1973.
15. Prien, R. F., Gillis, R. D., and Caffey, E. M.   Intermittent pharmacotherapy in chronic schizophrenia. *Hosp. Commun. Psychiatry* 24: 317–322, 1973.
16. Van Putten, T.   Why do schizophrenic patients refuse to take their drugs? *Arch. Gen. Psychiatry* 31:67–72, 1974.
17. Morgan, R. and Cheadle, J.   Maintenance treatment of chronic schizophrenia with neuroleptic drugs. *Acta Psychiatr. Scand.* 50:78–85, 1974.
18. Denham, J. and Adamson, L.   Long-acting phenothiazines in the prevention of relapse of schizophrenic patients. *Can. Psychiatr. Assoc. J.* 18:235–237, 1973.
19. Crawford, R. and Forrest, A.   Controlled trial of depot fluphenazine in outpatient schizophrenics. *Br. J. Psychiatry* 124:385–391, 1974.
20. Hogarty, G. E. and Goldberg, S. C.   Drug and sociotherapy in the

149

aftercare of schizophrenic patients. *Arch. Gen. Psychiatry 28:*54–64, 1973.

21. Hollister, L. E. *Clinical Use of Psychotherapeutic Drugs.* Springfield: Thomas, 1973.

22. Hollister, L. E. Adverse drug effects. *In: Drug Treatment of Mental Disorders.* L. L. Simpson, ed., New York: Raven Press, 1976, pp. 267–288.

23. Alvarez-Mena, S. C. and Frank, M. J. Phenothiazine-induced T-wave abnormalities. *J. Am. Med. Assoc. 222:*1730–1733, 1973.

24. Fann, W. E., Davis, J. M., and Janowsky, D. S. The prevalence of tardive dyskinesias in mental hospital patients. *Dis. Nerv. Syst. 33:* 182–186, 1972.

25. ACNP-FDA Task Force. Medical intelligence—drug therapy. *N. Eng. J. Med. 289:*20–24, 1973.

26. Klawans, H. L., Jr. The pharmacology of tardive dyskinesias. *Am. J. Psychiatry 130:*82–86, 1973.

27. Gerlach, J., Reisby, N., and Randrup, A. Dopaminergic hypersensitivity and cholinergic hypofunction in the pathophysiology of tardive dyskinesia. *Psychopharmacologia 34:*21–35, 1974.

28. Kazamatsuri, H., Chien, C-P., and Cole, J. O. Therapeutic approaches to tardive dyskinesia. *Arch. Gen. Psychiatry 27:*491–499, 1972.

29. Miller, E. M. Deanol: a solution for tardive dyskinesia? *N. Eng. J. Med. 291:*796, 1974.

10 | Biochemical Hypotheses of Affective Disorders

PHILIP A. BERGER and JACK D. BARCHAS

INTRODUCTION

An early biochemical hypothesis of depression came from ancient Greek physicians, who believed that the liver purged food of its toxic humours, including black bile (*melan-* + *cholē*). If the liver malfunctioned, severe depression, or melancholia, resulted from the excessive accumulation of black bile. Today, mania and depression are still thought to be related to excesses or deficiencies of "humours," i.e., the brain neurotransmitters, particularly norepinephrine and 5-hydroxytryptamine (serotonin). Studies of the biochemical correlates and pharmacological treatments of depression and mania have increased our understanding of these disorders and of normal brain function. However, a biochemical basis for affective disorders has not been established. Furthermore, the mechanisms by which efficacious medications alleviate these psychiatric conditions remain unknown, although there are some important hypotheses about their pharmacological activity.

Recent research on the affective disorders has focused on two major hypotheses. The first proposes that affective disorders result from functional changes in the central noradrenergic systems. The second postulates that, in some subgroups of these disorders, the primary abnormality is in central serotonergic pathways.

The catecholamine hypothesis of affective disorders was based, in part, upon the pharmacological actions of reserpine and iproniazid, which are described below. Everett and Tolman (1) may have made the first recorded statement of the catecholamine hypothesis in 1958, when they suggested that an excess of the amines might lead to increased activity and hostility, while a deficiency might produce depression and lassitude. Several other groups also independently used the catecholamine hypothesis to organize their research into the pharmacology of depression. However, two major review articles, both appearing in 1965, deserve credit for providing widely read and clear statements of the evidence supporting this hypothesis. One article, written by Joseph Schildkraut, appeared in the November 1965 issue of the *American Journal of Psychiatry;* the other, written by William Bunney and John Davis, can be found in the December 1965 issue of the *Archives of General Psychiatry.*

During this same period, investigators in England were concentrating upon the possible involvement of 5-hydroxytryptamine in the affective disorders. Since both reserpine and iproniazid affect indoleamines and catecholamines in an essentially analogous fashion, much of the early data could be used to support either hypothesis (2). In fact, these two hypotheses, together, have been called the biogenic amine hypothesis of affective disorders. Despite contradictory data, the biogenic amine hypothesis continues to offer the best available framework for understanding the biological substrates of depression and of manic psychosis.

PHARMACOLOGICAL SUPPORT FOR THE BIOGENIC AMINE HYPOTHESIS

Basic Evidence

Rauwolfia serpentina is a plant which, for many centuries, was used to treat illness in India. The active alkaloid, reserpine, was isolated from it in the early 1950's and used as a treatment for schizophrenia and hypertension (Chapter 9). Two important pharmacological effects of the drug soon emerged. First, reserpine was shown to produce a "depression-like" syndrome in animals, including sedation and motor retardation. Second, a subgroup of patients who received reserpine were found to develop a syndrome which resembles depression (Chapter 29). The subsequent discovery that reserpine depletes central stores of 5-hydroxytryptamine, norepinephrine, and dopamine (Chapters 2 and 3) suggested a possible connection between these systems and the behavioral effects.

In the early 1950's, iproniazid was synthesized for the treatment of tuberculosis. Clinically, it was reported to produce euphoria and over-active behavior in some patients, while pharmacologically it was shown to be a potent inhibitor of the enzyme monoamine oxidase (MAO) and to produce increased brain concentrations of norepinephrine and 5-hydroxytryptamine. Iproniazid was then tried in depressed patients. In 1957, two independent groups of investigators reported successful trials of iproniazid in depression (3). Thus, again, there was suggestive evidence which linked these biogenic amines and the affective disorders.

Tricyclic antidepressants (tricyclics) resulted from a modification of the phenothiazine molecule, which changed the clinical activity from antipsychotic to antidepressant (Chapter 11). The tricyclic anti-depressants are thought to act by preventing reuptake inactivation of biogenic amines through nerve endings, thus potentiating the amine action at postsynaptic receptors (Chapters 2 and 3).

Lithium has been demonstrated to be effective for the treatment of acute manic episodes in many controlled clinical trials (Chapter 12). The mechanism of action of lithium in mania has not been determined; however, lithium does affect biogenic amines in some test systems. In general, the effects of lithium appear to be opposite to those of the tricyclics. Thus, with lithium, both catecholaminergic and serotonergic activity decreases in some test systems (4,5).

In summary, pharmacological support for the biogenic hypothesis of affective disorders is found in the action of four agents. Reserpine depletes biogenic amines and may cause depression in some patients. MAO inhibitors and tricyclics increase the amount of biogenic amines at the synapse by two different mechanisms, and drugs in both classes are useful in treating depressed patients. Finally, lithium, which is ex-tremely effective in treating mania, may decrease the quantity of bio-genic amines available at the postsynaptic receptor.

PROBLEMS WITH THE EVIDENCE

Closer inspection of the pharmacological support for the biogenic amine hypothesis of affective disorders does reveal some discrepancies. These are summarized in Table 10-1.

As discussed in Chapter 29, reevaluation of the original reports of reserpine-induced depression has suggested that many of the patients

TABLE 10-1.

QUESTIONS ABOUT THE PHARMACOLOGICAL SUPPORT FOR THE BIOGENIC AMINE HYPOTHESIS

Does reserpine cause true depression?

Do MAO inhibitors act by inhibiting monoamine oxidase?

Why don't tricyclics and MAO inhibitors act immediately?

Why is iprindole an effective antidepressant?

Why is cocaine not an effective antidepressant?

Why does lithium work in both mania and depression?

---

experienced psychomotor retardation rather than clinical depression. Reserpine does seem to precipitate depression in patients with prior episodes of the disorder. This may be a primary effect, but it may also reflect a secondary depression resulting from the effects of reserpine-induced psychomotor retardation upon individuals who are reassured by psychomotor activity (6). The use of reserpine sedation as an animal model of human depression has also been criticized (cf. Chapter 1). Reserpine-induced motor retardation in animals results from depletion of dopamine and can be reversed by administration of L-DOPA, its amino acid precursor. Although L-DOPA also produces motor activation and, sometimes, hypomania in depressed patients, it has no useful antidepressant activity (7).

The pharmacological actions of MAO inhibitors may also be more complex than originally thought. These substances also inhibit catecholamine reuptake, and their clinical efficacy may correspond more closely to their ability to block reuptake than to their potency as MAO inhibitors (8). This would suggest that these drugs and tricyclics share a common mechanism of action.

Unfortunately, there are also problems with the data on uptake inhibitors. Cocaine is a potent inhibitor of monoamine reuptake at the synapse but has no significant antidepressant activity (Chapter 20). On the other hand, iprindole, a tricyclic related to imipramine, does not appear to be a good reuptake inhibitor; and yet it has been found to be an effective antidepressant (9). A second problem with the hypothesis that antidepressants act by blocking biogenic reuptake arises from the delayed onset of their antidepressant action: the antidepressant effects of these medications take two weeks to become apparent, while the inhibition of biogenic amine reuptake is seen soon after acute administration in laboratory studies.

The pharmacological and clinical effects of lithium and the tricyclics seem to fit nicely with the biogenic amine hypothesis of affective disorders. They produce opposite effects on biogenic amine activity; and the tricyclics are active in depressed patients, while lithium is used in the treatment of mania. This picture is complicated, however, by the recent finding that lithium is also useful in the treatment and prevention of some depressive episodes, particularly in patients with a history of both mania and depression (Chapter 11).

Data from psychopharmacological agents are further confounded by the possible involvement of several neurotransmitters. Reserpine, MAO inhibitors, tricyclics, and lithium all seem to act on both catecholamines and indoleamines. Thus, any one, or even some combination, of these monoamines may play the prominent role in the action of these drugs on affective disorders. As described below, this problem can be circumvented, in part, by using other pharmacological agents to deliberately manipulate a specific neurotransmitter system. In addition, careful investigation of tricyclics reveals that they differ in their relative potencies for a given neurotransmitter. Thus, imipramine and amitriptyline are more potent against serotonergic reuptake, while desipramine is more effective against catecholaminergic systems (10). Some support for clinical relevance of these differences comes from a preliminary study with depressed patients who showed an antidepressant response to imipramine. This response was sustained during treatment with α-methyl-p-tyrosine (AMPT), which inhibits catecholamine synthesis; but depression returned with p-chlorophenylalanine (PCPA), which inhibits synthesis of 5-hydroxytryptamine, suggesting that the the serotonergic system may have been involved in the antidepressant action of imipramine in these patients (11).

Finally, it is important to distinguish between neuronal systems which affect a disease process and those which produce it. The necessity for this distinction is illustrated by the efficacy of anticholinergics in the treatment of Parkinson's disease. Although anticholinergics were long known to help to control some symptoms, it would not have been correct to conclude that the primary defect in Parkinson's disease was an overactivity of the cholinergic nervous system. With the demonstration that dopaminergic underactivity is the basic defect in Parkinsonism, the role of the cholinergic system had to be reassessed. Similarly, even if current psychotherapeutic agents do act through biogenic amines, the etiology of depression and mania may result from a different physiological mechanism.

PHARMACOLOGICAL ATTEMPTS TO TEST THE BIOGENIC AMINE HYPOTHESIS

Since the biochemical effects of clinically active agents have not provided an unequivocal answer about which systems are involved in the affective disorders, investigators have attempted to examine these systems more directly. Several approaches have been used (Table 10-2). The "precursor-loading" strategy is an attempt to correct the postulated deficiency of biogenic amines by providing metabolic precursors. This indirect approach is necessitated by the inability of the amines themselves to cross the blood-brain barrier. Enzyme inhibitors and receptor blockers have been used in efforts to decrease neurotransmitter activity in patients with affective disorders. For more specific information about the actions of these pharmacological agents, see Chapters 2 and 3.

CATECHOLAMINERGIC SYSTEMS

Precursor-Loading

L-DOPA (L-dihydroxyphenylalanine) is the immediate amino acid precursor for the catecholamines. Unlike either dopamine or norepinephrine, L-DOPA readily crosses the blood-brain barrier. Early studies with depressed patients used low doses of L-DOPA. Generally, the results were disappointing. One problem with these studies is that L-DOPA is rapidly metabolized in the periphery. A peripheral decarboxylase inhibitor can be used to prevent the peripheral conversion of L-DOPA to dopamine without blocking this reaction centrally (12).

TABLE 10-2.
PHARMACOLOGICAL TESTS OF THE BIOGENIC AMINE HYPOTHESIS*

NEURO-TRANSMITTER SYSTEM	SUBSTANCE	PRESUMED PHARMACOLOGICAL ACTION	EXPECTED BIOCHEMICAL RESULT	EXPECTED CLINICAL RESULT
*Catecholaminergic***				
	L-DOPA	Catecholamine precursor	↑ Dopamine and Norepinephrine	↓ Depression
	α-Methyl-*p*-tyrosine	Tyrosine hydroxylase inhibitor	↓ Dopamine and Norepinephrine	↓ Mania
	Fusaric acid	Dopamine-β-hydroxylase inhibitor	↓ Norepinephrine	↓ Mania
*Serotonergic****				
	L–Tryptophan	5-Hydroxytryptamine precursor	↑ 5-Hydroxytryptamine	↓ Depression
	5-Hydroxytryptophan	5-Hydroxytryptamine precursor	↑ 5-Hydroxytryptamine	↓ Depression
	p-Chlorophenylalanine	Tryptophan hydroxylase inhibitor	↓ 5-Hydroxytryptamine	↓ Mania
	Methysergide Cinanserin	5-Hydroxytryptamine receptor blocker	↓ Serotonergic Activity	↓ Mania

* For actual result, see text.
** See Chapter 2 for a description of this system.
*** See Chapter 3 for a description of this system.

In one major study, high oral doses of L-DOPA were given to twenty-six depressed patients with and without a peripheral decarboxylase inhibitor (13). Under this regimen, five patients who had prominent psychomotor retardation may have improved. The remainder of the patients failed to show improvement, with some exhibiting increased anger and psychotic symptoms: eight of nine patients who had a history of bipolar illness developed hypomania during the study. Another recent double-blind study which also used high doses of L-DOPA found no significant antidepressant effects in six depressed patients (14). The failure of patients to respond to even high doses of L-DOPA may result from a concomitant decrease in central serotonergic activity. However, an attempt to correct this theoretical deficit by simultaneously administering L-tryptophan and L-DOPA did not produce a significant therapeutic response in a small sample of depressed patients (15).

Inhibitors

α-Methyl-p-tyrosine (AMPT) is a potent, competitive inhibitor of tyrosine hydroxylase, which is the rate-limiting enzyme in catecholamine biosynthesis (Chapter 2). It reduces brain catecholamine levels in animals and decreases the urinary excretion of catecholamine metabolites in man. α-Methyl-p-tyrosine has been used in treating hypertension. Some patients have developed transient depression while using the drug, and transient hypomanic reactions have been described when it is discontinued. One study has examined the effects of this inhibitor in both manic and depressed patients (16). The treatment produced decreased levels of urinary catecholamines, indicating that it did affect the activity of these systems. During treatment, five of the seven manic patients showed some improvement, and two of these five responders relapsed when placebo was given. All three depressed patients had increased symptoms of depression.

Fusaric acid is an inhibitor of the enzyme dopamine-β-hydroxylase, which converts dopamine to norepinephrine (Chapter 2). Thus, fusaric acid should decrease norepinephrine synthesis. When fusaric acid was given to eight manic patients, it decreased the urinary levels of the norepinephrine metabolite 3-methoxy-4-hydroxyphenylethylene glycol (MHPG); it also increased psychosis in patients with pre-existing psychotic features but caused slight improvement in a few patients with mild hypomania (17).

SEROTONERGIC SYSTEMS

Precursor-Loading

Attempts to treat depression with L-tryptophan have recently been reviewed (14). Tryptophan is reported to potentiate the effects of MAO inhibitors in depression; however, the relative contributions of the two treatments is unclear. Tryptophan alone has produced variable results: some investigators have found it to be as effective as imipramine in the treatment of depression; others were unable to find an effect. It has also been used as an experimental treatment for mania, and it is reported to reduce symptoms of manic patients. These effects of tryptophan lead to two problems for the biogenic amine hypothesis of affective disorders. First, results with tryptophan in depression have been inconsistent, at best. Second, the suggestion that tryptophan may relieve mania is opposite to prediction, since if manic patients have overactive biogenic amine activity, tryptophan should cause an exacerbation of manic symptoms, not an improvement.

5-Hydroxytryptophan, the immediate metabolic precursor of 5-hydroxytryptamine, has also been given to depressed patients. One report stated that 5-hydroxytryptophan potentiated the effects of MAO inhibitors, while others have found no beneficial effects from this combination. 5-Hydroxytryptophan alone has also been found to be useful in some depressed patients. van Praag (18) has suggested that only patients with decreased serotonergic activity will respond to 5-hydroxytryptophan. One recent study on depressed patients who were refractory to other treatments is consistent with this suggestion (19).

Inhibitors

p-Chlorophenylalanine inhibits tryptophan hydroxylase, the enzyme which catalyzes the first and rate-limiting step in the synthesis of 5-hydroxytryptamine (Chapter 3). Although it decreased synthesis of 5-hydroxytryptamine in humans, p-chlorophenylalanine did not decrease symptoms in three manic patients (20). Both methysergide and cinanserin are thought to antagonize serotonergic activity by blocking the receptor. Early reports that methysergide was useful in the treatment of mania were not confirmed in several controlled clinical trials (21). In another study, cinanserin was reported to have some antimanic activity, but this report will require confirmation (22).

METABOLIC STUDIES IN PATIENTS
WITH DEPRESSION AND MANIA

The problems with the pharmacological support for the biogenic amine hypothesis and the contradictory results of pharmacological attempts to test that hypothesis led to more direct efforts to detect alterations in biogenic amine metabolism in affective disorders. This approach involves the measurement of neurotransmitters and their metabolites in blood, urine, cerebrospinal fluid, and, when possible, brain tissue. Recently, the enzymes involved in the synthesis and degradation of the biogenic amines have also been assayed in patients with mania and depression. Again, information about these enzymes and metabolites is provided in Chapters 2 and 3. These metabolic studies have been the subject of several recent reviews (20, 21, 23, 24).

CATECHOLAMINERGIC SYSTEMS

The most extensive studies of the catecholamines and related substances have involved urinary excretion patterns. The compounds are concentrated in the urine, so that measurement problems are less of a concern than is the case with either plasma or cerebrospinal fluid samples. However, studies of the urinary catecholamine metabolites are seriously complicated by the large contribution by peripheral sources, making uncertain their relevance to central catecholaminergic processes.

Several studies have suggested that urinary excretion of both dopamine and norepinephrine is decreased in patients during depression and increased during mania, although not all investigators have confirmed these results. Activity may be a factor, since some patients with agitated depression have increased, rather than decreased, urinary norepinephrine. Arguing against a simple connection with activity, however, are reports that norepinephrine increases the day before bipolar patients switch from depression to mania. Urinary excretion of the norepinephrine metabolite normetanephrine essentially parallels that of norepinephrine itself, decreasing during depression and increasing during mania. Excretion of another metabolite, vanillylmandelic acid, also increases during mania.

One urinary metabolite which has aroused considerable interest in recent years has been 3-methoxy-4-hydroxyphenylglycol (MHPG), the deaminated, O-methylated metabolite of norepinephrine and normetanephrine. Although conclusive evidence in man is not yet available, animal studies suggest that MHPG may provide a reasonably good reflection of central noradrenergic activity (23). Recently, two groups of investigators have suggested that the response of depressed patients to certain tricyclics can be predicted by their excretion of urinary MHPG. Patients with low baseline excretion of MHPG were subsequently found to respond better to imipramine than did those whose initial MHPG excretion was high (23). In another investigation, MHPG excretion was higher in those who responded to amitryptyline than in those who did not (25). In agreement with these results, a third study has shown that depressed patients who respond to imipramine have lower urinary MHPG excretion than do those who respond to amitriptyline (26). This has led to an hypothesis that depressed patients can be divided into two groups based on their urinary excretion of MHPG, with low MHPG reflecting a defect in central noradrenergic systems and high MHPG resulting from a defect in another neurotransmitter, such as 5-hydroxytryptamine (25). This is consistent with studies indicating that imipramine is a better inhibitor of noradrenergic reuptake, while amitriptyline is a better inhibitor of serotonergic uptake (Chapter 11).

Studies of plasma catecholamines have been hindered by the technological difficulties of measuring very small concentrations of the substances of interest. As a result, most studies have examined either the catecholamine precursor, tyrosine, or norepinephrine. There is some suggestion that the normal diurnal rhythm of tyrosine may be altered in patients with depression, but results from studies of plasma concentrations of norepinephrine have been contradictory.

Investigations of cerebrospinal fluid metabolites have been restricted primarily to studies of MHPG and of the dopamine metabolite homovanillic acid (HVA). Depressed patients have not been found to have abnormal concentrations of MHPG. Some manic patients have increased levels of MHPG, but they have not yet been otherwise distinguishable from manics who do not. Some bipolar patients also show a definite shift in MHPG levels which parallels their mood swings, again suggesting that catecholamines might be involved in the switch process between depression and mania (24). To date, most studies of cerebrospinal fluid concentrations of homovanillic acid suggest that there are no consistent changes with either depression or mania. Several recent studies have estimated dopamine activity by examining the rate of production of homovanillic acid after its transportation from the spinal cord is blocked by probenicid. Increased and decreased production has been found in both depressed and manic patients. Possible explanations for these inconsistencies include differential effects of the probenicid and changes in the gradient of homovanillic acid down the spinal canal (21).

Enzymes

Dopamine-β-hydroxylase is present in the synaptic vesicles of adrenergic nerves and is released with norepinephrine when these nerves are stimulated. A portion of this released enzyme appears in the general circulation. Even in normal subjects, there are wide variations in basal serum activity of the enzyme, reflecting not only peripheral sympathetic activity but also genetic influences. Available studies suggest that measurement of the enzyme activity by current methods neither helps to differentiate among patients with affective disorders nor lends support to the biogenic amine hypothesis of depression (21,27).

Monoamine oxidase (MAO), which inactivates monoamines by deamination, is widely distributed throughout the body and is important in the metabolic degradation of both catecholamines and indoleamines (Chapters 2 and 3). Several studies have reported increased activity of both plasma and platelet MAO activity in a heterogeneous population of depressed patients. Some patients with bipolar depression were found to have decreased, rather than increased, platelet enzymatic activity, while some patients with unipolar depression had activities which did not differ significantly from control subjects. There is strong evidence that MAO exists in multiple forms, with each form having different substrate and inhibitor specificities (Chapters 2 and 3). The role and relative importance of each of the multiple forms of the enzyme in physiological and pathological states will be an important area for future research (3).

Catechol-O-methyl transferase (COMT) O-methylates both dopamine and norepinephrine. This enzyme is found in the central nervous system and in many peripheral tissues, including the erythrocyte. As with the other enzymes, there are reports that catechol-O-methyl transferase activity is both lower (28) and higher (29) in depressed patients than in normal controls. These contradictory results suggest that further studies of the factors that control levels of catechol-O-methyl transferase are needed. Recently, another form of the enzyme has been described. This form may have substrate affinities which differ from those of the original, soluble catechol-O-methyl transferase. If this second enzyme is found in human erythrocytes, it will be interesting to determine its activities in patients with mania and depression.

Cyclic Nucleotides

There is increasing evidence that the cyclic nucleotide adenosine $3'5'$-monophosphate (cyclic AMP) mediates the postsynaptic action of some brain neurotransmitters (Chapters 2 and 3). In the brain, this system has been best described for dopaminergic synapses. The postsynaptic action of dopamine includes the activation of a specific adenylate cyclase that participates in the conversion of adenosine triphosphate (ATP) to cyclic AMP. The cyclic AMP is then thought to activate a protein kinase which phosphorylates one or more proteins. Details remain to be determined, but this phosphorylated protein probably initiates the process that leads to the depolarization of the postsynaptic neuron. A similar mechanism may mediate the postsynaptic receptor action of norepinephrine and serotonin. The characterization of this so-called intracellular second messenger system is an important new direction for neurophysiological research (30).

Cyclic AMP concentrations have been measured in the urine and cerebrospinal fluid of depressed patients (31). In some, but not all studies, urinary cyclic AMP has been reported to be low in depressed patients and elevated in mania. The measurement of urinary cyclic AMP is complicated by the contribution of cyclic AMP from the kidney under the influence of endocrine factors. However, studies of cerebrospinal fluid concentrations of cyclic AMP are also inconclusive.

Another approach to the study of cyclic AMP has concentrated upon receptor responsiveness. In platelets, norepinephrine inhibits the induction of cyclic AMP formation by prostaglandin E_1. Such a system may offer a model in which to examine possible changes in receptor properties. In preliminary studies, however, no differences were found between depressed patients and controls (32). It can be expected that as the role of cyclic AMP and other secondary messengers, such as cyclic GMP, is defined more precisely, further studies of these compounds will be undertaken.

SEROTONERGIC SYSTEMS

Cerebrospinal Fluid

Most of the studies of serotonergic activity in depression and mania have involved measurements of cerebrospinal fluid levels of 5-hydroxy-indoleacetic acid (5-HIAA), the major metabolite of 5-hydroxy-tryptamine (Chapter 3). Both low and normal levels have been found in depressed patients. Those investigators who found decreased levels in patients disagree about the effects of remission, with some reporting that 5-HIAA levels return toward normal and others reporting that they remain low. Similarly, manic patients have been reported to have low, normal, and elevated levels of 5-HIAA (20, 21, 23).

Explanations for these inconsistencies are varied. If only a subgroup of depressed patients have an abnormality in serotonergic systems, then it is not surprising that studies might have either low or normal levels of 5-HIAA, depending upon the patient population. Furthermore, the acid metabolite forms a gradient down the spinal column, and mechanical disruption of this gradient during lumbar puncture could markedly affect the results. In addition, cerebrospinal fluid levels of 5-HIAA are affected by changes in activity and may be altered with age.

There are several other reasons for urging caution in interpretations of measurement of baseline 5-HIAA levels. Spinal cord metabolism of 5-hydroxytryptamine may contribute to the pool. In addition, there may be individual variation in the rate of its active removal from the cerebrospinal fluid. At least one tricyclic, imipramine, in usual therapeutic doses, lowers 5-HIAA concentrations; considering the long action of the tricyclics, low values could, therefore, reflect prior use of antidepressants. Despite these problems, the evidence from baseline studies is suggestive enough to have stimulated the development of further techniques for evaluating serotonergic activity in mania and depression.

Probenecid will inhibit the exit of 5-HIAA from the spinal fluid. Thus, after such blockade the levels of 5-HIAA rise. From the rate of rise, one can estimate the rate of formation of 5-HIAA, providing a measure of serotonergic activity. The accumulation of 5-HIAA in depressed patients has been lower than that in control subjects in several recent reports. Again, these studies must be interpreted with caution, since it is possible that probenecid produces different levels of transport inhibition in different patients (20,21).

Brain Tissue

Another approach to studies of the serotonergic system in depressed patients has entailed studies of brains from suicide victims. The reports have been contradictory, with increases, decreases, and no change in levels of 5-hydroxytryptamine and 5-HIAA (21). Interpretations of these postmortem differences in content is difficult. The age differences between suicide victims and controls might explain some of these results, as might differences in diet and drug use prior to death. The lengths of time between death and assay could also cause differences in levels of 5-hydroxytryptamine and its metabolites. Finally, psychological autopsy on both the accident and suicide victim is important. Some deaths which are classified as accidents may actually be suicide attempts. In general, appropriate controls for such studies are virtually impossible to obtain, for both ethical and practical reasons. As a result, their usefulness is strictly limited to detecting massive differences. To date, differences of that magnitude have not been found.

NEUROENDOCRINE STUDIES IN PATIENTS WITH AFFECTIVE DISORDERS

Several neuroendocrine abnormalities have been described in patients with affective disorders. In depressed patients, these abnormalities include hyperactivity of the pituitary-adrenal system, a blunted thyrotropin response to thyrotropin-releasing hormone (TRH), and a blunted growth hormone response to hypoglycemia. Some evidence suggests that these neuroendocrine abnormalities may be related to altered biogenic amine neurotransmitter metabolism. Thus, studies of neuroendocrine abnormalities in depressed patients may be another strategy for evaluating the biogenic amine hypothesis of affective disorders.

PITUITARY-ADRENAL ACTIVITY IN DEPRESSION

A subgroup of depressed patients has been found to have increased activity of the pituitary-adrenal axis. Elevated plasma cortisol levels, increased excretion of cortisol metabolites, increased excretion of urinary free cortisol, and elevated spinal fluid content of cortisol have all been reported. Some depressed patients have also been found to have disturbed diurnal patterns of cortisol output (33). The increase in pituitary-adrenal activity in some depressed patients resembles increased pituitary-adrenal activity in Cushing's disease, in that it is resistant to feedback suppression by dexamethasone (34). It is possible that depressed patients with altered pituitary-adrenal activity may overlap with the proposed groups of depressed patients who have defects in central catecholaminergic or serotonergic systems.

There is increasing, but somewhat contradictory, evidence that pituitary-adrenal activity is regulated by brain biogenic amines. Pharmacological investigations in animals have been interpreted to support the existence of a central noradrenergic system which exerts tonic inhibitory activity on the pituitary-adrenal system (21). There is also evidence from animal and human studies that brain 5-hydroxytryptamine plays a role in regulating this system. Depletion of this latter neurotransmitter enhances the pituitary-adrenal stress response in rats, while administration of precursors decrease or inhibit the stress response. 5-Hydroxytryptamine may mediate or modulate the negative feedback mechanism which regulates pituitary-adrenal stress response (35). However, this hypothesis is controversial, since other studies suggest that a central serotonergic system may stimulate pituitary-adrenal activity, rather than inhibit it. Thus, while further studies are needed to clarify relationships among 5-hydroxytryptamine, catecholamines, and the pituitary-adrenal system, it is possible that the increased activity of the pituitary-adrenal system may be secondary to a central biogenic amine defect.

PITUITARY-THYROID ACTIVITY AND DEPRESSION

Thyrotropin-releasing hormone (TRH) is a tripeptide which is produced in the hypothalamus and stimulates the secretion of pituitary thyrotropin. Secretion of thyroid hormones is subsequently stimulated by thyrotropin. The relationship between depression and the pituitary-thyroid axis may have first been suggested by the appearance of depressive symptoms in some patients with either hyperthyroidism or hypothyroidism. Administration of TRH to depressed patients was suggested by studies reporting that either TSH or thyrotropin enhanced both the speed of onset and the efficacy of imipramine in the treatment of women with primary depression. TRH was also shown to potentiate the activity of pargyline and L-DOPA in animals, a property it shares with some drugs which have antidepressant activity (36).

Despite some initial optimism, TRH is probably not a clinically useful antidepressant. However, trials of this substance in depression revealed a subgroup of depressed patients who had normal thyroid function and a blunted thyrotropin response to TRH challenge. The mechanism for the blunted thyrotropin response to TRH is not clear. Circulating levels of glucocorticoids have been found to alter the pituitary thyrotropin response to TRH. Thus, it is possible that depressed patients with altered pituitary-adrenal activity may overlap with the subgroup of patients with blunted thyrotropin responses (36).

PITUITARY GROWTH HORMONE IN DEPRESSION

A blunted pituitary growth hormone response to hypoglycemia has been reported for a significant percentage of postmenopausal women with depression. There is evidence that pituitary growth hormone activity is regulated or modulated by central noradrenergic and dopaminergic mechanisms, although serotonergic systems may also play a regulatory role. Future investigation may reveal that the proposed subgroup of depressed patients with altered pituitary growth hormone activity overlaps with those who demonstrate abnormalities in one or another neurotransmitter activities (37).

CONCLUSION

A striking feature of the pharmacological and biochemical data relating to the biogenic amine hypothesis is their inconsistency. Certainly the biogenic amine hypothesis cannot be accepted as established fact; and yet the large number of observations which support the hypothesis cannot be easily dismissed. It seems appropriate, therefore, to discuss some explanations for the inconsistent results. As discussed throughout the chapter, the multiple action of available pharmacological agents and the wide individual variability of specific metabolic measurements unquestionably contribute to the problem. More general explanations include the variability of study conditions, the lack of specificity and sensitivity of biological assays, the failure to distinguish between the acute and long-term actions of pharmacological agents, and the heterogeneity of patients with mania and depression.

Future studies of metabolic processes in patients with affective disorders can be improved by more careful control of clinical experimental conditions. In studies of hospitalized patients, important parameters include diagnostic criteria, diet, activity, medication, and longitudinal measurements of the severity of illness. The assays of physiological metabolites can be improved by the use of new techniques, such as gas liquid chromatographic/mass spectrometric, radioenzymatic, and radioimmunologic assays. Further, studies on the chronic effects of the medications used to treat affective disorders are important, because of their slow onset of clinical action. These studies must consider effects of pharmacological agents on neurotransmitter synthesis, storage, release, and inactivation. Particularly important will be investigations of receptor interaction processes through time.

While control of experimental conditions and improvement of experimental techniques is essential, successful categorization of the heterogeneous population of patients with affective disorders is also important. Depressive illness can be divided into subtypes using several different criteria. Clinical, pharmacological, and biochemical distinctions have been made among patients who previously were given the same diagnosis. One important distinction is between unipolar depressed patients, without a history of mania, and bipolar patients, with a history of at least one manic episode. This division is interesting because it separates depressed patients into clinically distinct groups which may have different genetic, biochemical, and pharmacological characteristics (Chapter 11). As described in this chapter, other biochemically distinguishable subgroups of depressed patients may also exist.

Additional studies may lead to modifications of the biogenic amine hypothesis for several reasons. Other neuroregulators may be involved in affective disease. Tissue content of octopamine, tryptamine, phenylethylamine, and other amines are increased by MAO inhibitors and, conceivably, could explain the antidepressant effects of these medications. Aldehyde metabolites of biogenic amines may also have pharmacological effects, and their alteration by antidepressant medications might have a role in antidepressant drug activity.

Mania and depression might reflect an altered balance between two or more neurotransmitters, rather than a change in activity of a single system. Thus, depression might result from cholinergic predominance over some other neurotransmitter, while mania could result from a reversed pattern. Such an imbalance hypothesis is supported by the transient reversal of manic symptoms by physostigmine, which increases central cholinergic activity by inhibiting the enzyme that metabolites acetylcholine (38). Partial reversal of this physostigmine-induced improvement in mania by methylphenidate, which increases central catecholamine activity, further supports the hypothesis of an imbalance between acetylcholine and catecholamines in mania (38). In addition, tricyclics are anticholinergics, suggesting that inhibition of central cholinergic activity could also be important for their antidepressant effects (21).

Further information about the relationships between behavioral and biochemical processes will be important in studies of depression. Ultimately, we will need to understand the relationship between processes such as loss and subsequent depression. For example, why do some grief reactions resolve, while others lead to depression? Some depressions may reflect inner-directed aggression. We now know that aggression and different patterns of coping markedly alter central transmitter mechanisms (Chapter 15). Some depressions may result from biochemical or genetic defects, with little influence from environmental or other processes; other forms may reflect an interaction between biochemical and behavioral processes, in which behavior alters biochemistry and the resultant biochemical change influences behavior.

In conclusion, future studies on the role of neurotransmitters in depression and mania can be improved in several ways. Careful control of clinical experimental conditions, improved techniques for biological assay, and studies on the chronic effects of pharmacological agents on the dynamic, rather than static, aspects of neurotransmitter mechanisms will be important. Studies of behavioral neurochemistry interactions should provide valuable information. The search for clinical and biochemical subtypes of mania and depression is another promising direction of current research. Consideration of other metabolic factors in affective disorders and of possible imbalances between several neuroregulators should also prove fruitful. These studies should lead to a better understanding of pathophysiology of affective disorders and, possibly, to more effective treatments for patients suffering with depression or mania.

REFERENCES

1. Everett, G. M. and Tolman, J. E. P. Mode of action of Rauwolfia alkaloids and motor activity. *In: Biological Psychiatry*. J. Masserman, *ed.*, New York: Grune and Stratton, 1959, pp. 75–81.
2. Pletscher, A., Shore, P. A., and Brodie, B. B. Serotonin as a mediator of reserpine action in brain. *J. Pharmacol. Exp. Ther. 116*:84–89, 1956.
3. Berger, P. A. and Barchas, J. D. Monoamine oxidase inhibitors. *In: Psychotherapeutic Drugs*. E. Usdin and I. S. Forrest, *eds.*, New York: Marcel Dekker, 1977.
4. Katz, R. I., Chase, T. N., and Kopin, I. J. Evoked release of norepinephrine and serotonin from brain slices: inhibition by lithium. *Science 162*:466–467, 1968.
5. Schanberg, S. M., Schildkraut, J. J., and Kopin, I. J. The effects of psychoactive drugs on norepinephrine-^{3}H metabolism in brain. *Biochem. Pharmacol. 16*:393–399, 1967.
6. Mendels, J. and Frazer, A. Brain biogenic amine depletion and mood. *Arch. Gen. Psychiatry 30*:447–451, 1974.
7. Murphy, D. L., Brodie, H. K. H., Goodwin, F. K., and Bunney, W. E., Jr. Regular induction of hypomania by L-DOPA in "bipolar" manic-depressive patients. *Nature 229*:135–136, 1971.
8. Hendley, E. D. and Snyder, S. H. Relationship between the action of monoamine oxidase inhibitors on the noradrenaline uptake system and their antidepressant efficacy. *Nature 220*:1130–1131, 1968.
9. Gluckman, M. I. and Baum, T. The pharmacology of iprindole, a new antidepressant. *Psychopharmacologia 15*:169–185, 1969.
10. Carlsson, A., Jonason, J., and Lindqvist, M. On the mechanism of 5-hydroxytryptamine release by thymoleptics. *J. Pharm. Pharmacol. 21*:769–773, 1969.
11. Shopsin, B., Gershon, S., Goldstein, M., Friedman, E., and Wilk, S. Use of synthesis inhibitors in defining a role for biogenic amines during imipramine treatment in depressed patients. *Psychopharmacol. Comm. 1*:239–249, 1975.
12. Matussek, N., Benkert, O., Schneider, K., Otten, H., and Pohlmeier, H. Wirkung eines Decarboxylasehemmers (Ro-4-4602) in Kombination mit L-dopa auf gehemmute Depressionen. *Arzneim.-Forsch. 20*:934–937, 1970.
13. Goodwin, F. K., Murphy, D. L., Brodie, H. K. H., and Bunney, W. E., Jr. L-dopa, catecholamines, and behavior: a clinical and biochemical study in depressed patients. *Biol. Psychiatry 2*:341–366, 1970.
14. Mendels, J., Stinnett, J. L., Burns, D., and Frazer, A. Amine precursors and depression. *Arch. Gen. Psychiatry 32*:22–30, 1975.
15. Dunner, D. L. and Fieve, R. R. Affective disorder: studies with amine precursors. *Am. J. Psychiatry 132*:180–182, 1975.
16. Brodie, H. K. H., Murphy, D. L., Goodwin, F. K., and Bunney, W. E., Jr. Catecholamines and mania: the effect of alpha-methyl-para-tyrosine on manic behavior and catecholamine metabolism. *Clin. Pharmacol. Ther. 12*:218–224, 1971.
17. Sack, R. L. and Goodwin, F. K. Inhibition of dopamine-β-hydroxylase in manic patients. *Arch. Gen. Psychiatry 31*:649–654, 1974.

172 | Berger, Barchas

18. Van Praag, H. M., Korf, J., and Schut, D. Cerebral monoamines and depression: an investigation with the probenecid technique. *Arch. Gen. Psychiatry* 28:827–831, 1973.
19. Zarcone, V., Berger, P. A., Brodie, H. K. H., Sack, R., and Barchas, J. The indoleamine hypothesis of depression: a pilot study and overview. *Dis. Nerv. Sys.*, in press.
20. Goodwin, F. K. and Murphy, D. L. Biological factors in affective disorders and schizophrenia. *In: Psychopharmacological Agents.* M. Gordon, *ed.*, New York: Academic, 1974, pp. 9–37.
21. Berger, P. A. Neurotransmitters and affective disorders. *In: Neurotransmitter Function: Basic and Clinical Aspects.* W. Fields, *ed.*, New York: Stratton Intercontinental, 1977, pp. 305–336.
22. Kune, F. J. Treatment of mania with cinanserin, an antiserotonin agent. *Am. J. Psychiatry* 126:1020–1023, 1970.
23. Schildkraut, J. J. Biogenic amines and affective disorders. *Ann. Rev. Med.* 25:333–348, 1974.
24. Shopsin, B., Wilk, S., Suthananthan, G., Gershon, S., and Davis, K. Catecholamines and affective disorders revised: a critical assessment. *J. Nerv. Ment. Dis.* 158:369–383, 1974.
25. Maas, J. W. Biogenic amines and depression: biochemical and pharmacological separation of two types of depression. *Arch. Gen. Psychiatry* 32:1357–1361, 1975.
26. Beckmann, H. and Goodwin, F. K. Antidepressant response to tricyclics and urinary MHPG in unipolar patients: clinical response to imipramine or amitriptyline. *Arch. Gen. Psychiatry* 32:17–21, 1975.
27. Shopsin, B., Freedman, L. S., Goldstein, M., and Gershon, S. Serum dopamine-β-hydroxylase (DBH) activity and affective states. *Psychopharmacologia* 27:11–16, 1972.
28. Dunner, D. L., Cohn, C. K., Gershon, E. S., and Goodwin, F. K. Differential catechol-O-methyltransferase activity in unipolar and bipolar affective illness. *Arch. Gen. Psychiatry* 25:348–353, 1971.
29. Gershon, E. S. and Jonas, W. Z. Erythrocyte soluble catechol-O-methyltransferase activity in primary affective disorder: a clinical and genetic study. *Arch. Gen. Psychiatry* 32:1351–1356, 1975.
30. Greengard, P., McAlfee, D. A., and Kebabian, J. W. On the mechanism of action of cyclic AMP and its role in synaptic transmission. *Adv. Cyc. Nucleotide Res.* 1:337–355, 1972.
31. Robison, G. A., Coppen, A. J., and Whybrow, P. C. Cyclic AMP in affective disorders. *Lancet* 2:1028–1029, 1970.
32. Murphy, D. L., Donnelly, C., and Moskowitz, J. Catecholamine receptor function in depressed patients. *Am. J. Psychiatry* 131:1389–1391, 1974.
33. Sachar, E. J., Hellman, L., Roffwarg, H. P., Halpern, F. S., Fukushima, D., and Gallagher, T. F. Disrupted 24-hour patterns of cortisol secretion in psychotic depression. *Arch. Gen. Psychiatry* 28:19–24, 1973.
34. Carroll, B. J. Control of plasma cortisol levels in depression: studies with the dexamethasone suppression test. *In: Depressive Illness: Some Research Studies.* B. Davies, B. J. Carroll, and R. M. Mowbray, *eds.*, Springfield: Thomas, 1972, pp. 87–148.

35. Berger, P. A., Barchas, J. D., and Vernikos-Danellis, J. Serotonin and the pituitary adrenal system. *Nature 248:*424–426, 1974.
36. Hollister, L. E., Davis, K. L., and Berger, P. A. Thyrotropin releasing hormone and psychiatric disorders. *In: Neuroregulators and Psychiatric Disorders.* E. Usdin, D. A. Hamburg, and J. D. Barchas, *eds.*, New York: Oxford University Press, 1977, pp. 250–257.
37. Gruen, P. H., Sachar, E. J., Altman, N., and Sassin, J. Growth hormone responses to hypoglycemia in post-menopausal depressed women. *Arch. Gen. Psychiatry 32:*31–33, 1975.
38. Janowsky, D. S., El-Yousef, M. K., Davis, J. M., and Sederke, H. J. Antagonistic effects of physostigmine and methylphenidate in man. *Am. J. Psychiatry 130:*1370–1376, 1970.

11 | Antidepressant Medications and the Treatment of Depression

PHILIP A. BERGER

INTRODUCTION

The term depression is used to describe a normal mood, a medical symptom, and a collection of psychiatric syndromes. As a normal mood, depression is a common human reaction to a significant loss. As a medical term, it is also used to describe the sadness seen in patients who have other severe medical and psychiatric disorders. For the purposes of this chapter, however, depression refers to a group of psychiatric syndromes or illnesses with well-defined symptoms, only one of which is sadness.

Depression syndromes are probably universal. There are accounts of depressive illness throughout history from almost every human society. The universality of depressive illness is also reflected in the frequency of depression as a theme of the world's great literature. Pharmacological attempts to relieve depression also have a long history. The use of cocaine in South America, of opium in Europe and Asia, and of alcohol in most cultures may often reflect an attempt at self-medication for depression. These pharmacological agents probably do offer some temporary relief. However, it was the development of monoamine oxidase (MAO) inhibitors and tricyclic antidepressants (tricyclics) in the 1950's which first provided truly effective antidepressants for medical use.

This chapter is divided into five sections. The first gives a brief history of the antidepressants. The second reviews the pharmacology of two major classes of antidepressant medications, the tricyclics and the MAO inhibitors. The third details the diagnosis and classification of depression for pharmacological treatment, followed by a discussion of the practical aspects of drug treatment of depressed patients. The

174

final section describes some experimental treatments for depressive illness.

HISTORY

In 1889, Thiele and Holzinger synthesized iminodibenzyl and described its chemical character. However, it was not until 1948 that Häfliger synthesized derivatives of iminodibenzyl for pharmacological use. One of these derivatives was imipramine. The story continued in Switzerland, in 1950, when Domenjoz of the Geigy Company approached Kuhn with an "antihistamine" for clinical testing as an hypnotic. The results were essentially negative. About four years later, however, after chlorpromazine's antipsychotic effects were reported (Chapter 9), Kuhn decided to test the Geigy antihistamine further. The compound had the triple ring of imipramine but a different sidechain. It had no antidepressant activity. The next substance they tested was imipramine itself, which has the same sidechain as chlorpromazine. After a careful study of three hundred patients, Kuhn reported upon the antidepressant activity of imipramine at the 2nd International Congress of Psychiatry in Zurich in September 1957, before an audience of about twelve people. Since that time, imipramine and other tricyclics have become the most important pharmacological treatment for depressed patients (1, 2).

The antidepressant activity of the MAO inhibitors was discovered during this same time period. The development of MAO inhibitor antidepressants follows the common pattern of a medication synthesized for one disease and then found to be useful for another pathological condition. The first antidepressant MAO inhibitor, iproniazid, was synthesized by Fox at Roche Laboratories for the treatment of tuberculosis. Investigators soon noted that some patients on iproniazid developed euphoria and overactive behavior. At about the same time, Zeller, who had been studying MAO for some time, found that iproniazid inhibited the activity of this enzyme. Trials of iproniazid in depression quickly followed. In 1957, on the basis of independent studies, Kline and Crane reported that this medication was a useful treatment for some depressed patients. At first, it was debated whether the antidepressant activity of iproniazid was related to its ability to inhibit MAO or to the hydrazine moiety in its molecular structure. The development of nonhydrazine MAO inhibitors which also had antidepressant activity put an end to this debate (2).

The MAO inhibitors taught psychopharmacologists an important lesson about the importance of clinical observation for understanding drug side effects. This lesson is contained in the "tyramine-cheese" story, which began with Blackwell's review in *Lancet* of six cases of subarachnoid hemorrhage in patients on MAO inhibitors. Rowe, a hospital pharmacist, saw this review and wrote a letter to Blackwell describing a hypertensive episode in his wife, who was on an MAO inhibitor. The episode occurred after she ate some cheese, and Rowe wondered if the hypertension could be due to an amino acid in the cheese. Blackwell and his fellow residents at the Maudsely had a hearty laugh. But a drug salesman then told Blackwell that his company had received two other letters reporting the same phenomenon. Soon after, Blackwell reviewed the dietary history of a man who died while on an MAO inhibitor and of a woman who had a hypertensive crisis while on one. Both patients had eaten cheese. Blackwell then tried a cheese challenge in a patient on MAO inhibitors and produced hypertension. Shortly after, Milne reported that the intake of certain cheeses led to the appearance of tyramine in the blood. Blackwell then did some animal studies to confirm that the hypertensive reaction seen in MAO-inhibited patients who eat cheese is due to excess tyramine in the blood (2).

PHARMACOLOGY OF ANTIDEPRESSANTS

TRICYCLIC ANTIDEPRESSANTS

Structure-Activity Relationships

The tricyclics resulted from a modification of the phenothiazine nucleus. Imipramine is identical to promazine, except that the sulfur between the two aromatic rings has been replaced by an ethylene bridge (Fig. 11-1). This modification changes the structure from planar tricyclic rings to a skewed, three-dimensional, iminodibenzyl ring system. Amitriptyline differs from imipramine in that its ring nitrogen has been replaced by a carbon atom. The removal of methyl groups on the terminal nitrogen of imipramine yields desipramine, while elimination of the same N-methyl group from amitriptyline yields nortriptyline. Both desipramine and nortriptyline are secondary amines. Protriptyline is a secondary amine tricyclic differing from nortriptyline only by the position of a double bond (3) (Fig. 11-1).

Metabolism

The tricyclics are rapidly absorbed after parenteral or oral administration, and relatively high concentrations are found in the brain and

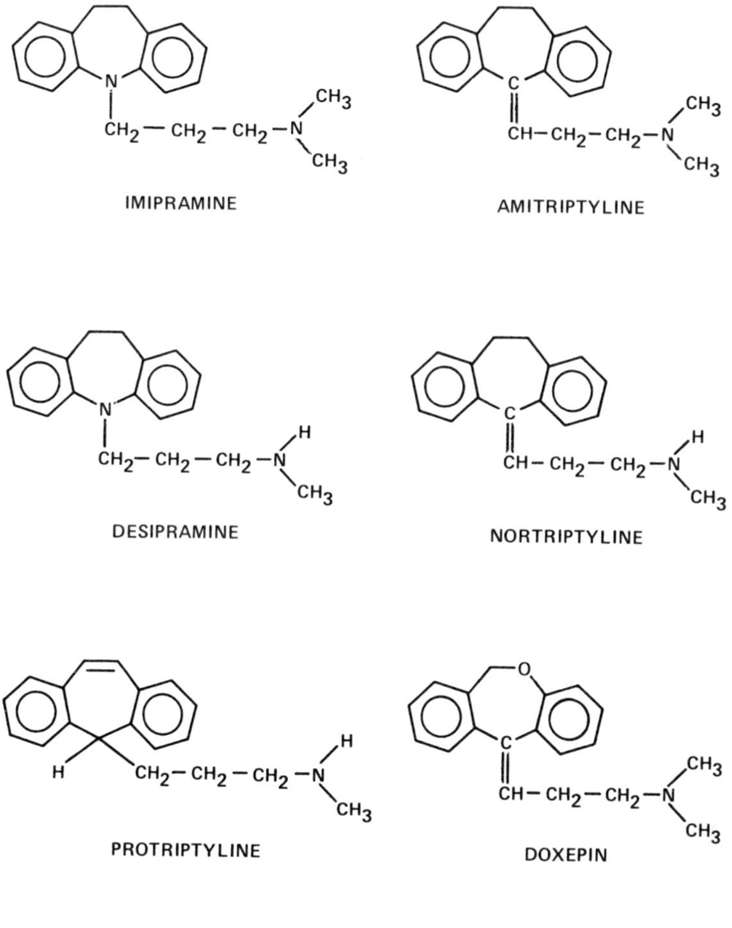

FIGURE 11-1. Structures for Common Tricyclic Antidepressants

several other organs. The most important metabolic routes for the tricyclics include oxidative demethylation, N-oxidation of the sidechain, hydroxylation, and conjugation, mainly with glucuronic acid. Some of these metabolites are also active. For example, amitriptyline is N-demethylated to form nortriptyline. Most of the metabolites are excreted in the urine, with about 33 percent eliminated through the intestinal route (4).

Several compounds seem to affect the metabolism of the tricyclics. Chlorpromazine (Thorazine) and methylphenidate (Ritalin) elevate plasma levels of imipramine and desipramine. Aspirin and haloperidol (Haldol) appear to increase plasma concentrations of nortriptyline, while oral contraceptives reduce nortriptyline levels in patients receiving its N-methylated analogue, amitriptyline (5).

Biological Effects

The tricyclics have both peripheral and central effects. In addition to their anticholinergic activity, the tricyclics also cause important alterations in central catecholaminergic and serotonergic activity and metabolism. In animal studies, the tricyclics have been shown to antagonize some of the actions of reserpine and to potentiate the effects of amphetamine-like compounds and of neurotransmitter precursors such as 5-hydroxytryptophan and L-DOPA.

Currently, inhibition of synaptic reuptake mechanisms for catechol- and indoleamines (biogenic amines) is considered to be important in the antidepressant activity of the tricyclics (Chapters 2 and 3). This inhibition presumably increases the neurotransmitter concentration at the receptor and thus enhances the activity of the neuronal circuit. In support of this hypothesis, many studies show that the tricyclics inhibit the uptake of norepinephrine into tissues which are innervated by noradrenergic sympathetic nerves. The tricyclics also decrease the uptake of intraventricularly administered norepinephrine by the rat brain. Similar results have been obtained for reuptake of 5-hydroxytryptamine. Also consistent with the prevention of amine reuptake, the tricyclics increase extraneuronal metabolism of norepinephrine and decrease its intraneuronal metabolism (Chapter 10).

Two important structure-activity relationships have emerged from biochemical and clinical studies of the tricyclics. Biochemically, the tertiary amine tricyclics such as chlorimipramine and amitriptyline generally are more potent inhibitors of 5-hydroxytryptamine reuptake, while secondary amines such as desipramine and nortriptyline are more potent in blocking norepinephrine uptake. Clinically, the tertiary amine tricyclics tend to be more sedating, while the secondary amines have a greater tendency toward stimulating activity (3,6).

Despite the variety of findings supporting the hypothesis that reuptake inhibition is important for the antidepressive action of tricyclics, there are two medications whose clinical actions do not fit with this theory. As described in Chapter 10, iprindole is structurally related to imipramine but does not appear to block biogenic amine reuptake; however, iprindole has been shown to be an effective antidepressant in several clinical trials. On the other hand, cocaine, like the tricyclics, is a potent blocker of biogenic amine reuptake but is probably not an effective antidepressant.

The latency of antidepressant activity of the tricyclics is also difficult to explain. The blockade of biogenic amine reuptake is rapidly evident in laboratory test systems. And yet, it usually takes from four days to three weeks for the antidepressant effects of these medications to develop. Thus, future studies with the tricyclics must consider chronic effects on *in vivo* biogenic amine metabolism.

It is possible that other aspects of the pharmacological activity of the tricyclics play a role in their antidepressant effects. They are all potent anticholinergic agents. Some investigators have suggested that this anticholinergic effect may correlate with antidepressant activity. There is also some evidence that an increase in cholinergic activity can induce depression in some bipolar patients (Chapter 10). However, anticholinergic agents such as atropine or antiparkinsonian drugs have not been shown to be useful antidepressants (7).

MAO INHIBITORS

Structure-Activity Relationships

Any drug which interferes with the function of the enzyme monoamine oxidase (MAO) is an MAO inhibitor, regardless of its other pharmacological properties. Not surprisingly, therefore, the MAO inhibitors are a rather heterogeneous group of compounds. It is convenient to distinguish between those substances which inhibit MAO more readily or exclusively *in vitro* from those which are also active or only active *in vivo*. Substances which are only effective *in vitro* require relatively high concentrations to produce inhibition. These substances include d-amphetamine, cocaine, ephedrine, procaine, and diphenhydramine (8). None of these agents has been used clinically as an MAO inhibitor, and it is not now generally believed that the pharmacological activity of cocaine or amphetamine (Chapter 21) is significantly related to its ability to inhibit MAO.

The potent *in vivo* MAO inhibitors are also a diverse group of compounds including hydrazines, cyclopropylamines, propargylamines, aminopyrazines, substituted indolealkylamines, and β-carbolines. Many of these compounds also strongly inhibit MAO *in vitro*. However, the hydrazines, propargylamines and cyclopropylamines require prior incubation with tissue extract, presumably to allow transformation to active metabolites. The MAO inhibitors can also be subdivided into short-acting, or reversible, inhibitors and long-lasting, or mainly irreversible, inhibitors. The substituted indolealkylamines and β-carbolines can be classified as short-acting MAO inhibitors; long-acting MAO inhibitors include the hydrazine derivatives, propargylamines, cyclopropylamines and aminopyrazines (8).

The MAO inhibitors used clinically include the hydrazine derivatives phenelzine and isocarboxazid (Fig. 11-2). The nonhydrazine derivatives used clinically include the cyclopropylamine tranylcypromine, which results from a cyclization of the isopropyl sidechain of amphetamine, and the propargylamine pargyline, which is used for hypertension rather than depression. The structure-activity relationships of the hydrazine and nonhydrazine MAO inhibitors have been reviewed in detail (9,10).

Recently, several groups of investigators have reported that MAO may exist in two forms, with different substrate and inhibitor specificities (Chapters 2 and 3). The MAO inhibitor clorgyline preferentially inhibits Type A MAO, while the MAO inhibitor deprenyl is more potent against Type B (Fig. 11-2). Since the proportion of MAO Types A and B varies with tissue, it is conceivable that such drugs could lead to the development of better MAO inhibitor antidepressants. Ideally, such substances would retard the breakdown of a specific amine in a given brain region, where it is deficient in a particular disorder; at the same time, it would allow metabolism of other amines whose accumulation might be responsible for a toxic side effect in another tissue (11).

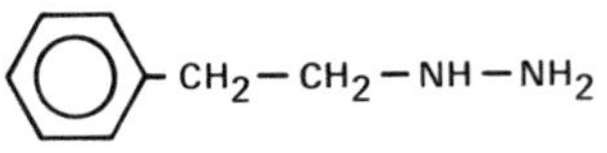

PHENELZINE

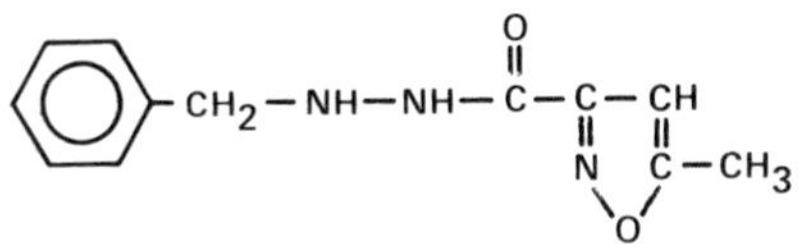

ISOCARBOXAZID

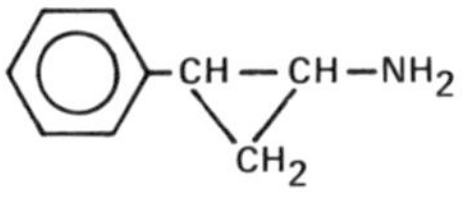

TRANYLCYPROMINE

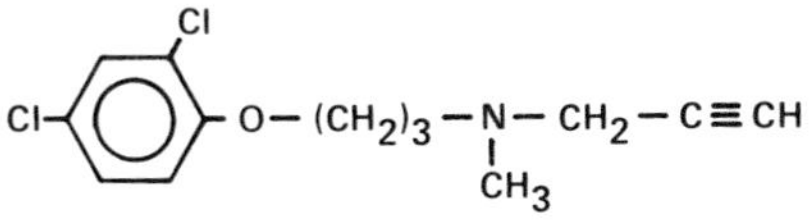

CLORGYLINE

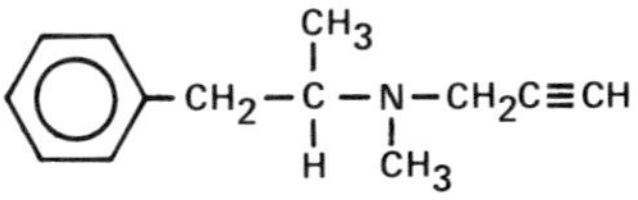

DEPRENYL

FIGURE 11-2. Structures for Important MAO Inhibitors

Biological Effects

The MAO inhibitors have both peripheral and central actions, at least some of which are probably caused by MAO inhibition. They increase the concentration of endogenous amines such as norepinephrine and 5-hydroxytryptamine and of exogenous monoamines such as tyramine. They also enhance the biological or pharmacological actions of these substances. Increases in brain amines do not show a smooth, dose-response relationship for MAO inhibitors: MAO must be almost completely inhibited before brain amine content rises. MAO inhibitors also inhibit enzymes other than MAO, including L-aromatic amino acid decarboxylase and oxidases of diamine, methylamine, and choline (11,12).

The metabolic degradation of barbiturates, aminopyrine, acetanalid, cocaine, and meperidine is altered by some MAO inhibitors. Thus, MAO inhibitors may prolong the effects of these other drugs. Other drug interactions are also important. For example, MAO inhibitors potentiate the action of amphetamine-like compounds, sympathomimetic amines used in the treatment of allergies, and anticholinergic agents used in the treatment of parkinsonism. On the other hand, MAO inhibitors antagonize some of the pharmacological and biochemical effects of reserpine (13).

Peripherally, some MAO inhibitors cause hypotension and some relief from angina pectoris. The fact that not all MAO inhibitors cause hypotension suggests that enzyme inhibition may not be the mechanism. Other hypotheses about this effect have been made. Hypotension may reflect sympathetic ganglionic blockade produced either by the accumulation of false transmitters, such as octopamine, or by feedback inhibition of tyrosine hydroxylase activity (Chapter 2). Similar mechanisms may produce the symptomatic relief of angina pectoris (14).

Centrally, MAO inhibitors cause stimulation in animals and have an antidepressant effect in man. The mechanism of action of the MAO inhibitors in human depression is not known. However, there is reason to speculate that it is related to MAO inhibition, since many of the chemically heterogeneous groups of substances called MAO inhibitors apparently have in common only their inhibitory action on MAO and their antidepressant activity. MAO inhibitors may act by decreasing the metabolism of norepinephrine, dopamine, or 5-hydroxytryptamine in the brain, making more catechol- or indoleamines available for release at the synapse. Indirect evidence supporting this mechanism of action comes from a study on terminally ill depressed patients treated with MAO inhibitors. At autopsy, brain biogenic amine levels in such patients were maximal at two weeks. This correlates with the time of onset of the antidepressant effect of MAO inhibitors (15). A recent study with the MAO inhibitor tranylcypromine suggests that 5-hydroxytryptamine may play a role in this compound's antidepressant action, since its antidepressant effect were reversed by the 5-hydroxytryptamine synthesis inhibitor p-chlorophenylalanine (PCPA) (16).

Other hypotheses for the antidepressant activity of MAO inhibitors have also been offered. Some investigators suggest that the inhibition of biogenic amine reuptake may be more important than enzyme inhibition (Chapter 10). Even if MAO inhibition is the mechanism of antidepressant action, it is possible that amines other than norepinephrine, dopamine, or 5-hydroxytryptamine are involved, since phenylethylamine, octopamine, and many other amines are also increased by MAO inhibitors (11).

Efficacy of Antidepressant Drugs

Antidepressant drugs improve the prognosis for patients with depression. However, this is not easy to demonstrate rigorously. Part of the difficulty arises from the high rate of "spontaneous remission" in depression. In the era before pharmacological or electroconvulsive therapies, studies reported an improvement rate of 44 percent recovery or social improvement of hospitalized depressed patients during the first year, with a 56 percent recovery rate after longer periods of treatment (17). This reported recovery rate may actually be low, because stricter criteria were used at that time, resulting in the hospitalization of only the most severely depressed patients. More recently, with the advent of controlled studies, the response of depressed patients to placebo has been estimated more precisely. Averages pooled from several studies suggest that about 16 percent of chronically depressed inpatients and outpatients improve on placebo, while 46 percent of acutely ill patients respond to placebo (18).

Because of this high remission rate on placebo, it is important that trials of an antidepressant include a placebo control group. In fact, the best studies also include a random-assignment, double-blind design (Chapters 31 and 32). Two recent review articles summarize the results of numerous controlled studies comparing antidepressant medications to placebos (19,20).

Tricyclic Antidepressants

In one recent literature review which summarized only random-assignment, double-blind studies, the tricyclics were found to be more effective than placebo in 61 of 93 treatment groups studied (19). While numerous studies have compared one tricyclic to another, none of the major ones has yet been shown to be consistently superior or inferior to any other.

Another aspect of the efficacy of the tricyclics concerns their use as a maintenance treatment for preventing a reoccurrence of depression. In two small studies, they were shown to significantly decrease the relapse rate of depressed patients who were initially treated with electroconvulsive therapy. Three large collaborative studies—two in the United States and one in England—have found that the tricyclics also significantly reduced the relapse rate in patients initially treated with a tricyclic (21).

MAO Inhibitors

Well-controlled studies of MAO inhibitors are not as plentiful. In three out of four studies tranylcypromine was superior to placebo. Phenelzine was superior to placebo in five out of nine, but isocarboxazid was superior in only one of eight. In comparisons of the tricyclics and MAO inhibitors, three studies found tranylcypromine to be equal to imipramine. Phenelzine was inferior to imipramine in five investigations but equal to imipramine in four (19).

Summary

The tricyclics are superior to placebo in about two-thirds of well-controlled studies. The MAO inhibitors are also superior to placebo in some studies; but, except for tranylcypromine, they are somewhat less effective than the tricyclics for treating a heterogeneous population of depressed patients. One interpretation of these results is that antidepressants are only effective for some depressed patients. This is consistent with the clinical observations of physicians. It is also consistent with the original reports of the efficacy of the tricyclics, which suggested that these medications were most useful in endogenous depressions. Furthermore, it emphasizes the need for an appreciation of the heterogeneity of depressive illness when considering pharmacological treatment.

THE DIAGNOSIS OF DEPRESSION FOR DRUG TREATMENT

Depressive illness can present with many symptoms, one of which is often sadness. However, sadness is neither a necessary nor a sufficient part of the syndrome. Other symptoms include pessimism; loss of interest in usual activities; feelings of low self-esteem, worthlessness or guilt; and the loss of the ability to feel pleasure. Some depressed patients may also be anxious or agitated, while others are retarded, with extremely slow thinking and activity. Somatic symptoms can also be part of the syndrome: sleep disturbance, decreased appetite and weight loss, gastrointestinal distress, constipation, backaches, and hypochondriasis are all seen in patients with depressive illness. Thought disturbances, which can include delusions and hallucinations, are present in some depressed patients. Of course, the most immediately dangerous symptom of depressive illness is suicidal ideation. Since not every patient has all of these symptoms, the clinical presentation of depressive illness is quite variable. Although depressive illness is recognized as a clinically heterogeneous syndrome, there is no universally accepted classification scheme for depressive subtypes. Recent attempts to classify depression have led to a revival of interest in earlier depression dichotomies and the development of new dichotomies, along with other classification schemes (Table 11-1) (22,23).

Dichotomies are based upon both origins and symptoms. The *neurotic-psychotic* division distinguishes depressed patients without psychotic symptoms from those with them. The psychosis usually presents as a profound alteration in the patient's relation to reality because of delusions or hallucinations or illogical thinking. The *reactive-endog-*

TABLE 11-1.
PROPOSED SUBTYPES IN DEPRESSION

Dichotomies
Neurotic-psychotic
Reactive-endogenous
Personal-vital
Agitated-retarded
Primary-secondary
Unipolar-bipolar

Three-Dimensional Subtypes
Hostile-anxious-retarded

Age Related
Involutional melancholia
Pseudosenile depression

Reactive Depressions
Grief reactions
Chronic characterological
Depression in hysterical personalities
Demoralization

Atypical Depressions

Masked Depressions

---

enous depressive dimension reflects the importance of precipitating events in the onset of depressive symptoms. Reactive depressions are responses to identifiable precipitating factors; endogenous depressions occur without obvious precipitants. The distinction between *vital* and *personal* depression is more commonly made in Europe. *Vital depressions* are characterized by somatic symptoms, while patients with *personal depressions* experience primarily sadness. Clearly, these three dichotomies can overlap. In common usage, the neurotic-psychotic, reactive-endogenous, and personal-vital dichotomies all reflect at least three dimensions of depression—severity, the importance of precipitating factors, and the importance of somatic symptoms in the presenting syndrome.

The distinction between *primary* and *secondary depression* is based on the presence or absence of other medical or psychiatric illness. *Secondary depressions* occur in patients with serious medical or psychiatric illnesses, while patients with *primary depressions* have no pre-existing psychiatric or other illnesses. The *bipolar* and *unipolar depression* dichotomy is increasingly emphasized. *Bipolar* patients have a history of at least one episode of mania or hypomania, while patients with *unipolar* depression may have previous episodes only of depression.

The *agitated-retarded* and *hostile, anxious,* or *retarded* classifications define aspects of the pattern of depressive symptomatology. *Agitated depressed* patients are anxious and often in constant but purposeless motion, while patients with *retarded depression* are slowed down in both thought and action. The division of depressed patients into *anxious, retarded,* and *hostile* is based on a factor analysis of the symptoms of depressed patients using the Brief Psychiatric Rating Scale (5). The distinction between *anxious* and *retarded* depressed patients clearly overlaps with the distinction between *agitated* and *retarded* patients. *Hostile depressed* patients, however, have anger or irritability as a dominant symptom. The term *atypical depression* is used for depressed patients who present with fatigue, somatic complaints, phobias, and anxiety. Patients with *masked depression* present with somatic, rather than psychological, symptoms of depression.

Age-related depressive diagnoses have also been suggested. Many clinicians have pointed to the distinction between depression in younger and older patients. *Involutional melancholia* is a depression diagnosis given to women in their late forties or fifties and to men in their fifties or sixties who develop an anxious or agitated endogenous depression. *Pseudosenile depression* refers to a syndrome in patients in their sixties and older who present with apathy and confusion and other symptoms of senility; unlike senile patients, these individuals respond to treatment. Since the presenting picture sometimes resembles true senility, this diagnosis is often retrospectively applied to patients who get well with antidepressant treatment.

Reactive depressions have been further subdivided. *Grief reactions* occur in response to a significant loss in normal individuals and pathological reactions to a loss in patients with preceding neurotic or character disorders. The patients with neurotic or character disorders include the hysterical personalities who have wide but transient mood swings from joyfulness to profound unhappiness, which respond to environmental conditions. These individuals belong to a larger group called *chronic characterological depressives,* whose depression is part of a life-long personality problem in which minor stresses may lead to depressive symptoms. *Demoralization* is another term given to a type of reactive depression. Patients with demoralization experience a change in self-image, such as feeling ineffective or incapable after a serious setback in life.

The term "reactive" has two different meanings when applied to depression. One meaning refers to depressions which are a "reaction" to a life stress, as opposed to endogenous depressions, which have no obvious precipitants. "Reactive" is also used to describe the capacity of some depressed patients to respond to the environment and to experience pleasure under certain circumstances, despite profound unhappiness. This second usage is contrasted to "autonomous" depressions, in which the patient's mood is independent of fluctuations in environment. This double use of "reactive" is not commonly noted, because both adjectives often apply to the same patient. Thus a patient with depression from a grief "reaction" may also be able to "react" to attempts to cheer him up.

THE DRUG TREATMENT OF DEPRESSION

Clearly, the terms used in the diagnosis and classification of depression define a complex group of overlapping syndromes. A detailed analysis and criticism of these classifications is beyond the scope of this chapter. Such analysis is also of questionable relevance to the pharmacological treatment of psychiatrically depressed patients. Nevertheless, the clinician should be familiar with these diagnostic classifications to promote consistent communications among fellow physicians. However, the priority for the clinician is to determine whether a specific patient should be treated with medication and, if so, which medication is most likely to be helpful.

APPROACH TO THE PATIENT

Fortunately, there are some generally accepted guidelines to help physicians make decisions about appropriate therapy for depressed patients. Rather than use the complicated diagnostic categories suggested above, the physician can often evaluate the patient by answering the questions in Table 11-2.

Is there a medical or pharmacological illness causing the depressive symptoms?

A careful medical work-up is an essential feature of treating any depressed patient. If depressive symptoms are caused by an underlying medical disease or are the result of a drug action, then treatment of this medical or pharmacological condition should be the first priority. Depressive symptoms can result from a variety of medical illnesses.

TABLE 11-2.
MAJOR QUESTIONS FOR EVALUATING A DEPRESSION

- Is there a medical or pharmacological illness causing the depressive symptoms?
- How severe is the depression?
- What is the pattern of depressive symptomatology?
    Is the patient suicidal?
    Are there symptoms of psychosis?
    Is the patient anxious, agitated, retarded, or hostile?
- Is there a history of a previous episode of depression or mania?
- Does the patient have a history of a previous positive or negative response to any trial of psychiatric medication?
- Are there important precipitating factors?

Any severe somatic disease can lead to a reactive depression, but certain diseases have been specifically associated with depression. Mononucleosis, hepatitis, and viral pneumonia sometimes cause depressive symptoms during the active or the recovery phase of the illness. Carcinoma of the pancreas has also been reported to cause depression, as have some epilepsies. Over- or underactivity of almost every endocrine organ may lead to depression. Both pituitary-adrenal hyperactivity (Cushing's Syndrome) and hypoactivity (Addison's disease) are often associated with depression. Hyperthyroidism can be accompanied by agitated or anxious depression, while hypothyroidism can be associated with retarded depression. Hyperparathyroidism can also result in depression and psychosis. Depression can occur following pregnancy, after the ovaries are removed, and during the premenstrual period. Patients with diabetes mellitus may appear to be depressed when blood sugar levels are poorly controlled.

Numerous pharmacological substances can also contribute to depressive symptoms. Antihypertensive medications, corticosteroids, contraceptive steroids, thyroid hormone, antianxiety medications, and sedative hypnotics have all been associated with depressive symptoms (Chapter 29). The abuse of amphetamines, cocaine, barbiturates, heroin, and alcohol also can lead to depression or may be associated with pre-existing depression; therefore, a careful drug history should be taken from every patient with depression. Some of these pharmacological agents and the syndromes they can produce are described in more detail in Chapters 23 and 24.

How severe is the depression?

Mild depression of short duration should probably not be treated with antidepressants. Mild depression with anxiety will often respond to treatment with an antianxiety agent (Chapter 13). More severe depressive syndromes should be treated with antidepressants. Severe depressive syndromes include: psychotic depression, endogenous depression, vital depression, involutional melancholia, and pseudosenile depression. Any depressive syndromes that significantly interfere with a patient's ability to function in interpersonal relationships or in employment should be treated with medication.

One method for evaluating and recording the initial severity of depression is to complete a depression rating scale after an interview with the patient or to have the patient complete a self-rating scale. The

Hamilton Scale for depression, the Zung or Bunney-Hamburg Rating Scales, the D scale of Minnesota Multiphasic Personality Inventory (MMPI), and numerous other scales can be used for this purpose (24–27). These scales also provide a convenient way of following a patient's illness after treatment is started. Using a weekly depression rating scale, a physician can follow overall improvement as well as changes in the symptom pattern of a depressed patient.

What is the pattern of depressive symptomatology?

When suicide risk is present, hospitalization and treatment with antidepressants are necessary. Other symptoms may help the physician to determine which antidepressant medication is most appropriate. If there are symptoms of psychosis, e.g., delusions, hallucinations, or formal thought disorder, the patient should probably be treated with an antipsychotic. If the patient is extremely anxious, hostile, irritable, or agitated, an antipsychotic-tricyclic combination may be helpful. The combination of perphenazine and amitriptyline is available in a single pill and, therefore, with a fixed dose ratio; however, this combination can also be obtained by prescribing both individual drugs, which allows for a flexible ratio. This drug combination has been used extensively with safety, but other combinations are also possible. Combinations of a tricyclic and thiorizadine should be avoided because of the possibility of additive, cardiac side effects.

The pattern of symptoms can also help the physician choose among the available tricyclics. While these drugs do not appear to differ markedly in clinical efficacy, they do differ in their ability to produce sedation. Doxepin and amitriptyline are the most sedative; imipramine falls somewhere in the middle; and nortriptyline, desipramine, and protriptyline are much less sedative.

Is there a history of previous episodes of depression or mania?

A patient with bipolar depression, i.e., depression with a history of one or more episodes of mania or hypomania, should be treated with lithium carbonate (Chapter 12). If the bipolar patient has a severe retarded depression or depression with psychosis, a tricyclic or antipsychotic can be used in addition to lithium carbonate during the acute phase of treatment. However, lithium carbonate should then be used in maintenance doses to prevent further episodes of illness.

Patients with a previous history of unipolar depression should be treated acutely with either a tricyclic or an antipsychotic, depending upon the initial presenting symptoms. If unipolar depression occurs in repeated, severe episodes, the tricyclics can be used in maintenance doses to decrease the risk of future episodes. Lithium carbonate has also been used as a maintenance treatment for recurrent unipolar depression. To date, neither approach has shown superiority in preventing recurrent episodes of unipolar depression. Antipsychotics should probably not be used as a maintenance treatment in depressed patients, since prolonged treatment can lead to tardive dyskinesia (Chapter 9).

Does the patient have a history of a previous positive or negative response to any trial of psychiatric medications?

The history of a past positive response to a particular antidepressant treatment suggests that this treatment should be tried again. A patient who had an adverse side effect or no response to a prior treatment will require a careful historical evaluation. A significant adverse reaction to one medication suggests the trial of a different antidepressant. A failure to respond to adequate doses of an antidepressant medication should also lead the physician to try a different pharmacological agent.

Are there important significant precipitating factors?

A patient with a history of a significant precipitating factor, such as the death of a relative, may present with a normal grief reaction which can have symptoms similar to some depressive syndromes. Most grief reactions are self-limited and do not require treatment with antidepressants. However, if a grief reaction is severe or prolonged or if it is out of proportion to the loss, then antidepressant treatment may be necessary.

Patients with chronic characterological depressions or demoralization after a life stress are probably less likely to respond to antidepressant medication. However, even in these patients, if the symptoms are severe or prolonged, antidepressant treatment with tricyclics should be tried, since these medications may be of benefit.

Use of Drug Categories

Drug treatment for depression may also be viewed in terms of major drug classes. Although the information is essentially identical to that given above, this second organization does help to emphasize the major indications for a particular drug.

Tricyclic Antidepressants

The tricyclics are the most important treatments for depressive syndromes. Endogenous, vital, unipolar, retarded, and pseudosenile depression should all be treated with tricyclics. They should also be used in severe or prolonged reactive depression or in pathological grief reactions. In addition, they can be used for the seriously depressed bipolar patient, while the lithium work-up and lithium blood levels are established.

Some anxious, hostile, agitated, or irritable depressed patients, often seen in involutional melancholia, respond to tricyclics; others respond better to antipsychotics. The flexible combination of amitriptyline and perphenazine can also be used in these patients. Tricyclics should also be used in maintenance therapy for patients with recurrent unipolar depression, at about half the dose that obtained initial antidepressant response.

There is little difference among the several tricyclics. However, as mentioned earlier, desipramine, nortriptyline and protriptyline have less sedative activity than other tricyclics. Imipramine is in the middle, and doxepin and amitriptyline cause the most sedation.

Antipsychotics

The antipsychotics are also useful agents for treating depression (cf. Chapter 9). They are most important in psychotic depression. In this case the term psychotic depression is not used as a synonym for severe depression but to denote depression with delusions, hallucinations, or thought disorders. Antipsychotics can also be used in severe agitated, hostile, or anxious depressions, in combination with a tricyclic. They should not be used in mild depression, should not be used as antianxiety agents, and should not be used in the maintenance treatments of depression, because of the danger of tardive dyskinesia.

Lithium Carbonate

Lithium is an increasingly important antidepressant and should be used in patients with bipolar illness, both as an acute treatment in combination with tricyclics and as a maintenance treatment alone (Chapter 12).

Antianxiety Agents
These can be used for mild depression with anxiety (Chapter 13).

MAO Inhibitors
This second major class of antidepressants should probably not be used as the first treatment for any patient with depression, with the important exception of a patient with a past history of a previous response to MAO inhibitors. However, when a patient has not responded to the tricyclics in adequate doses and adequate trials, then an MAO inhibitor can be used. Phenelzine and tranylcypromine are probably the most effective. British investigators have suggested that MAO inhibitors are the treatment of choice for atypical depressions.

PRACTICAL ASPECTS OF TREATMENT

TRICYCLIC ANTIDEPRESSANTS

Proper Dose and Maintenance
It is difficult to judge the proper dose of tricyclics, since the antidepressant effect takes about two weeks to appear in severe depression. Experimental approaches to determining proper doses are discussed in the last section of this chapter. Empirically, the dose should be increased gradually to near the maximal range or until the presence of unwanted side effects makes further increase in dose intolerable (Table 11-3). For imipramine, 25 mg twice daily plus 50 mg at bedtime is a suitable starting treatment. Dividing the dose lessens the impact of the anticholinergic and other side effects. The dose can then be increased by 25 mg every day or every other day, until a dose of about 150 mg is achieved. In severe depression, 200–300 mg may be necessary. In the elderly or underweight, 100–125 mg may be sufficient (Chapter 28). An adequate trial for a tricyclic is about four weeks of maximal dosage. If no response is seen, a second tricyclic should then be given a similar trial. If a tertiary amine tricyclic was used for the first trial, a secondary amine might then be tried. The second trial can be started immediately after the first. A second failure to respond suggests that either MAO inhibitors or electroconvulsive therapy (Chapter 33) should be considered.

TABLE 11-3.
ANTIDEPRESSANTS

NAMES		APPROXIMATE INPATIENT DOSE RANGE (MG/DAY)	APPROXIMATE OUTPATIENT OR MAINTENANCE RANGE (MG/DAY)
GENERIC	REPRESENTATIVE BRAND		
Tricyclics			
Imipramine	Tofranil	150–300	75–150
Desipramine	Norpramin Petrofrane	150–250	75–150
Amitriptyline	Elavil Endep	150–300	75–150
Nortriptyline	Aventyl	75–150	50–100
Protriptyline	Vivactyl	15–60	10–40
Doxepin	Sinequan	150–300	75–150
MAO Inhibitors			
Phenelzine	Nardil	15–75	15–30
Isocarboxazid	Marplan	10–50	10–30
Tranylcypromine	Parnate	20–40	20–30

Once a therapeutic dose is reached, the daytime dose can be gradually transferred to evening doses. It is possible to give a single bedtime dose, although this should be a mutual decision between patient and physician. For some, this is convenient; for others, it leads to too much morning confusion or sedation. Since tricyclics can produce fatal overdoses, a week's supply is probably the maximum amount a patient with depression should be given at one time (5).

When maintenance doses of a tricyclic are indicated because of recurrent episodes of depression, the patient should be continued for four to six weeks on full dosage. Following this period, approximately half of this dose can be used for maintenance. For example, 75–100 mg of imipramine or a comparable dose of another tricyclic is the usual daily maintenance dose (Table 11-3). For a patient who does not require maintenance tricyclics, full dose can also be reduced by 50 percent after four to six weeks. After an additional four to six weeks, they can be gradually withdrawn. Gradual withdrawal is used because mild withdrawal reactions, including nausea and vomiting, have been reported following abrupt withdrawal from imipramine. If depressive symptoms return on withdrawal, maintenance tricyclics can be used for an additional period of time, perhaps three months. Withdrawal can then be attempted again (20).

Toxicity and Side Effects

Overdose. The tricyclics can be dangerous drugs when ingested as an overdose—a fact that may not always be appreciated by non-psychiatrists. The tricyclics are particularly toxic to the heart. Consequently, the cardiac problems are typically the most difficult to manage. After an overdose, the patient is generally restless, agitated, and delirious. This may progress into coma. Anticholinergic signs may be prominent, and seizures may also occur. The first sign of cardiac toxicity is usually a prolongation of intraventricular conduction, followed by atrioventricular conduction abnormality and then a variety of other arrhythmias.

Central Nervous System Effects. Tricyclics can occasionally precipitate hypomania or mania in a patient with bipolar illness or psychosis in a patient with a history of schizophrenia. Toxic psychosis, probably related to central anticholinergic activity, is also seen, particularly in older patients. Some tricyclics, particularly amitriptyline and doxepin, may produce drowsiness or excessive sedation. On the other hand, insomnia, restlessness, and agitation are sometimes seen. The tricyclics do not produce the Parkinson-like symptoms of the antipsychotics, but a fine tremor can occur. Seizures have also occasionally been reported to occur in patients with a predisposition to epilepsy.

Peripheral Anticholinergic Effects. The anticholinergic activity of the tricyclics can cause dry mouth, pupillary dilitation, and blurred vision. It can also exacerbate narrow-angle glaucoma and cause urinary retention, constipation, decreased sexual performance and, rarely, paralytic ileus. Some of the cardiac toxicity described below is probably due, in part, to anticholinergic activity.

Cardiovascular Toxicity. The tricyclics can cause tachycardia and orthostatic hypotension. They also produce changes in cardiac electrical conduction. The electrocardiogram (ECG) sometimes shows prolonged QT intervals, depressed ST segments, and flattened T waves, which may precede the onset of ventricular tachyarrhythmias. Occasionally, an association of tricyclics with the sudden death of cardiac patients has been reported but will require further investigation.

Miscellaneous Side Effects. Occasionally, mild cholestatic jaundice has been reported with imipramine. Sometimes, allergic skin reactions are seen, although excessive sweating is more common. Fortunately, agranulocytosis is rare. A mild withdrawal syndrome, characterized by nausea and vomiting, can also occur.

Incompatibility Reactions. Patients on high doses of the tricyclics have been reported to have hypertensive reactions when they were also taking high doses of MAO inhibitors. Tricyclics also add to the effects of other anticholinergic drugs. In addition, tricyclics can prevent the antihypertensive action of guanethidine (4,5,20).

Management of Toxicity and Side Effects

Because the tricyclics are detoxified rather rapidly by the liver, the period of coma following severe toxicity is relatively short. However, since much of the drug is bound to plasma protein or to body tissues, forced diuresis and dialysis are of little value. Late fatalities following initial improvement have been observed. Severe anticholinergic effects can be treated by physostigmine in doses of from 1–3 mg, infused slowly intravenously, while the patient is on a cardiac monitor (Chapter 24). Physostigmine, rather than neostigmine, is preferable since it crosses the blood-brain barrier and may reverse some of the central anticholinergic effects.

When the tricyclics precipitate mania or schizophrenia or cause severe agitation or toxic psychosis, they should be withdrawn. The symptoms of toxic psychosis and agitation usually subside within a few days. Schizophrenia and manic psychosis may require treatment with antipsychotics (Chapters 9 and 12). Autonomic side effects rarely necessitate discontinuation of tricyclics. Dry mouth and blurred vision should be predicted. Constipation usually responds to a laxative. If anticholinergic side effects are severe, the cholinergic agonist, bethanechol, 25 mg two to three times a day has been recommended (28). If urinary retention is severe or paralytic ileus develops, the tricyclics should be discontinued.

Cardiac side effects can be a major problem. An ECG and careful cardiac history should be obtained in all patients. Patients with cardiac disease can be treated with tricyclics: the risk of suicide must be weighed against the possibility of adverse reactions. If a tricyclic is necessary for a patient with cardiac disease, the dosage should be started lower than normal and increased gradually, in consultation with a cardiologist.

MAO INHIBITORS

Proper Dose and Maintenance

Like the tricyclics, MAO inhibitors may take two to three weeks to produce antidepressant effects, making it difficult to determine the proper dose (Table 11-3). Methods to measure the extent of inhibition of the enzyme MAO might make it easier to ensure adequate dosage, but such techniques are only experimental and are not available to the clinician. As described earlier in this chapter, tranylcypromine and phenelzine have been reported to be the most effective MAO inhibitors. Tranylcypromine has some amphetamine-like stimulating activity. But since tranylcypromine can produce hypertension, phenelzine may be preferable. Phenelzine can be started at 15 mg, two times a day and gradually increased to 60 mg per day. For inpatients, this dose can be increased to a maximum of 75 mg per day, if no response is seen after two to three weeks on 60 mg. After two weeks at 75 mg per day, phenelzine should probably be discontinued if no response is seen. If a clinical response is achieved, the doses can be gradually consolidated into a single daily dose, because of the long duration of enzyme inhibition (5,11).

Toxicity and Side Effects

The MAO inhibitors are a heterogeneous group of substances. Therapy with MAO inhibitors can be associated with numerous side effects and adverse reactions, some of which are probably related to MAO inhibition.

Overdose. While the antidepressant effect of MAO inhibitors is slow to develop, acute toxic effects can be manifested within hours. Overdose can produce agitation, hallucinations, hyperpyrexia, hyperreflexia, blood-pressure changes, and convulsions. Treatment of hypotension with sympathomimetic amines or of agitation with barbiturates can further complicate this picture, because of drug interactions. Conservative management of temperature, blood pressure, and fluid and electrolyte balance has been successfully utilized in reported cases (13).

Central Nervous System Effects. MAO inhibitors have central side effects that can be viewed as extensions of their central stimulating properties. Insomnia, irritability, motor restlessness, and agitation are reported. MAO inhibitors have also been reported to convert a retarded depression into an agitated or anxious depression. The appearance of hypomania or the precipitation of psychosis in patients with a history of schizophrenia is also described.

Autonomic Side Effects. Autonomic side effects caused by MAO inhibitors are variable but include dry mouth, constipation, delayed bladder and bowel function, impotence, delayed ejaculation, dizziness, and orthostatic hypotension. Tranylcypromine, particularly, has been reported to occasionally cause a hypertensive syndrome.

Hepatic Toxicity. Toxic liver reactions were more common with iproniazid and pheniprazine than with current MAO inhibitors. The clinical syndrome produced is similar to viral hepatitis, with jaundice, diffuse hepatocellular damage, elevated serum liver enzymes, and bile stasis. Apparently, hepatic toxicity is not correlated with duration of therapy or dosage. The liver toxicity has not yet been related to MAO inhibition; thus, it remains possible that MAO inhibitors could be developed without such side effects.

Miscellaneous Side Effects. Blood dyscrasias have rarely been reported during treatment with MAO inhibitors. Cases of red-green color blindness, secondary to pheniprazine, have been described. Pathological skin reactions are rare, but maculopapular rashes do occur.

Incompatibility Reactions. The "tyramine-cheese" reaction is possibly the most important of the incompatibility reactions. Hypertensive crises and headaches were probably first described in patients being treated for tuberculosis. The hypertensive crisis usually begins with a severe headache of sudden onset, usually occipital in location. Vomiting, hyperpyrexia, chest pain, muscle twitching, and restlessness are also part of the syndrome. The attack usually disappears in a few hours, without sequelae; but it may cause intracranial bleeding, which can be fatal.

As described earlier, these hypertensive attacks are related to diet and drug interactions. Tyramine, a pressor amine usually oxidized by MAO, is probably a frequent cause; it occurs in many foods as a by-product of certain fermentation processes. Foods which are rich in phenylethylamine or L-DOPA may also interact with MAO inhibitors to produce hypertensive attacks. The syndrome has been reported to be produced by cheeses (e.g., Camembert, Gorgonzola, Cheddar, or Stilton), certain beers, Chianti wine, chicken livers, yeast products (e.g., Bovril, Marmite), pickled products such as herring, some chocolate, broad beans, pods, and canned figs. In other cases, the hypertensive syndrome has been initiated by amphetamines, methylphenidate, sympathomimetic amines such as ephedrine, methyldopa, and high doses of tricyclics. Patients should be told that some local anesthetics contain epinephrine and should be avoided. It has not yet been determined whether there is a predisposing factor in certain patients (11).

Management of Toxicity and Side Effects

The treatment of the side effects produced by MAO inhibitors depends on the type and severity of the reaction. The acute overdose may require gastric lavage and maintenance of cardiopulmonary function. The dangers of barbiturates for agitation and sympathomimetic amines for hypotension have been mentioned, but these treatments may be necessary in severe cases. Conservative management, with external cooling for fever and maintenance of fluid and electrolyte balance has been suggested (13).

Central stimulation, if severe, may require withdrawal of MAO inhibitors. Psychosis may necessitate the addition of phenothiazines. Autonomic side effects rarely lead to discontinuation of MAO inhibitors. In a majority of cases, excessive stimulation and autonomic reactions respond to a reduction in the dose of MAO inhibitors. Liver toxicity is more serious, however; MAO inhibitors should be withdrawn and replacement therapy begun at any indication of sustained abnormality of liver-function tests, because of the danger of irreversible changes (11).

The prevention of the hypertensive reaction is an extremely important part of the appropriate use of MAO inhibitors. Lists of dietary items and drugs that may lead to this reaction should be supplied to patients and family members. If a hypertensive crisis does develop, the MAO inhibitor should be withdrawn immediately. Conservative management for mild cases may be sufficient, but severe cases may require antihypertensive agents such as phentolamine (11).

EXPERIMENTAL APPROACHES TO TREATMENT

Predicative Laboratory Tests for Tricyclics

Ideally, a simple clinical laboratory test would determine which patients will respond to the tricyclics and which tricyclic is most appropriate for each patient. A second useful laboratory test, or possibly the same test done at intervals, would ensure an adequate but nontoxic drug level. Unfortunately, such tests do not exist. However, several investigators are following research directions that may lead to their development.

Metabolic Tests

The measurement of urinary 3-methoxy-4-hydroxyphenylglycol (MHPG) in depressed patients may prove to be a useful predictor of response to imipramine and amitriptyline. As described in Chapter 10, patients who excrete lower amounts of this catecholamine metabolite (Chapter 2) may respond better to imipramine than to amitriptyline, while depressed patients with higher MHPG excretion seem to show the reverse response pattern. Measurement of urinary MHPG is still a research procedure and not yet available to the practitioner. However, preliminary results are encouraging. If this finding is confirmed in more extensive investigations, it may eventually be useful to the clinician.

Other potentially useful metabolic tests are also suggested by basic research in depression (Chapter 10). Spinal fluid levels of 5-hydroxyindoleacetic acid (5-HIAA) may identify a subgroup of depressed patients. The dexamethasone suppression tests, the tyrotropin-stimulating hormone response to thyrotropin-releasing hormone (TRH), and growth hormone response to insulin may also distinguish patients with a particular response to antidepressants (29).

Metabolic tests may also prove helpful in achieving a therapeutic level of a tricyclic. The tricyclics alter the metabolic patterns of norepinephrine. In a preliminary study, this change correlated somewhat with clinical improvement (30). Techniques similar to this one may eventually prove clinically useful. Since the mechanism of action of the tricyclics is thought to involve inhibition of reuptake mechanisms for biogenic amines, it may be possible to develop a plasma or spinal fluid index of the reuptake blockade. Perhaps, the ability of a quantity of serum or cerebrospinal fluid to prevent synaptosomal uptake of radiolabeled norepinephrine or 5-hydroxytryptamine would correlate with clinical response.

Plasma Levels

A more straightforward approach to clinical monitoring of treatment is the measurement of plasma tricyclic levels. Unfortunately, the usefulness of this technique for the clinician remains a subject of controversy. Almost every possible relationship between plasma tricyclic levels and clinical response has been reported. One group of investigators found that nortriptyline concentrations below 50 ng per ml or above 150–175 ng per ml are associated with poor responses (31). Other investigators reported that increased plasma levels of amitriptyline were associated with increased therapeutic responses (32). In one study, no significant correlation was found between plasma concentrations of nortriptyline and therapeutic response (33).

The issue of plasma levels may be further complicated by protein binding. Tricyclics are tightly bound to protein, and it is possible that only the unbound portion is pharmacologically active. If the portion of the tricyclic which is protein-bound varies from patient to patient, this could account for the discrepancies in the attempts to correlate tricyclic plasma levels with clinical response (34). Thus, further research is necessary before the measurement of plasma levels of tricyclics can be recommended for routine clinical use.

INTRAVENOUS USE OF TRICYCLICS

Chlorimipramine is a tricyclic which is, as yet, unavailable for non-investigational use in the United States, although it is widely used in other countries. Chlorimipramine appears to be a potent reuptake inhibitor of 5-hydroxytryptamine. There are several preliminary reports which suggest that intravenously administered chlorimipramine can produce a rapid antidepressant effect, sometimes as early as the second day of treatment. The speed and efficacy of this treatment has been suggested to be comparable to that of electroconvulsive therapy (ECT) (35). If these preliminary reports can be confirmed, the rapid response to intravenous administration could greatly reduce morbidity and mortality for severely ill or suicidally depressed patients (3).

EXPERIMENTAL DRUG COMBINATIONS

Combined MAO Inhibitors and Tricyclics

An important treatment approach that merits further study is the combined use of MAO inhibitors and tricyclics. The question of this combination of treatments is the subject of two recent reviews (36,37). The combination is frequently used in Great Britain but less so in the United States. A series of reports suggesting morbidity and even mortality prompted the United States Food and Drug Administration and the manufacturers of antidepressants to warn against their concomitant use. Anecdotal reports of combined antidepressant therapy describe fever, blood-pressure changes, convulsions, and even death; however, a careful review of the twenty-six case reports revealed no clear evidence that the oral combination of MAO inhibitors and tricyclics in therapeutic doses, in absence of other drugs active on the brain, was responsible for the morbidity reported (36).

In a recent study, the records of 150 inpatients and 51 outpatients treated with tricyclics and MAO inhibitors were examined. The incidence and severity of side effects of the combination were reported to be essentially the same as control groups of the same size taking drugs from either class alone. Commonly used combinations were amitriptyline and phenelzine or imipramine and isocarboxazide (37).

The question of the safety of combined tricyclics and MAO inhibitors will require further research, as will the question of therapeutic advantage. There is some theoretical basis for increased effectiveness, since the MAO inhibitors and tricyclics could each increase the functional level of biogenic amines by different mechanisms. There have also been some positive reports by investigators of the use of this combination in refractory depressions. However, none of these reports was based on the controlled, double-blind protocol which is so important for such a study.

Tricyclics and Thyroid Medications

There have been several studies which report that adding small doses of triiodothyronine (T_3) accelerates and potentiates the antidepressant activity of tricyclics (38). The mechanism of this effect may involve sensitization or activation of catecholamine receptors or a change in tricyclic protein binding. Unfortunately, further studies with the combination of thyroid hormone and a tricyclic have only found beneficial effects in female but not in male patients. Other studies have been unable to demonstrate any value for this combination in either depressed men or depressed women (39). Studies with thyroid-stimulating hormone (TSH) and tricyclics are also encouraging but inconclusive. Thus, the combination of tricyclics and thyroid hormones should still be considered to be experimental. The possibility of additive, adverse cardiac effects may limit the usefulness of this combination, even if it is shown to be effective in some patients.

Tricyclics and Methylphenidate

Methylphenidate increases the plasma levels of tricyclics, presumably by blocking their metabolism. This combination has been reported to be useful in a small number of patients who were refractory to tricyclics alone. It is not clear, however, whether using higher doses of tricyclics would achieve the same results in most patients. Careful double-blind studies will be necessary before this use of methylphenidate can be routinely recommended.

The use of methylphenidate has also been proposed for the first few weeks of treatment with tricyclics. Since tricyclics take one to three weeks to produce clinical response, depressed patients often get discouraged. The immediate, but transient, mood-elevating effects of methylphenidate on some patients can be reassuring. However, further studies are also necessary before this use of methylphenidate and tricyclics can be shown to be safe and useful for a majority of patients. It is possible that the risk of hypertensive episodes outweighs any benefits from this practice.

Antidepressants and Biogenic Amine Precursors

The biogenic amine hypothesis of depression led to numerous trials of biogenic amine precursors in depressed patients (Chapter 10). L-DOPA was used in an attempt to increase central catecholamine levels, and tryptophan and 5-hydroxytryptophan (5-HTP) were administered in an attempt to increase brain serotonergic activity. Biogenic amine precursors have also been used in combination with tricyclics and MAO inhibitors. Studies with biogenic amine precursors in heterogeneous populations of depressed patients have produced inconsistent but somewhat disappointing results. L-DOPA does not seem to be an effective antidepressant and can precipitate psychosis in some patients. Tryptophan and 5-hydroxytryptophan are also ineffective for many depressed patients. However, in a subgroup of depressed patients with a defect in 5-hydroxytryptamine metabolism, tryptophan or 5-hydroxytrytophan may be useful alone or in combination with standard antidepressants. Careful double-blind studies with these 5-hydroxytryptamine precursors in patients who demonstrate decreased accumulation of 5-hydroxyindoleacetic acid in their spinal fluid would be interesting (29).

CONCLUSION

Depressive syndromes are common disorders. They can be severely disabling and, too often, may lead to suicide. Antidepressant medications, when used appropriately, improve the prognosis for some patients with depressive illness. These drugs are not ideal. They are slow acting, have side effects, can cause fatal overdoses, and do not help every patient. The ideal antidepressant treatment regimen would be different in several ways. A more immediate onset of drug action could decrease the risk of suicide and diminish the severe life disruptions that long illnesses can cause. Less toxic medications could also decrease their utilization for suicide attempts. Predictive laboratory tests could lead to more accurate matching of antidepressant medications and depressed patients. Laboratory methods would also make it easier to safely achieve adequate levels of antidepressant activity. Finally, and perhaps most important, a better understanding of the possible metabolic origins of some depressive syndromes could lead to the first rational development of antidepressants to correct these metabolic defects.

REFERENCES

1. Byck, R. Drugs and the treatment of psychiatric disorders. *In: The Pharmacological Basis of Therapeutics*, 5th ed. L. S. Goodman and A. Gilman, *eds.*, New York: Macmillan, 1975, pp. 152–200.
2. Ayd, F. J. and Blackwell, B., *eds.*, *Discoveries in Biological Psychiatry.* Philadelphia: Lippincott Co., 1970.
3. Biel, H. J. and Bopp, B. Antidepressant drugs. *In: Psychopharmacological Agents.* M. Gordon, *ed.*, New York: Academic Press, 1974, pp. 302–309.
4. Ban, T. A. Tricyclic antidepressants. *In: Psychopharmacology.* Thomas A. Ban, Baltimore: Williams and Wilkins Co., 1969, pp. 270–289.
5. Hollister, L. E. *Clinical Use of Psychotherapeutic Drugs.* Springfield: Thomas, 1973.
6. Carlsson, A., Corrodi, H., Fuxe, K., and Hökfelt, T. Effect of antidepressant drugs on the depletion of intraneuronal brain 5-hydroxytryptamine stores caused by 5-methyl-α-ethyl-*meta*-tyramine. *Eur. J. Pharmacol.* 5:357–366, 1969.
7. Davis, K. L., Hollister, L. E., Berger, P. A., and Barchas, J. D. Cholinergic imbalance hypotheses of psychosis and movement disorders: a strategy for evaluation. *Psychopharmacol. Comm.* 1:533–543, 1975.
8. Brücke, F. T., Hornykiewicz, O., and Sigg, E. B. Monoamine oxidase inhibitors. *In: The Pharmacology of Psychotherapeutic Drugs.* New York: Springer-Verlag, 1969, pp. 78–102.
9. Biel, J. H., Horita, A., and Drukker, A. E. Monoamine oxidase inhibitors (hydrazines). *In: Psychopharmacological Agents.* M. Gordon, *ed.*, New York: Academic Press, 1964, pp. 354–443.
10. Biel, J. H. Monoamine oxidase inhibitor antidepressants. Structure activity relationships. *In: Principles of Psychopharmacology.* W. G. Clark and J. delGuidice, *eds.*, New York: Academic Press, 1970, pp. 279–287.
11. Berger, P. A. and Barchas, J. D. Monoamine oxidase inhibitors. *In: Psychotherapeutic Drugs.* E. Usdin and I. Forrest, *eds.*, New York: Marcel Dekker, 1977.
12. Pletscher, A., Gey, K. F., and Zeller, P. Monoaminoxidase-Hemmer. *Arzneim-Forschung.* 2:417–590, 1960.
13. Jarvik, M. Drugs used in the treatment of psychiatric disorders. *In: The Pharmacological Basis of Therapeutics*, 5th ed. L. S. Goodman and H. Gilman, *eds.*, New York: Macmillan Co., 1970, pp. 151–203.
14. Nickerson, M. and Ruedy, J. Antihypertensive agents and the drug therapy of hypertension. *In: The Pharmacological Basis of Therapeutics*, 5th ed. L. S. Goodman and A. Gilman, *eds.*, New York: Macmillan Co., 1970, pp. 705–726.
15. Pare, C. M. B. Some clinical aspects of antidepressant drugs. *In: The Scientific Basis of Therapy in Psychiatry.* J. Marks and C. M. B. Pare, *eds.*, New York: Pergamon Press, 1965, pp. 103–113.
16. Shopsin, B., Friedman, E., and Gershon S. Parachlorophenylalanine reversal of tranylcypromine effects in depressed patients. *Arch. Gen. Psychiatry* 33:811–822, 1976.

17. Alexander, L. *Treatment of Mental Disorders.* Philadelphia: W. B. Saunders, 1953.
18. Klerman, G. L. Drug therapy of clinical depressions—current status and implications for research on the neuropharmacology of affective disorders. *J. Psychiatr. Res. 9*:253–270, 1972.
19. Morris, J. B. and Beck, A. T. The efficacy of antidepressant drugs: a review of research 1958 to 1972. *Arch. Gen. Psychiatry 30*:667–674, 1974.
20. Davis, J. M. Tricyclic antidepressants. *In: The Drug Treatment of Mental Disorders.* L. Simpson, *ed.*, New York: Raven Press, 1976, pp. 127–146.
21. Davis, J. M. Overview: maintenance therapy in psychiatry. II. Affective Disorders. *Am. J. Psychiatry 133*:1–13, 1976.
22. Feighner, J. P., Robins, E., Guze, S. B., Woodruff, R. A. J., Winokur, G., and Munoz, R. Diagnostic criteria for use in psychiatric research. *Arch. Gen. Psychiatry 26*:57–68, 1972.
23. Schildkraut, J. J. and Klein, D. F. The classification and treatment of depressive disorders. *In: Manual for Psychiatric Therapeutics.* Boston: Little, Brown, 1975, pp. 37–61.
24. Hamilton, M. A rating scale for depression. *J. Neurol. Neurosurg. Psychiatry 23*:56–62, 1960.
25. Zung, W. A self rating depression scale. *Arch. Gen. Psychiatry 12*: 63–70, 1965.
26. Bunney, W. E. and Hamburg, D. A. Methods for reliable longitudinal observation of behavior. *Arch. Gen. Psychiatry 9*:280–294, 1963.
27. Dahlstrom, W. G. and Welsh, G. S. *An MMPI Handbook.* Minneapolis: The University of Minnesota Press, 1960.
28. Everett, H. C. The use of bethanechol chloride with tricyclic antidepressants. *Am. J. Psychiatry 132*:1202–1204, 1975.
29. Berger, P. A. Neurotransmitters and affective disorders. *In: Neurotransmitter Function: Basic and Clinical Aspects.* W. Fields, *ed.*, New York: Stratton Intercontinental, 1977, pp. 305–336.
30. Rosenblatt, S. and Chanley, J. D. Measuring the pharmacological action of imipramine in the treatment of depression. *Arch. Gen. Psychiatry 30*:456–460, 1974.
31. Kragh-Sørensen, P., Asberg, M., and Eggert-Hansen, C. Plasmanortriptyline levels in endogenous depression. *Lancet 1*:113–115, 1973.
32. Braithwaite, R. A., Goulding, R., Theano, G., Bailey, J., and Coppen, A. Clinical significance of plasma levels of tricyclic antidepressant drugs in the treatment of depression. *Lancet 1*:556–558, 1973.
33. Burrows, G. D., Davies, B., and Scoggins, B. A. Plasma concentration of nortriptyline and clinical response in depressive illness. *Lancet 2*: 619–623, 1972.
34. Glassman, A., Hurwic, M., and Perel, J. M. Plasma binding of imipramine and clinical outcome. *Am. J. Psychiatry 130*:1367–1369, 1973.
35. Becker, A. L. A new adjunct to the treatment and management of depression: intravenous infusion of chlorimipramine (Anafranil). *S. Afr. Med. J. 45*:168–170, 1971.
36. Schuckit, M., Robins, E., and Feighner, J. Tricyclic antidepressants and monoamine oxidase inhibitors: combination therapy in the treatment of depression. *Arch. Gen. Psychiatry 24*:509–514, 1971.

37. Spiker, D. G. and Pugh, D. D. Combining tricyclic and monoamine oxidase inhibitor antidepressants. *Arch. Gen. Psychiatry* 33:828–830, 1976.
38. Wilson, I. C., Prange, A. J., Jr., and McClune, T. K. Thyroid hormone enhancement of imipramine in non-retarded depressions. *N. Engl. J. Med.* 282:1063–1067, 1970.
39. Feighner, J. P., King, L. J., Schuckit, M. A., Croughan, J., and Briscoe, W. Hormonal potentiation of imipramine and ECT in primary depression. *Am. J. Psychiatry* 128:1230–1238, 1972.

12 | Lithium and the Treatment of Mania

ROBERT L. SACK and EMANUEL De FRAITES

INTRODUCTION

Although lithium carbonate was not approved for general use in the United States until 1969, the discovery by John Cade, in 1949, that it is an effective antimanic agent marks the advent of modern psychopharmacology. This long delay from discovery to general, widespread use in the United States was the result of initial skepticism, followed by conservative federal drug policy and, possibly, lack of economic incentive.

Lithium is unique in several respects. It is highly specific in its alleviation of manic symptoms, normalizing the mood of manic patients rather than compensating for the excesses of the manic state through sedation or "tranquilization." In addition, it is the only drug in psychiatry for which clear prophylaxis against disease recurrences and deterioration has been demonstrated. Finally, it is a simple inorganic salt that has no known function in normal metabolism. Two recent monographs summarize the current state of knowledge about lithium treatment of psychotic disorders (1,2).

HISTORY

Lithium salts were used in 1859 in the treatment of gout, because lithium urate was shown to be the most soluble salt of uric acid. The medication was sold as "Lithia tablets," which were noted to cause "cardiac depression and even dilation and [to] upset the stomach." Lithia tablets soon fell into disuse. In the 1940's, lithium chloride was used as a salt substitute in cardiac cases. There were serious toxicity problems, and its use was abandoned in 1949.

The story of the revival of lithium is a strange one. John Cade, in Australia, thought that manic-depressive illness, like thyrotoxicosis and myxedema, might be caused by an excess of a normal body substance. Cade decided to look at the urine of manic patients in a rather primitive way—by injecting it into guinea pigs. It killed them. However, the urine of some manic patients seemed to kill guinea pigs at lower doses than did urine from normals. The toxic agent appeared to be urea, which causes death by convulsions. This explanation was complicated by the fact that manics had the same concentration of urea as controls, suggesting that another factor was involved. Cade next found that creatinine reduced the toxicity of urea and even protected against seizures produced by pentylenetetrazol. Again, there was no difference in creatinine between manics and controls. Thus Cade sought a third substance which might neutralize the protective effect creatinine had in manics and found that uric acid increased urea toxicity. Consequently, he pretreated the animals with the most soluble urate salt, lithium urate. Unexpectedly, the animals were somewhat sedated. Cade wisely used controls in the experiment by administering other lithium salts to distinguish whether this was an effect of the urate or the lithium. He found that lithium was the sedative agent. On the basis of these rather meager animal data, he administered the drug to himself, experiencing no untoward effects. He then gave it to manic patients in a dosage range very close to what is now considered to be optimal and found that ten out of ten patients responded positively.

These initial observations were extended in several uncontrolled studies in Australia. However, the major credit for verifying and elaborating the effects of lithium carbonate goes to the Danish investigators headed by Mogens Schou. Although lithium therapy had become commonplace in Europe by 1965, it was considered to be an experimental treatment in the United States until 1969, when it was released from investigational status (3).

PHARMACOLOGICAL PROPERTIES OF LITHIUM

ABSORPTION AND EXCRETION

Lithium is completely absorbed from the gastrointestinal tract. It accumulates in some organs; for example, the thyroid gland concentration is three to four times that of plasma. Lithium is somewhat irritating to the gastrointestinal tract and may cause transient nausea after ingestion. It is excreted almost entirely by the kidney, with a half-life of about twenty-four hours. Lithium excretion varies with the sodium intake. Consequently, the addition of salt to the diet increases the excretion, while patients on a low salt diet or diuretic retain lithium. Similarly, patients who perspire heavily in hot weather, with exercise, or with a high fever will lose sodium and retain lithium (4).

Biological Effects

Lithium is distributed ubiquitously and interacts with many biological systems. It has been shown to alter exchangeable and residual sodium, total body potassium, and urinary excretion of sodium and other electrolytes. It also alters hormones which regulate electrolyte balance, such as aldosterone. Since all of these effects can alter membrane excitability, they may account for lithium's antimanic effect (4). Generally, lithium decreases the amount of catecholamines at the receptor. For example, lithium enhances the reuptake of norepinephrine from the synaptic cleft, causes a decrease in norepinephrine release, and increases its intracellular turnover (4).

Lithium also alters serotonergic function. In rats, chronic administration of lithium seems to produce an initial increase in tryptophan uptake, followed by a reduction in the activity of tryptophan hydroxylase in the brain. The result is a rate of 5-hydroxytryptamine synthesis which is similar to control animals but with increased tryptophan uptake. In these animals, the usual decrease in 5-hydroxytryptamine synthesis produced by amphetamines is prevented, as is the usual amphetamine-induced increase in locomotor activity. This lithium-produced "stability" to amphetamine-induced changes in both 5-hydroxytryptamine synthesis and behavior has been proposed to relate to lithium's stabilizing action in the treatment of mania and depression (5). Clearly, this hypothesis remains speculative, but it indicates the importance both of chronic studies and of the consideration of the net effect of pharmacological actions on several biogenic processes simultaneously.

DIAGNOSIS OF MANIC-DEPRESSIVE ILLNESS

The treatment of the acute manic episode and the prophylaxis of manic-depressive illness constitute the only fully verified indications for lithium use. There is a continuing search to identify other syndromes or symptoms which might benefit from lithium therapy, including certain subtypes of schizophrenia, premenstrual tension, hyperaggressiveness, alcoholism, and seizure disorders. However, the major use of lithium is in the treatment of manic-depressive illness. In fact, the efficacy of lithium has stimulated efforts at greater diagnostic precision in this previously somewhat loosely defined entity.

Kraepelin coined the term "manic-depressive" psychosis and delineated it from dementia praecox. He proposed that a unitary etiology underlay the many forms of affective illness, including mania, depression, melancholia, and other "periodic and circular insanities." In the early twentieth century, the apparent unity of the manic-depressive illness concept gave way to the proliferation of multiple subcategories of affective disorder. Particularly vigorous debates involved the subcategories of depression, with their associated etiological connotations, such as psychotic, neurotic, reactive, endogenous, involutional, and post-partum (Chapter 11). However, in recent years, the concept of "bipolar affective illness," encompassing patients with both depressive and manic episodes, has served to factor out a relatively homogeneous group and has gained considerable acceptance as a nosological entity. Genetic and pharmacological evidence has accumulated to support this homogeneity. The remaining group of "unipolar" depressed patients appears to be more heterogeneous.

In its classical manifestations, the manic episode is characteristic and reliably diagnosable. Manic episodes may begin in a symptom-free period or after a depressive episode. Typically, an episode begins with an elevation of mood and an increase in activity. In the early stages, this may be difficult to differentiate from normal euphoria. As the mania intensifies, insomnia develops. This is not experienced as noxious but rather as the result of increased energy and involvement in increasingly compelling activity. Great plans are laid. Projects begin to proliferate. Good humor, optimism, and generosity abound. The pace of talking picks up, and the patient may be difficult to interrupt. He becomes more sexually oriented and flirtatious and may begin indulging in casual affairs. Money is no object: many manic patients have squandered a life's savings in a few weeks. Physical movement increases, ranging from restlessness to frantic activity. Although the manic individual may be "feeling no pain," his family and friends find his behavior increasingly distressing. Attempts to reason, to set limits, and to advise treatment are often met with a nonplussed reaction, finally progressing to outright hostility with occasional physical violence. As the episode intensifies, the manic may become frankly psychotic, with racing, disorganized speech, agitation, paranoid ideation, delusions, and hallucinations. In extreme cases, the patient may become self-destructive, hostile and violent, and may even die of exhaustion.

The more severe form of mania may be difficult to differentiate from other types of psychoses. The most helpful diagnostic information comes from a careful review of the progression of the illness, rather than from a cross-sectional view of the patient as he presents to the psychiatrist. This kind of information may be obtained largely from family or other informants. Since the prophylactic benefits of lithium are so dramatic, it is a serious diagnostic error to label a hyperactively agitated patient as "schizophrenic," until the possibility of manic illness is eliminated.

The first manic episodes typically begin in the thirties, but well-documented cases are reported with an onset as early as the teens and as late as the seventies. The natural course of an uninterrupted manic episode is about two months, although the range is great.

When examining the manic patient, the physician must be firm but sympathetic. Often, one can empathetically reflect to the patient how difficult it is to give up his "high" feeling. With some patience, one can often uncover an unspoken fear that if the mania stops, the patient may drop into depression. For example, one manic described herself as "in a giant squirrel cage like they have at carnivals where you are plastered to the side by centrifugal forces. If someone turned off the switch, I would fall to the bottom."

PRACTICAL ASPECTS OF PHARMACOLOGICAL TREATMENT

After the diagnosis is reasonably sure, one can begin pharmacotherapy. If the patient is only hypomanic and is cooperative with treatment, therapy can begin on an outpatient basis. More typically, the patient will require hospitalization, at times against his wishes. During the manic period intensive psychotherapy with the patient and the family is extremely difficult. The physician must do his best to see that no further damage is done to the already strained relationships with family, employers, and legal authorities. The emphasis is on setting firm, understandable limits and in focusing the patient on cooperating with drug treatment. The therapist will usually have to resign himself to a great deal of testing and verbal abuse. Short, frequent visits with the patient are more mutually gratifying than are extended ones.

Acute Treatment

Antipsychotic drugs are the first pharmacological mode of treatment, unless the patient is manageable enough to wait the seven to ten days it takes for lithium to exert its antimanic effect. A sedating phenothiazine has the advantage of slowing the patient down, although claims have been made for haloperidol (Haldol) as a more specific antimanic agent (cf. Chapter 9). Occasionally, the manic episode is "broken" by the use of phenothiazines alone, but more usually the patient retains an essentially manic outlook underneath the sedating and calming effects.

Once the patient is under control, a prelithium "work-up" is needed. Routine physical examination, blood studies, and urinalysis are important in defining any cardiovascular or renal disease. A baseline white blood cell count is important, since lithium can cause a transient leukocytosis, which may lead one into an unnecessary search for infection. A baseline thyroid function test is also important, since patients with borderline thyroid reserve may become clinically hypothyroid while on lithium. An electrocardiogram (ECG) should be obtained in anyone who is suspected of having or is in the age range for cardiac disease. Renal excretion is the primary route of lithium metabolism, so renal function should be assessed by measuring blood urea nitrogen (BUN), creatinine, and creatinine clearance.

A wide range of lithium dosage can produce the therapeutic blood level currently considered to be optimal, i.e., 0.8 to 1.2 mEq/L. Most clinicians initiate treatment with a dose of 900–1200 mg per day in divided doses and adjust dosage until a therapeutic blood level is reached. If one is interested in speeding the onset of response, a "loading" dose of 1500–1800 mg can be given over the first few days and then adjusted, usually downward, on the third or fourth day. A more systematic approach, using a standard 600 mg test dose of lithium and measuring a lithium level twenty-four hours later, is outlined in Table 12-1 (6).

There is good evidence that patients will require more lithium during an acute manic phase of their illness than when they are in remission. Consequently, as the mania comes under control, the dose may have to be adjusted downward. Likewise, a patient on prophylactic lithium may require an increase in dose when an incipient manic attack begins, in order to reestablish an adequate blood level.

It is best to begin with a divided dose schedule, until a therapeutic

TABLE 12-1.
DOSAGES REQUIRED TO ACHIEVE OPTIMAL SERUM LEVELS OF LITHIUM*

THE 24-HOUR SERUM LITHIUM (mEq/L) AFTER A SINGLE LOADING DOSE (600 MG)	PREDICTED DAILY DOSAGE	
	TOTAL DOSE (MG/DAY)	No. OF DIVIDED DOSES
<0.05	3600	3
0.05–0.09	2700	3
0.10–0.14	1800	3
0.15–0.19	1200	4
0.20–0.30	600	2
>0.30	600	2**

* From Cooper et al. (6).
** Use extreme caution.

serum level is reached. Then, one can switch to a twice-daily or even to a single nighttime administration, if the total dose is not over about 1500 mg per day. It should be remembered, however, that a blood level obtained in the morning after a single nighttime dose will be 20–30 percent higher than that obtained on a divided schedule. Slow-release forms of lithium, which should allow once-a-day therapy without excessive surges in blood levels, are under development. Lithium should never be administered parenterally.

Serum levels of lithium should be measured by flame spectrophotometry. It is important for the clinician to have confidence in the quality of laboratory data. Delivering a duplicate sample to the lab on occasion is a useful way of determining replicability. It is very important to draw the samples at a similar time each day. Usually, this is done before the morning dose. However, for those patients who find it inconvenient to get to the lab at this time, levels can be drawn at any time during the day, as long as it is about eight hours after the last dose. Saliva lithium levels are about twice those of plasma and have been suggested as a method for routine testing, although this will require further study.

Initially, lithium levels should be measured three times a week, gradually extending the interval to weeks or even months if the serum level remains constant and the reliability of the patient is assured. Since it is the intracellular and not the extracellular lithium concentration which is presumably responsible for the therapeutic effect, there has been some interest in correlating the intracellular red blood cell concentration with clinical effect. Correlations of plasma and red blood cell concentrations are not high, and the latter may be a better index of appropriate therapy (7). This approach remains a research technique and is not done routinely. However, if the intracellular red blood cell lithium level can be obtained, it may be a useful approach to the patient who appears to be refractory to lithium despite adequate serum levels.

PROPHYLACTIC TREATMENT

Considerable research has gone into determining the prophylactic effects of lithium (8,9). The use of the term "prophylaxis" in psychiatry has been criticized because psychotropic medications do not immunize an individual against the acquisition of disease. In psychiatry, the term has generally come to mean prevention of the recrudesence of psychopathology. It remains uncertain whether lithium's prophylactic properties are related to actual prevention or to pretreatment of recurring disease.

Lithium's prophylaxis against bipolar affective episodes is supported by over one hundred single-blind studies and at least nine double-blind studies (9). In addition, studies have indicated that the rate of relapse in patients before receiving lithium and after its withdrawal are approximately equal. Thus, one should be cautious about stopping prophylactic lithium in a bipolar patient with a history of frequent relapse, irrespective of the duration of prophylactic treatment.

Studies comparing lithium's effectiveness against the manic and depressive phases of bipolar illness have drawn different conclusions. One group of studies indicates that lithium is equally effective against both phases; another group indicates that lithium is more effective against mania. Demonstration of prophylaxis against the depressive phase usually requires a long trial period. Additional evidence suggests that depressive and manic episodes occurring during lithium maintenance therapy may be attenuated in severity and duration. However, the number of patients studied to date remains too small for definitive conclusions.

LITHIUM IN OTHER DISEASE STATES

The success of lithium in manic states has led to lithium trials in a variety of disease states (10,11). The most intense work involves acute depression and schizoaffective illness; however, a few controlled studies and a large anecdotal literature exist about lithium's effects on a variety of other conditions.

Depression

Since lithium is definitely useful in the treatment of manic states, it might be conceptually difficult to understand how it could also be useful in depression. Superficially, these two states seem to be polar opposites. However, mixed states of mania and depression were described by Kraepelin and have been confirmed by more modern systematic observation, as well as by extensive clinical lore. This conceptualization is consistent with the dominant psychodynamic concept of affective disorder, in which mania is viewed as a defense against depression. Furthermore, the two states share some similar biological abnormalities.

In his original trial, Cade (3) treated three depressed patients and reported no beneficial effects. However, some subsequent investigations suggested that lithium may be useful in acute depressive states. Despite increasingly sophisticated research designs addressed to this issue, it has not yet been resolved.

Because of the heterogeneity of depressive illness and because of its high spontaneous remission rate, the establishment of antidepressant action is always difficult (cf. Chapter 11). Some of the criteria for the effectiveness of lithium which have been utilized include:

- Improvement on lithium followed by deterioration on placebo.
- Improvement on lithium after having been unresponsive to other treatment modalities.
- Synergy of lithium with known antidepressant treatments.
- Treatment of two consecutive depressive episodes in the same patient, one with tricyclic antidepressants and the other with lithium.
- Comparison with tricyclic antidepressants both in grouped comparisons and cross-over design.

Research trials utilizing these criteria have yielded both positive and negative reports.

Currently, the major emphasis has turned toward the identification of a lithium-responsive subgroup of depressed patients. There is some evidence that a positive response to lithium is associated with a history of manic-depressive illness or a premorbid cyclothymic personality, a positive family history of affective illness, a lack of precipitating causes for depression, or vegetative signs of depression.

At the present time, the tricyclic antidepressants (tricyclics) remain the major therapeutic agents for serious depression. However, lithium is indicated in acute depression for patients who are unresponsive to other somatic treatments and for those bipolar patients who are at serious risk for a manic episode if treated with tricyclics.

While the usefulness of lithium in the treatment of acute depressive episodes remains unsettled, considerable evidence suggests that it may be as useful in the prophylaxis of unipolar depression as it is in preventing bipolar affective illness. The smaller number of unipolar patients studied to date and the greater heterogeneity of this population require that these results be interpreted with caution. Lithium may prove to be most useful only in certain subpopulations of unipolar affective illness.

SCHIZOAFFECTIVE ILLNESS

It is generally believed that lithium is prophylactic in schizoaffective illness but less so than in either bipolar or unipolar affective illness. Naturally these studies are complicated by the difficulty of defining reliable criteria for distinguishing schizoaffective illness from atypical presentations of manic or depressive illness. Some investigators believe that lithium may be more useful against the affective than the schizophrenic features of the illness. Evidence is accumulating for the use of a combination of lithium and antipsychotics in the treatment of these patients (12).

EPILEPSY

Lithium has been reported to cause improvement in up to 60 percent of epileptics. In addition to a reduction of the frequency of seizures, a "normalizing effect" on the electroencephalogram (EEG) and improved behavior between seizures have been reported. Benefits in temporal lobe epilepsy, a subtype particularly resistant to conventional treatment, have been reported. However, a small number of patients have increased seizure activity or the induction of status epilepticus while on lithium.

AGGRESSION

Based upon the assumption that paroxysmal abnormal brain activity may underlie aggressive states, the effect of lithium on violence in prison populations has been studied. Statistically significant results were achieved, showing a reduction in disciplinary action for aggressive outbursts, a reduction in aggressive feelings, and an impression, on the part both of the prisoners and of those observing them that, the individual prisoner had greater self-control (Chapter 15).

CHILDHOOD AND ADOLESCENCE DISORDERS

Lithium has been tried in a number of illnesses in children and adolescents. Most of these studies suffer from a lack of nosologic clarity and uncertainty about proper lithium dosage in children. Probably the most promising results to date have been in the treatment of maladaptive teenagers with labile mood and acting-out behavior. Lithium has generally been found not to be useful in hyperactive children, except for the hyperactive children of lithium-responsive parents.

ALCOHOLISM

Alcoholics without a diagnosable affective disease have been treated with lithium. In some instances, lithium-treated patients had significantly fewer episodes of disabling drinking than did those given a placebo.

MOVEMENT DISORDERS

A small number of preliminary reports have claimed success in using lithium to treat the abnormal movements of Huntington's chorea and tardive dyskinesia and the hyperkinetic movements seen in L-DOPA-treated parkinsonian patients.

PERIODIC PSYCHOSES AND OTHER PSYCHIATRIC DISORDERS

Lithium has been tried in a small number of periodic psychoses with mixed results. Anecdotal reports have claimed usefulness in sociopathic personality. A small number of studies have reported positive effects of lithium on the periodic mood disorder associated with premenstrual tension. A careful study of lithium in obsessive-compulsive personality failed to confirm earlier claims of efficacy in this disorder.

SIDE EFFECTS OF LITHIUM CARBONATE

EARLY MANIFESTATIONS

The most common early, reversible, side effects of lithium are: gastrointestinal distress, including nausea, vomiting, diarrhea; fine hand tremor; muscular weakness; urinary frequency; dry mouth and thirst; pretibial and hand edema. These side effects usually occur with a serum level of about 1.0–1.5 mEq/L, but may be more associated with the steepness of the rise in lithium concentration than with the steady-state level. Often these side effects will diminish without reducing the dose; however, they deserve close attention, since more serious toxicity may follow.

The nausea, vomiting, and diarrhea produced by lithium are difficult to distinguish from common "flu" symptoms. Consequently, if the patient complains of these symptoms, it is advisable to stop the medication and obtain a measurement of blood lithium at the earliest convenience. The hand tremor can often be controlled, if persistent, with propranolol, 15–60 mg per day. The edema is usually not incapacitating, but patients with a predisposition to pulmonary embolus can be at some risk. Diuretic therapy for the edema is ineffective and may result in problems with lithium toxicity. The combination of lithium and diuretics is generally contraindicated. Where overriding considerations necessitate combined therapy, the patient's electrolyte balance and renal function must be closely monitored.

OVERDOSE

Manifestations of serious lithium toxicity, usually associated with blood levels over 1.5 mEq/L, are ataxia, persistent drowsiness, muscular fasciculations, choreoathetotic movements, hyperactive deep tendon reflexes, incontinence, slurred speech, blurred vision, cardiac arrhythmias, and seizures. These symptoms are often associated with a diffusely slowed electroencephalogram (EEG). There is no specific antidote. Treatment consists of discontinuation of the drug, general supportive measures, and perhaps forced diuresis.

CARDIAC TOXICITY

In view of lithium's known effects on electrolyte and catecholamine metabolism, and of its ability to produce T-wave flattening and inversion in the ECG, the issue of cardiotoxicity has been of concern. Despite these effects, serious morbidity or mortality from cardiac arrhythmias has not presented a major problem in patients whose levels have remained in the therapeutic range. "Hypotension and cardiovascular collapse," alleged cardiotoxic manifestations of lithium, invariably follow days of coma after an overdose. In patients with pre-existing cardiac disease, both cardiac state and lithium levels must be followed carefully. The risk of lithium therapy must be weighed against the risks of a recurrent manic episode.

THYROID EFFECTS

The occurrence of goiter in patients on lithium has been estimated to be about 4 percent. Individuals with pre-existing low thyroid reserve are particularly predisposed. Although the mechanism whereby lithium suppresses the thyroid gland has not been fully elaborated, the overall effect of lithium administration is to decrease circulating thyroid. This results in negative feedback, leading to increased thyroid-stimulating hormone (TSH) production, followed by autoregulatory mechanisms which usually produce a slow return to baseline thyroid parameters. Lithium therapy may be associated with a diffuse, nontender thyroid enlargement, hypothyroidism, or both. These effects can be reversed by discontinuation of the drug or by the administration of exogenous thyroid extract. Consequently, borderline hypothyroidism or other forms of thyroid illness do not constitute a contraindication to lithium therapy.

NEPHROGENIC DIABETES INSIPIDUS SYNDROME

Although a significant number of patients taking lithium will notice some mild polydipsia and polyuria, this is not ordinarily a major problem. Rarely, patients develop a profound polyuria and polydipsia which resembles diabetes insipidus. The syndrome is not sensitive to vasopressin and is presumed to be of renal origin. This bothersome side effect is fully reversible and is not accompanied by changes in other kidney functions or by renal damage. No change in lithium dose is required, nor is there any other danger of electrolyte disturbance. If the polyuria is over 4 L per day, it may be sufficiently bothersome to prompt discontinuation of lithium maintenance. The syndrome is not necessarily associated with high lithium levels; it may become intolerable with lithium levels as low as 0.4 mEq/L.

LITHIUM AND PREGNANCY

Several registries of lithium-treated pregnant women have been established and are continuing to collect data. Any case of lithium administered to a pregnant woman should be reported. To date, the incidence of congenital abnormalities does not appear to exceed that seen in the general population. However, studies in animals suggest that teratogenic effects from lithium are possible. Several guidelines for the use of lithium in pregnant women are suggested (Table 12-2).

EXPERIMENTAL APPROACHES TO THE TREATMENT OF MANIA

Experimental approaches to the treatment of mania have generally followed the leads provided by the biogenic amine hypothesis of affective disorders (Chapter 10). For example, the catecholamine hypothesis of affective disorders leads to the suggestion that mania is associated with a relative excess of norepinephrine at the postsynaptic receptor. It follows that amine-depleting drugs or catecholamine-synthesis in-

TABLE 12-2.

GUIDELINES FOR LITHIUM USE IN PREGNANT WOMEN

• Lithium should be continued or initiated in pregnant women only when there are strong indications.
• Contraception should be practiced by women in the childbearing years if they are taking lithium, and lithium should be discontinued if a pregnancy is desired or suspected.
• If lithium is necessary at all during pregnancy, it should be avoided during the first trimester.
• If lithium is necessary during pregnancy, careful attention should be paid to the control of levels and to the effects of salt depletion by dietary restriction or diuretics.
• Breast feeding should be avoided, since the concentration of lithium in breast milk approximates the plasma level.

---

hibitors should benefit manic patients. Of the amine-depleting drugs, reserpine is known to be antimanic. But it may be generally antipsychotic, and its biochemical effects are numerous and complicated (Chapters 2 and 3).

Several amine-synthesis inhibitors have been given trials in mania. α-Methyl-p-tyrosine (AMPT) inhibits the rate-limiting step in catecholamine synthesis, conversion of tyrosine to L-DOPA (Chapter 2). Of seven patients treated with this drug, five had a significant decrease in mania ratings, with several of the patients showing a rebound upon drug withdrawal (13). However, α-methyl-p-tyrosine is not a practical treatment for mania, since it is relatively toxic and the response is not nearly as satisfying as that to lithium.

Although α-methyl-p-tyrosine is a relatively specific inhibitor of catecholamine synthesis, it inhibits the formation of both dopamine and norepinephrine. In contrast, fusaric acid is a relatively specific inhibitor of dopamine-β-hydroxylase and, thus, blocks only norepinephrine synthesis (Chapter 2). In one study, fusaric acid inhibited norepinephrine synthesis in manic patients but did not produce marked improvement of manic symptoms (14). In fact, the patients may have developed increased psychosis.

Much of the evidence in support of catecholamine hypothesis of mania may also be used in support of an excess of 5-hydroxytryptamine in mania (Chapter 10). With this in mind, the putative serotonergic receptor blocker methysergide has been evaluated as an antimanic agent (15). Some of the early nonblind studies were encouraging; but with well-controlled double-blind studies, this agent has been found to be without antimanic activity.

An alternate approach to the relationship of neurotransmitters to the manic syndrome is derived from viewing these substances as operating in some kind of balance. For example, in Parkinson's disease, either an increase in dopaminergic activity or a decrease in cholinergic activity will modify the symptoms. A balance between acetylcholine and norepinephrine has been hypothesized to mediate mood disorders, and infusions of physostigmine, a potent cholinesterase inhibitor, reportedly ameliorates manic symptoms (16). Since physostigmine causes side effects of nausea and vomiting and produces some sedation, these findings will need further confirmation.

REFERENCES

1. Gershon, S. and Shopsin, B., eds., *Lithium: Its Role in Psychiatric Research and Treatment*. New York: Plenum Press, 1973.
2. Johnson, F. N., ed., *Lithium Research and Therapy*. New York: Academic Press, 1975.
3. Cade, J. F. J. The story of lithium. *In: Discoveries in Biological Psychiatry*. F. J. Ayd and B. Blackwell, eds., Philadelphia: Lippincott, 1970, pp. 218–219.
4. Byck, R. Drugs and the treatment of psychiatric disorders. *In: The Pharmacological Basis of Therapeutics*, 5th ed. L. S. Goodman and A. Gilman, eds., New York: Macmillan Co:, 1975, pp. 152–200.
5. Mandell, A. J. The bucket, the train, and the feedback loop in biochemical psychiatry. *In: Schizophrenia: Biological and Psychological Perspectives*. G. Usdin, ed., New York: Brunner/Mazel, 1975, pp. 38–55.
6. Cooper, T. B., Bergner, P. E., and Simpson, G. M. The 24-hour lithium level as a prognosticator of dosage requirements. *Am. J. Psychiatry 130*:601–603, 1973.
7. Mendels, J. and Frazer, A. Intracellular lithium concentration and clinical response. Towards a membrane theory of depression. *J. Psychiatr. Res. 10*:9–18, 1973.
8. Quitkin, F., Rifkin, A., and Klein, D. Prophylaxis of affective disorders —current status of knowledge. *Arch. Gen. Psychiatry 33*:337–341, 1976.
9. Davis, J. Maintenance therapy in psychiatry. I: Affective disorders. *Am. J. Psychiatry 133*:1–13, 1976.
10. Kline, N. S. and Simpson, G. Lithium in the treatment of conditions other than affective disorders. *In: Lithium: Its Role in Psychiatric Research and Treatment*. S. Gershon and B. Shopsin, eds., New York: Plenum Press, 1973, pp. 85–97.
11. Quitkin, F. M., Rifkin, A., and Klein, D. F. Lithium in other psychiatric disorders. *In: Lithium: Its Role in Psychiatric Research and Treatment*. S. Gershon and B. Shopsin, eds., New York: Plenum Press, 1973, pp. 295–315.
12. Small, J. G., Kellans, J. J., Milstein, V., and Moore, J. A placebo-controlled study of lithium combined with neuroleptics in chronic schizophrenic patients. *Am. J. Psychiatry 132*:1315–1317, 1975.
13. Brodie, H. K. H., Murphy, K. D., Goodwin, F. K., and Bunney, W. E., Jr. Catecholamines and mania: the effect of alpha-methyl-para-tyrosine on manic behavior and catecholamine metabolism. *Clin. Pharmacol. Ther. 12*:218–224, 1971.
14. Sack, R. L. and Goodwin, F. K. Inhibition of dopamine-β-hydroxylase in manic patients. *Arch. Gen. Psychiatry 31*:649–654, 1974.
15. Fieve, R. R., Platman, S. F., and Fleiss, J. L. A clinical trial of methysergide and lithium in mania. *Psychopharmacologia 15*:425–429, 1969.
16. Janowsky, D. S., El-Yousef, M. K., and Davis, J. M. A cholinergic-adrenergic hypothesis of mania and depression. *Lancet 1*:632–635, 1972.

13 | Antianxiety Medications and the Treatment of Anxiety

JARED R. TINKLENBERG

INTRODUCTION

Antianxiety agents encompass several different groups of drugs, including benzodiazepines, propanediols, antihistaminics, and some barbiturates. These drugs are also called anxiolytics, daytime sedatives, and calmatives. The term "minor tranquilizers," which is often used to refer to these drugs, is misleading, since it erroneously connotes that they are on the same spectrum as the antipsychotics or "major tranquilizers." The antianxiety drugs differ from the antipsychotics chemically, pharmacologically, and clinically. However, in certain settings, the antipsychotics and tricyclic antidepressants (tricyclics) are also used for their antianxiety properties.

HISTORY

The development of meprobamate, one of the first popular antianxiety agents, is a story of serendipity and careful observation. In 1945, Berger was searching for a chemical which could kill gram negative bacteria that were unaffected by penicillin. He and his co-workers decided to modify a phenylglycol ether which was marketed as a disinfectant. They tried these compounds on rodents to determine toxicity. One of these substances, mephenesin carbamate (Fig. 13-1), seemed to produce a profound muscle relaxation in rats without inducing total paralysis. In addition, it seemed to quiet the animals. Mephenesin carbamate (Tolseram) was marketed as a muscle relaxant. Several investigators noted that the drug also seemed to allay anxiety without much sedation, although the effect was transient and required high doses. Over the next five years attempts to increase the duration of these antianxiety effects by altering mephenesin carbamate led,

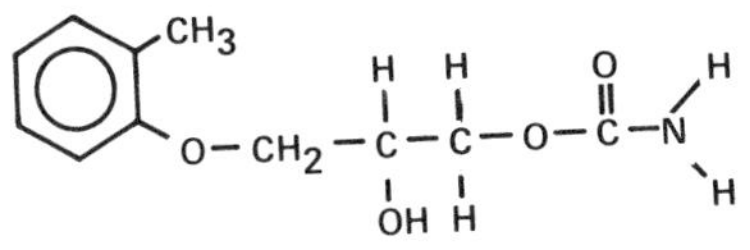

FIGURE 13-1. Mephenesin Carbamate

eventually, to meprobamate (see Fig. 13-2). This latter compound, a propanediol dicarbamate, has no obvious structural relationship to mephenesin carbamate, unless the steps in its development are described.
Thus, what began as an attempt to develop an antibiotic resulted
finally in a substance which reduced anxiety (1).

Currently, the most widely used antianxiety agents are the benzodiazepines. In the 1930's, Sternbach was a postdoctoral research assistant at the University of Cracow in Poland. He was interested in the
physical and theoretical rather than medical or pharmacological aspects of chemistry and synthesized several heptoxdiazines. Twenty
years later, Sternbach, then a medicinal chemist at Roche Laboratories,
followed a procedure common to much of medicinal chemistry: he decided to screen the heptoxdiazines for biological activity. He soon determined that the compounds were not heptoxdiazines (seven-member
rings) but quinazolone 3-oxides (six-member rings). This finding led
to the synthesis of forty derivatives, all of which were pharmacologically inert. The last in the series, a quinazolone treated with methylamine, was not tested. Instead, it was labeled RO 5–0690 and shelved,
because of other research priorities.

In May 1957, literally during a clean-up of the laboratory, one of
Sternbach's chemists suggested that they test this compound. Randall
found that, in cats, RO 5–0690 was similar to, but two to five times
more potent than, meprobamate. The compound was a 1,4 benzodiazepine, chlordiazepoxide. It is not a quinazoline 3-oxide derivative, as
were the forty compounds without biological activity. Methylamine
caused an unexpected ring enlargement, forming a seven-member ring—
a fact which was not definitely established until almost a year after
Randall's report of biological activity. Since then, several hundred benzodiazepine derivatives have been synthesized, including the more potent diazepam, which also has anticonvulsive activity. Chlordiazepoxide
and diazepam are currently the most widely used antianxiety agents in
the world and, except for alcohol, are probably the most frequently

used psychoactive substances (2). The biological actions of the benzo-diazepines are described in Chapter 19.

CHARACTERISTICS OF ANXIETY

Anxiety may be defined as a pervading feeling of apprehension or dread, which may or may not be associated with immediately stressful or fearful stimuli. Anxiety frequently overlaps with fear. However, with a fear response, an immediate cause is clearly discernible; and the response is rapid, marked, and congruous to the degree of threat. In contrast, anxiety generally refers to an overreaction to real danger or to an attenuated fear and dread response without any clear source of danger. Anxiety states rarely occur in isolation and are frequently mixed with other emotions, especially depression and anger. Anxiety takes such forms as: situational anxiety, related to a stressful event such as an examination; traumatic anxiety, following an unexpected, possibly tragic, event; toxic anxiety, resulting from high doses of psycho-active drugs; and free-floating anxiety, associated with no discernible event.

Both subjective and objective symptoms are associated with the anxiety state. In addition to having extreme dysphoria, the patient may manifest a variety of physical symptoms, such as muscular tension, palpitations, headache, dizziness, abdominal distress, chest pains, tremulousness, and nausea. Common behavioral concomitants include restlessness, irritability, fatigue, distractibility, and insomnia. Finally, anxiety may be associated with medical conditions, depression, psychosis, pervasive neurotic conflict, and fearful or stressful life situations.

TREATMENT OF ANXIETY

Usually, pharmacological treatment should be initiated if anxiety is severe enough to interfere with the patient's daily functioning. Anti-anxiety agents are particularly valuable in the control of acute anxiety resulting from transient inner or environmental stress or from a somatic illness. They are also useful when pretreatment sedation is required for medical or surgical procedures. These drugs are less clearly appropriate for treating chronic anxiety conditions or for ameliorating the tensions and anxieties of everyday living.

Ideally, drugs should be only an adjunct to psychotherapy and judicious alteration of the patient's environment. Clinicians generally agree that the proper use of antianxiety drugs does not retard psychotherapy. In fact, it may permit the patient to more effectively utilize psychotherapeutic help (Chapter 30). In prescribing these agents, the clinician should remember that moderate levels of anxiety have adaptive functions in mobilizing and directing energies and in providing the persistent motivation that is required to cope successfully with difficulties. Care should be taken that these constructive forces are not unduly negated by pharmacological agents.

When administering these drugs, physicians should remember that psychological variables are very important determinants of the "drug effect" (Chapter 31). Maximal confidence and enthusiasm about the pharmacological properties of the drug should be conveyed to the patient, to take advantage of nonspecific "placebo effects." The patient should be told about the course of pharmacological treatment as it is planned, including the clinical effects that can be expected, guides for adjustments in dosages, and the expected period of time during which the drug will be administered. With antianxiety agents, the duration of therapy is usually transient and limited to the period of extreme stress. In this way, the administration of drugs can be an effective means of increasing the patient's awareness of his own responses to various forms of stress.

Unfortunately, these drugs are so safe and generally effective that physicians often prescribe them for minor indications and without adequate supervision. For example, mild tension or appropriate situational anxiety is not an indication for any drug. Rather, the patient should learn how to handle such unpleasant states with appropriate psychological coping maneuvers.

PRACTICAL ASPECTS OF PHARMACOLOGICAL TREATMENT

Acute Treatment

Initial and daily dose ranges for antianxiety agents are presented in Table 13-1. The drug should be taken one to two hours before bedtime, if possible. The acute sedative effects can facilitate sleep, and the long plasma half-life of many antianxiety drugs provides continued mild sedation during the following day. The patient should be alerted to the dangers of sudden drowsiness and impaired psychomotor function, which can result from these drugs. He should also be cautioned against the concomitant use of other drugs, including alcohol.

The initial treatment of severely agitated states, such as those associated with acute psychotic reactions, toxic delirium, or drug withdrawal syndromes, may require the parenteral administration of antianxiety drugs. Although titration is required for the individual patient, doses are usually about one-half the oral dose. Following appropriate sedation by parenteral administration, continued medication is usually given by mouth.

The dosage schedule should be adjusted to accommodate the individual needs and responses of the patient. As with most drugs in psychiatry, dosage is determined by the clinical response of the patient and by his ability to tolerate any side effects. Most conditions requiring the use of antianxiety agents fluctuate with changes in the patient's life. Therefore, dosages of antianxiety agents require more frequent adjustments than do dosages of antipsychotic agents, where steady tissue levels are often required for months or years. The patient should be informed that anxiety is usually episodic and that medication will be changed in response to his needs. A daily diary of fluctuations in anxiety levels and associated environmental events can be very helpful in the development of psychological awareness and the identification of areas requiring special attention in psychotherapy. The practice of treating a patient for weeks or months at unchanged dosage schedules should be reviewed by the therapist. In the relatively rare instances when anxiety persists unchanged for more than a few weeks the diagnosis should be reconsidered, and more intensive psychotherapy or modification of the patient's life-style and environment should be implemented.

MAINTENANCE TREATMENT

There are some situations in which continuous maintenance on antianxiety agents may be appropriate. For example, some individuals have marked tendencies to develop drug dependencies and seem to be unable to deal with the difficulties of daily living without the use of some chemical with antianxiety properties. Such situations must be judged individually; but in some instances it may be preferable to prescribe a benzodiazepine on a continuous basis, if it enables the patient to reduce or to eliminate his use of more deleterious pharmacological agents and live a more socially acceptable life.

Maintenance therapy with antianxiety agents may also be indicated for selected patients with medical conditions that can be aggravated by high levels of anxiety, as with peptic ulcers or essential hypertension. In this situation, it is necessary to demonstrate that the primary disorder specifically responds to the antianxiety drug. Thus, in the case of hypertension, one should document that the use of antianxiety preparations induces a reduction in blood pressure which could not be accomplished with less intensive methods, such as sodium restriction, weight loss, and alteration of a harried life-style.

SIDE EFFECTS AND COMPLICATIONS

Drowsiness is the most common side effect reported with the antianxiety drugs. It usually subsides with continued use; however, a dosage reduction may be useful, as long as anxiety symptoms are appropriately managed. Other less common and usually mild side effects include tremor, ataxia, postural hypotension, lightheadedness, mental confusion, skin eruptions, and abdominal pain. Teratogenic effects have not been definitely established with antianxiety drugs, but the use of these or any other potent drug during pregnancy demands that potential therapeutic gains be judiciously weighed against the possible risk of fetal harm. Very recently, specific precautions have been issued about the use of diazepam during pregnancy.

TABLE 13-1.
ANTIANXIETY DRUGS

NAME		INITIAL ORAL DOSE (MG)	DOSE RANGE* (MG/DAY)
GENERIC	REPRESENTATIVE BRAND		
Benzodiazepines			
Chlordiazepoxide	Librium	10–50	15–200
Diazepam	Valium	5–20 (5–20, intramuscular or intravenous)	6–40
Oxazepam	Serax	15–60	30–120
Clorazepate	Tranxene	7.5–30	15–60
Propanediols			
Meprobamate	Miltown	200–600	600–2000
Tybamate	Tybatran	250–500	750–2800
Antihistamines			
Hydroxyzine	Vistaril	30–100 (25–50, intramuscular or intravenous)	75–400
Diphenhydramine	Benadryl	50–100 (10–50, intramuscular or intravenous)	75–300
Tricyclic Antidepressants			
Doxepin	Sinequan	25–50	75–300
β-Adrenergic Antagonists			
Propranolol	Inderal**	10–40	30–240

* Divided into 2–4 doses
** Not approved by FDA for treatment of anxiety

CONTRAINDICATIONS

In prescribing drugs, the physician should always assess possible allergic or idiosyncratic responses. The patient should be asked specifically about the drug under consideration and about unusual responses to other drugs. If the patient describes an unusual drug reaction, full details should be obtained. Some patients will initially state that they are allergic to a psychotropic drug, although a more complete descrip-

BENZODIAZEPINES

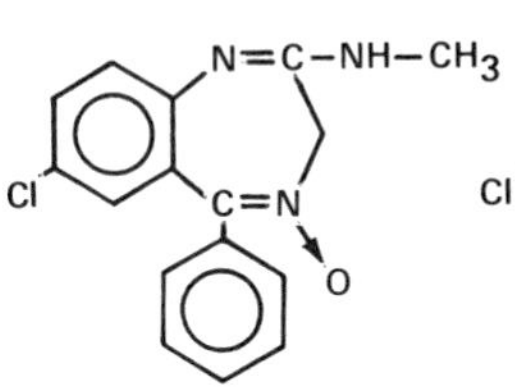
CHLORDIAZEPOXIDE

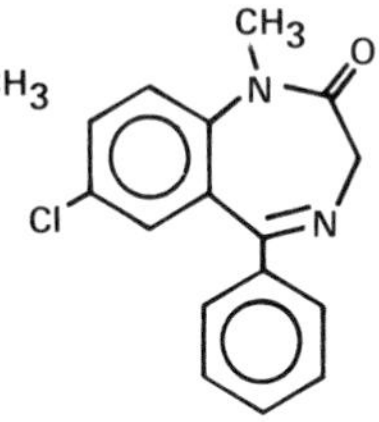
DIAZEPAM

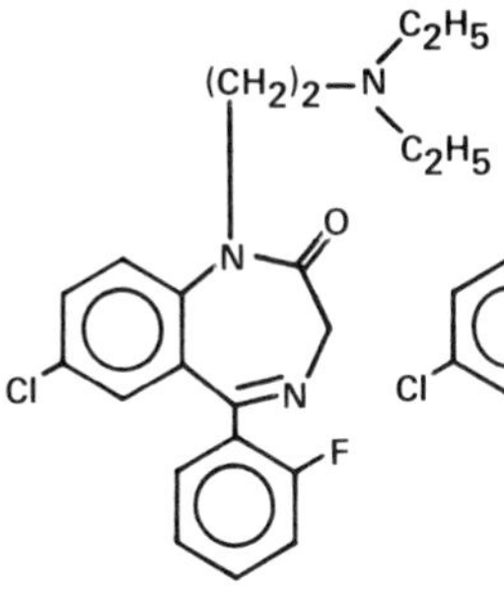
FLURAZEPAM

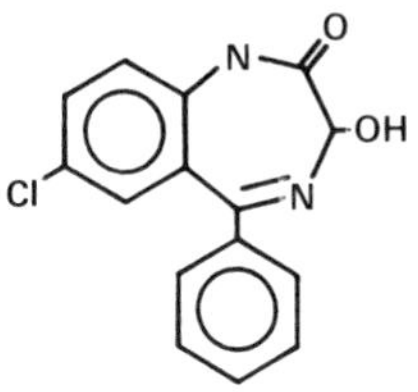
OXAZEPAM

PROPANEDIOLS

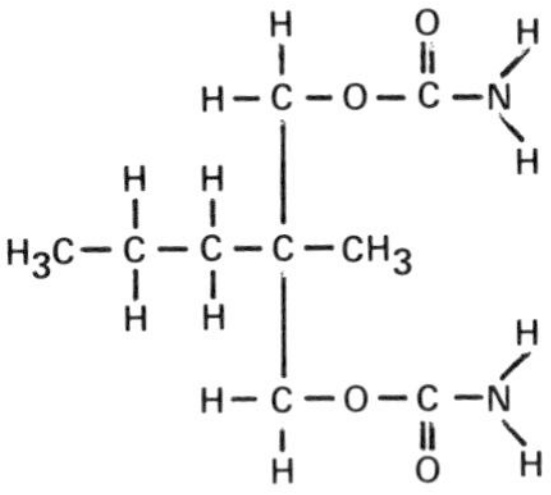
MEPROBAMATE

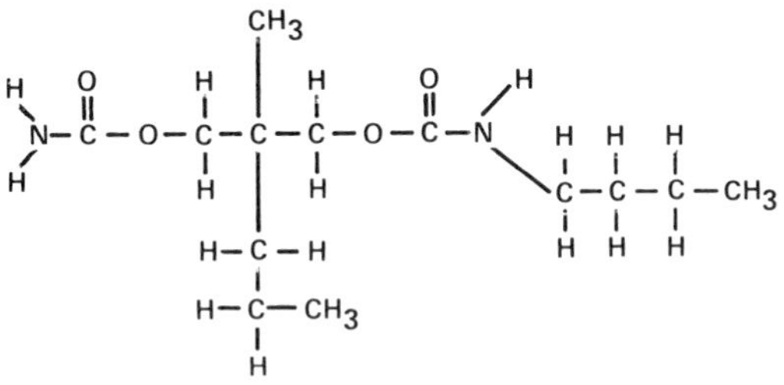
TYBAMATE

ANTIHISTAMINES

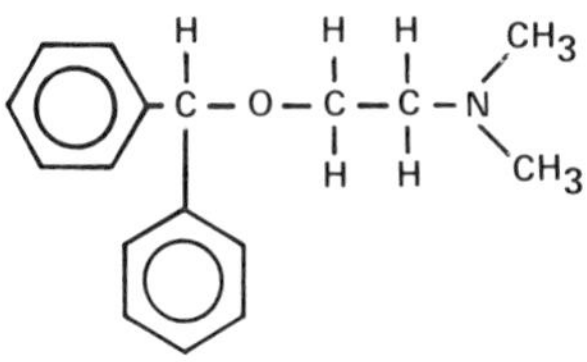
DIPHENHYDRAMINE

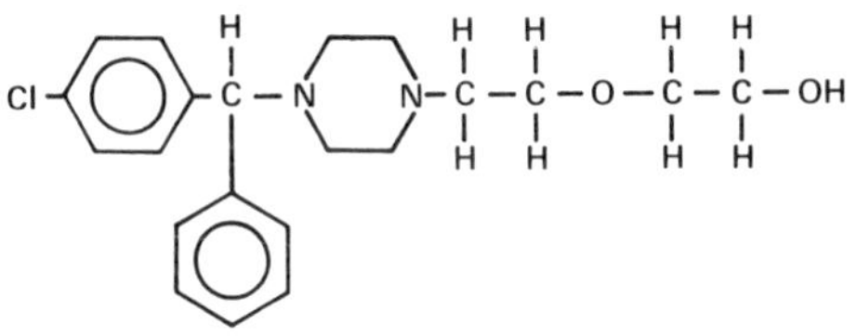
HYDROXYZINE

FIGURE 13-2. Chemical Structures for Common Antianxiety Agents tion clearly indicates that they merely experienced an unpleasant but expected side effect of that drug. In such instances, antianxiety agents can and should be used, if clinically indicated. On the other hand, in the very rare situations in which a specific antianxiety drug has been associated with urticaria, angioneurotic edema, breathing difficulties, hemolysis, or other signs of a generalized allergic reaction, that drug and closely related drugs are definitely contraindicated. Special caution should also be used in prescribing antianxiety drugs for patients who have histories of liver or renal impairment, blood dyscrasias, or depression of the central nervous system from any cause. Special surveillance is required for patients with histories of alcoholism or other forms of drug abuse (Chapter 23).

CHOICE OF SPECIFIC ANTIANXIETY AGENTS

Since most antianxiety agents are effective in reducing overall anxiety and muscle tension, the choice of which specific drug to use is based on considerations other than their antianxiety efficacy. If the patient has had a good response to a particular drug or has a definite preference, that drug would be a logical first choice. Occasionally, the side effects of a specific antianxiety agent can be utilized or avoided to the patient's advantage (3). For example, if the patient's anxiety is mixed with significant depression which requires therapy (cf. Chapter 11), a sedative-antidepressant such as doxepin would be a reasonable selection. On the other hand, if the patient has benign prostatic hypertrophy with intermittent urinary retention or if he is otherwise susceptible to anticholinergic effects, sedative-antihistamines and other antianxiety drugs with anticholinergic properties should be avoided. If none of these considerations obtains, the physician should prescribe an agent with which he is thoroughly familiar, so that he can administer the drug with confidence and exploit the placebo effect (Chapter 31).

BENZODIAZEPINES

For several reasons, many physicians prefer to use one of the benzodiazepines for the treatment of anxiety. First, unless combined with other drugs, oral benzodiazepines are virtually never lethal—an important factor in reducing the risk of intentional or accidental overdose (4,5). In contrast, the barbiturates and meprobamate have a relatively narrow margin between lethal and effective dosages. Second, unlike many other antianxiety agents, the benzodiazepines do not markedly stimulate hepatic microsomal metabolic enzymes (Chapter 19). Thus, they are less likely to lose their effectiveness when taken repeatedly or to interfere with the metabolism of other drugs, such as the coumarin anticoagulants, the tricyclic antidepressants, or the antipsychotic agents. Third, most benzodiazepines have a long duration of action. For example, the half-life of chlordiazepoxide is about eight to twenty-eight hours and that of diazepam is twenty to fifty hours. Finally, the benzodiazepines are at relatively low risk for the production of physical tolerance. Physical dependence does occur, but only with high doses over long periods of time. This low abuse potential for the benzodiazepines is in marked contrast to that of meprobamate and the barbiturates. Despite the low incidence of physiological tolerance, psychological dependency or habituation is a growing problem with benzodiazepines (Chapter 23).

Although there are no marked differences in the pharmacological effects of benzodiazepines, differences in their pharmacokinetics may provide reasons for preferred use (6,7). Chlordiazepoxide, diazepam, and clorazepate all have relatively long half-lives and produce one or more active metabolites. Daily administration of these drugs usually results in steady-state levels in four to six days. Thus, after the first or second day of treatment, the dosage schedule can often consist of a single dose two hours before bedtime. Commonly, benzodiazepines are prescribed for several times a day. This practice should be avoided, since the resulting accumulation of the drug can produce unnecessary side effects of excessive sedation, confused thinking, and ataxia. Excessive sedation is especially apparent when the patient also takes other central depressants, such as alcohol.

Oxazepam has no significant active metabolites and has a relatively short half-life of four to twenty hours. Steady-state levels are obtained in about two days. Since accumulation of oxazepam is less troublesome, it can be given more frequently and is a reasonable choice for clinical situations in which a relatively short-acting, rapidly terminating drug is required. For example, it might be more useful than other benzodiazepines in treating elderly patients, in whom drug impairment can be especially undesirable (Chapter 28). Systematic data on this issue are still needed, however (8,9). It should be also noted that, in some instances, the relatively rapid metabolism of oxazepam may limit usefulness for treating insomnia, since its hypnotic effects may dissipate too rapidly.

Psychological dependency or habituation to the benzodiazepines does occur, but the incidence of actual physiological dependency, as defined by withdrawal seizures or psychosis, is low (Chapter 19). This low incidence may reflect the pharmacokinetic characteristics of the drugs, since their active metabolites and long half-lives result in the very gradual reduction of tissue levels. When serious withdrawal phenomena do occur, they are associated with the prolonged consumption of high doses. The onset of these withdrawal signs is determined by the half-life of the specific drug. For example, since both diazepam and chlordiazepoxide have long half-lives, any serious withdrawal reactions would begin five to seven days after stopping drug ingestion (Chapter 23). By contrast, withdrawal seizures can occur within twenty-four hours after the abrupt cessation of chronic meprobamate or barbiturate consumption.

The most common side effects associated with the benzodiazepines are drowsiness, ataxia, paradoxical excitement, and dizziness or vertigo (10). These effects are more common in older patients; but all patients should be cautioned to avoid high-risk activity, such as driving or operating complex machinery, until they are accustomed to the drug. Heavy cigarette smokers tend to be less sedated with comparable doses of benzodiazepines when compared to nonsmokers (11). Usually these individual differences can be managed by adjusting the dosage as needed. Since the sedating effects of the benzodiazepines can be potentiated by central depressants, such as alcohol, antihistamines, and many over-the-counter remedies for colds or insomnia, the concomitant use of these latter drugs should be carefully monitored. Similarly, the benzodiazepines can potentiate the anticholinergic effects of the antipsychotics, the antidepressants, and other centrally active drugs.

PROPANEDIOLS

For several reasons, meprobamate, the best-known propanediol, and tybamate have been used less frequently in recent years than they were in the 1950's and 1960's. Unlike the benzodiazepines, the propanediols have a narrow margin between the therapeutic and lethal doses, and fatal overdoses do occur. In addition, meprobamate is associated with significant physical dependence. Tolerance can develop rapidly, and profound withdrawal reactions can occur. Meprobamate also seems to be somewhat less efficacious than the benzodiazepines as an anti-anxiety agent and has a significantly shorter duration of clinical action. Tybamate, a congener of meprobamate which has not been extensively studied, requires repeated doses. In some individuals, tybamate is erratically absorbed, leading to irregular effectiveness. Some clinicians only prescribe propanediols to individuals for whom these drugs have been effective in the past; others try to avoid their use entirely (12).

SEDATIVE ANTIHISTAMINICS

Sedative antihistaminics may be of special value in the treatment of anxiety-related skin conditions. Since their side effects, such as visual disturbances and dry mouth, provide intrinsic limitations against escalation of dosages, they are reasonable antianxiety agents for individuals who have demonstrated tendencies to abuse psychoactive drugs. On the other hand, dose-response characteristics are sometimes unpredictable: increasing the dosage may precipitate paradoxical excitement, rather than increase sedation. Some individuals are stimulated by even low doses of these drugs. Furthermore, tolerance can develop to their pharmacological effects.

SEDATIVE ANTIDEPRESSANTS

The sedative antidepressants are effective in certain patients who demonstrate both high levels of anxiety and clinical indications of depression, such as psychomotor retardation, early-morning awakening, and bowel disturbances (Chapter 11). Many other forms of depression respond to conventional antianxiety agents. As with the antihistaminics, the use of sedative antidepressants is sometimes limited by their anticholinergic side effects.

BARBITURATES

Although the barbiturates are the least expensive of the antianxiety agents, they have characteristics which limit their clinical usefulness. Since they depress the respiratory centers, fatal accidental or intentional overdose is a significant clinical problem (Chapter 23). Their use in the presence of asthma or other respiratory difficulties can be troublesome. The barbiturates stimulate hepatic microsomal enzymes, which leads to the development of metabolic tolerance and modifies the metabolism of certain other drugs, such as warfarin (coumarin) (Chapter 19). In addition, the short- and intermediate-acting barbiturates such as pentobarbital, secobarbital, and amobarbital have pronounced abuse potential and have been associated with life-threatening physical withdrawal reactions (Chapter 23). Finally, the barbiturates have fairly steep dose-response curves, so that in some patients it is difficult to find a dosage level that adequately reduces anxiety without excessive sedation. This characteristic tends to limit the use of barbiturates as antianxiety agents to settings in which the patient need not remain alert.

β-ADRENERGIC BLOCKING AGENTS

β-Adrenergic blocking agents such as propranolol seem to be effective in reducing at least the sympathetic discharge associated with anxiety (13). To date, propranolol has not been approved by the Food and Drug Administration (FDA) for the routine treatment of anxiety but might reasonably be used when anxiety is associated with a medical condition for which β-adrenergic blocking is indicated. These conditions include hypertension and certain paroxysmal tachycardias. As with all potent drugs, absolute and relative contraindications must be considered before treatment is initiated. Preliminary reports also suggest that propranolol may be an effective antipsychotic.

COMBINATIONS OF ANTIANXIETY AND OTHER PSYCHOACTIVE DRUGS

There are a number of trade preparations which combine an antianxiety drug with one or more other pharmacological agents, such as antispasmodics. Since these combinations are often characterized by inappropriate expense and fixed ratios of ingredients, they are seldom preferable to the individual drugs prescribed separately.

New Antianxiety Drugs

There are already far more antianxiety drugs on the market than the clinician can or should master. The time-honored principle is to become familiar with one or more drugs in each pharmacological class. The psychological advantages of effectively and confidently using a familiar drug usually outweigh the actual pharmacological differences among the various drugs within a given class. One must expect that new antianxiety drugs will continue to be introduced into the market as significant therapeutic advances. However, the history of clinical pharmacology is replete with examples of new drugs which are heralded as both safe and efficacious and prove to be neither. The probability that newly introduced drugs will be more effective than established drugs is small, whereas the risk of unforeseen adverse reactions is appreciable (14). Therefore, one should wait until new drugs have been demonstrated to offer significant advantages before adding them to the armamentarium.

ANTIANXIETY AGENTS IN OTHER DISEASE STATES

Panic Attacks and Other Phobic States

Panic attacks are characterized by extreme anxiety, leading to terror, disorganization, disorientation, and depersonalization. Often these phobic states are elicited by contact with certain people or by restriction of mobility, as occurs in elevators, airplanes, and crowded restaurants. In children, one such state is "school phobia" (Chapter 25). Patients who demonstrate panic attacks also frequently experience anticipatory anxiety and free-floating anxiety in a variety of situations. Phobic states can be treated with psychotherapy, in conjunction with the use of antianxiety agents. Systematic desensitization and other techniques of behavioral modification are often useful and are considered to be the treatment of choice by some clinicians (15). An interesting prospect in the treatment of panic attacks and other phobic states is the use of antidepressants such as imipramine (16). Although their use for panic attacks is not approved by the FDA and must be viewed as experimental at this time, antidepressants seem to be effective with certain panic-ridden individuals.

Insomnia

As discussed in greater detail in Chapter 14, the antianxiety agents are used in certain types of insomnia. Great care must be exercised, since insomnia is a common complication of excessive drug use (17).

Muscle Tension and Convulsions

In addition to their antianxiety effects, the benzodiazepines are effective muscle relaxants. They are often useful in various muscular dystrophies, spastic states, psychosomatic disorders, and physical diseases associated with high levels of tension. Benzodiazepines have some utility as anticonvulsants in treating status epilepticus, alcohol and barbiturate withdrawal, and eclampsia. However, they are not useful prophylactics for grand mal or psychomotor seizures. Diazepam is frequently used as a preanesthetic and before cardioversion.

SUMMARY

For many patients, antianxiety agents are extremely useful; at the same time the compounds present a number of problems from a therapeutic and philosophical standpoint. There are concerns associated with the long-term use of such agents and many individuals abuse the materials. Appropriately, there is debate as to the role of these pharmacological substances in therapy.

The mechanisms of action of the antianxiety agents remain unclear despite several intriguing leads. Such mechanisms pose extremely interesting questions as to the relationships between the development of anxiety and biochemical aspects of its treatment. In contrast to many of the psychological problems considered in this volume, anxiety is ubiquitous; hence an understanding of the various mechanisms associated with it is of broad concern.

REFERENCES

1. Berger, F. M.   Anxiety and the discovery of tranquilizers. *In: Discoveries in Biological Psychiatry*. F. J. Ayd and B. Blackwell, *eds.*, Philadelphia: Lippincott, 1970, pp. 115–129.
2. Cohen, I. M.   The benzodiazepines. *In: Discoveries in Biological Psychiatry*. F. J. Ayd and B. Blackwell, *eds.*, Philadelphia: Lippincott, 1970, pp. 130–141.
3. Shader, R. I. and DiMascio, A., *eds*. *Psychotropic Drug Side Effects. Clinical and Theoretical Perspectives*. Baltimore: Williams and Wilkins, 1970.
4. Hollister, L. E. *Clinical Use of Psychotherapeutic Drugs*. Springfield: Thomas, 1973.
5. Shader, R. I., Greenblatt, D. J., Salzman, C., Kochansky, G. E., and Harmatz, A. B.   Benzodiazepines: safety and toxicity. *Dis. Nerv. Sys. 36:*23–26, 1975.
6. Greenblatt, D. J. and Shader, R. I.   *Benzodiazepines in Clinical Practice*. New York: Raven Press, 1974.
7. Greenblatt, D. J., Shader, R. I., and Koch-Weser, J.   Pharmacokinetics in clinical medicine: oxazepam versus other benzodiazepines. *Dis. Nerv. Sys. 36:*6–13, 1975.
8. Blackwell, B.   A critical review of oxazepam: efficacy and specificity. *Dis. Nerv. Sys. 36:*17–22, 1975.
9. Merlis, S. and Koepke, H. H.   The use of oxazepam in elderly patients. *Dis. Nerv. Sys. 36:*27–29, 1975.
10. Svenson, S. E. and Hamilton, R. G.   A critique of overemphasis on side effects with the psychotropic drugs: an analysis of 18,000 chlordiazepoxide-treated cases. *Curr. Ther. Res. 8:*455–464, 1966.
11. Boston Collaborative Drug Surveillance Program.   Clinical depression of the central nervous system due to diazepam and chlordiazepoxide in relation to cigarette smoking and age. *N. Eng. J. Med. 288:*277–280, 1973.
12. Greenblatt, D. J. and Shader, R. I.   Meprobamate: a study of irrational drug use. *Am. J. Psychiatry 127:*33–39, 1971.
13. Easton, J. D. and Sherman, D. G.   Somatic anxiety attacks. *Arch. Neurol. 33:*689–691, 1976.
14. Modell, W.   The hazards of new drugs. *Science 139:*1180–1185, 1963.
15. Brady, J. P.   Systematic desensitization. *In: Behavioral Modification, Principles and Clinical Applications*. W. S. Agras, *ed.*, Boston: Little, Brown, 1972, pp. 127–150.
16. Gittelman-Klein, R. and Klein, D. F.   Controlled imipramine treatment of school phobia. *Arch. Gen. Psychiatry 25:*204–207, 1971.
17. Dement, W. C. and Guilleminault, C.   Sleep disorders: the state of the art. *Hosp. Prac. 8*(11)57–71, 1973.

14 | Pharmacological Treatment of Sleep Disorders

WILLIAM C. DEMENT and

VINCENT P. ZARCONE, JR.

INTRODUCTION

Psychopharmacological attempts to treat sleep disorders affect 40 to 60 million people in the United States. Hundreds of prescription and nonprescription medications are marketed for insomnia or to produce drowsiness. Despite the obvious importance of this area, information about sleep disorders still relies heavily upon old mythologies about both normal sleep and sleep problems. Fortunately, several centers in the United States have begun to develop solid, empirical data for defining sleep disorders and for evaluating specific treatments of those disorders. This chapter emphasizes the general principles which have begun to emerge from that work.

Sleep and wakefulness are alternating phases in the daily cycle of existence. For many years, sleep has been viewed as a period of physical or psychological restoration. This conceptualization has led many people to conclude that the way they feel during the day—their moods, their energy, their desire, even their appetite—can be attributed to the "way" they sleep at night. However, recent studies do not confirm this view. For example, if the wake/sleep cycle of normal volunteers is reversed, the resulting insomnia of the new sleeping hours can be treated pharmacologically, with no effect on the concomitant sleepiness during the waking hours (1). Furthermore, the requirement for sleep appears to vary widely, both among individuals and over time for any given individual. These and other considerations have prompted a current trend toward viewing sleep and wakefulness as parts of a biological rhythm, with both parts serving important functions.

Studies to date suggest that sleep disorder complaints can be divided into several categories (Table 14-1). Insomniacs perceive a relationship between a nocturnal sleep disturbance and daytime problems, such as

TABLE 14-1.
COMMON SLEEP DISORDERS

Insomnia
  Nocturnal myoclonus
  "Restless legs" syndrome
  Central sleep apnea
  Drug-dependency insomnia
  Circadian rhythm disturbances
  Insomnias secondary to other disorders
Excessive Daytime Sleepiness (Hypersomnia)
  Narcolepsy syndrome
  Upper airway sleep apnea
Abnormal Nocturnal Behaviors
  Enuresis
  Somnambulism
  Night terrors

---

sleepiness, anxiety, tiredness, irritability, and inability to concentrate. Sometimes such patients can relate the two on a longitudinal basis, noting that absence of the perceived nocturnal disturbance is accompanied by a sense of relief during the day. Patients with excessive daytime sleepiness (hypersomnia) typically feel overwhelmingly sleepy and fall asleep during the day. However, they are not aware of a nighttime disturbance; and, indeed, substantial sleep deprivation is required to produce such a problem. Abnormal nocturnal behaviors, such as enuresis, somnambulism, and night terrors are more common among children and are discussed in Chapter 25.

SLEEP STAGES

Sleep consists of two distinct patterns (2,3). One type is characterized by rapid eye movements and is, therefore, called "REM" sleep. The second has been called non-REM or slow-wave sleep. REM sleep may be further characterized by phasic and tonic events. Phasic events include rapid eye movements, while tonic events include a desynchronized electroencephalogram (EEG) and a loss of muscle tone. Non-REM sleep has a synchronized EEG. It has been divided into four stages of increasing sleep depth. Stage 4 sleep, the deepest stage of non-REM sleep, occurs predominantly in the early part of the night.

INSOMNIA

Individuals may present to their physicians with specific complaints about inability to fall asleep at a conventional bedtime, about frequent or early awakenings, or about a feeling that sleep is inadequate despite normal duration. Many patients may be unable to define what sleep is not doing for them or why they are sure that sleeping pills are needed. These issues should be explored carefully, and assumptions both of the patient and of the physician should be evaluated. For example, it is often assumed that hospitalization induces sleep disturbance, for which the patient should receive medication. The physician should also explore past use of hypnotic agents, many of which produce tolerance (cf. Chapter 19). Such discussions may uncover cycles of drug dependency in which the patient knows from repeated trial that if he does not take a bedtime medication his sleep will, indeed, be worse. Complaints should also be evaluated for chronicity and severity. As physicians have become reluctant to prescribe sleep medications and skeptical about the complaint of insomnia, patients have escalated the intensity of their complaining in order to obtain sleeping pills. A reasonable rule may be that insomnia should have been present for at least three months with sufficient frequency to ensure that any given night will be characterized by subjectively disturbed sleep.

RELATION OF SUBJECTIVE COMPLAINT TO OBJECTIVE SLEEP PARAMETERS

Polygraphic techniques, particularly electroencephalographic (EEG) recording (polysomnography), permit precise measurement of sleep parameters. Sleep is defined objectively as a reversible state in which the organism ceases to respond meaningfully to complex environmental stimuli, and the EEG signs of sleep are very reliably correlated with the cessation of the organism's ability to respond. However, a significant group of individuals deny that they have been asleep, despite objective evidence of sleep. For example, in a recent study of drug-free insomniacs who complained of not falling asleep, 40 percent fell asleep in ten minutes or less, 65 percent fell asleep within thirty minutes, and 98 percent were asleep within sixty minutes (4). The reason for this discrepancy is unclear, and issues about sleep adequacy remain highly controversial. Certainly it is questionable whether such patients benefit from the use of sleep medications to lengthen objective sleep time.

SPECIFIC CAUSES

Nocturnal Myoclonus

First described in 1953, nocturnal myoclonus consists of repetitive muscular jerks occurring predominantly in the lower limbs at the onset of sleep and at times during the sleep period (5). Although it was originally believed to be a form of epilepsy, extensive EEG studies have conclusively ruled out an epileptic etiology. The diagnosis of nocturnal myoclonus is established when electromyelographic (EMG) recordings of the anterior tibial muscles show sleep-related, repetitive contractions which last about two seconds each and repeat rhythmically at intervals of approximately thirty seconds over long periods of time. Such contractions are not related to the hypnic jerks often experienced at sleep onset, and they occur very infrequently in matched control subjects who do not complain of a sleep disturbance. The myoclonic jerk is consistently followed by arousal of varying duration. Often, the most obvious response is autonomic, with a change in heart rate and marked peripheral vascular constriction. The patient's arousal is temporally associated with the movement, and longitudinal data unequivocally show that the perceived sleep disturbance decreases dramatically when the actual frequency of the abnormal movements decreases. A sample of a typical polygraphic recording for nocturnal myoclonus is shown in Figure 14-1. This syndrome may account for 15–20 percent of drug-free insomnias.

"Restless" Legs Syndrome

As first reported in 1945, some patients describe distracting and uncomfortable sensations in their legs when they are at rest (6), as occurs when they prepare to fall asleep. The urge to move, in order to relieve

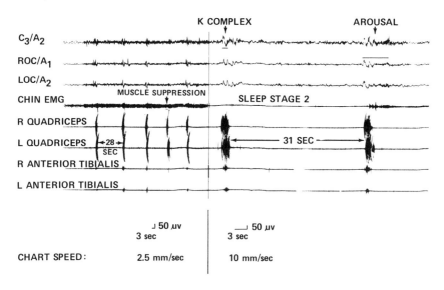

FIGURE 14-1. Nocturnal Myoclonus
Recorded at two different chart speeds; this tracing illustrates the periodic nature of the nocturnal movements and of the associated arousals.

the symptoms, can interfere with the onset of sleep. With time, this distressing pain may develop a glove- and boot-type distribution. Patients with "restless leg" syndrome uniformly have nocturnal myoclonus during sleep. In contrast, most patients with nocturnal myoclonus do not complain of restless leg at the time they are seen.

Central Sleep Apnea

A small number of patients show a failure of respiratory drive in association with the complaint of insomnia. This sleep apnea syndrome was first described in 1972 (7). In these patients, sleep-related repetitive apneas, involving the loss of contraction of the diaphragm and intercostal muscles, are followed by arousals of varying intervals. Hundreds of apneas a night lead to extremely disturbed sleep (Fig. 14-2). With "pathological sleep apneas," respiratory pauses are of more than ten seconds' duration, and thirty or more episodes occur in a single night. The incidence appears to be about 5 percent, although one study failed to identify any instances in a group of fifty insomniacs (8).

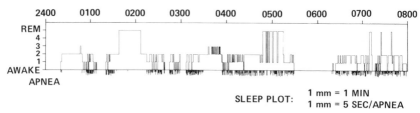

FIGURE 14-2. Effects of Apnea on Sleep

    This histogram of sleep stages demonstrates the disturbances related to sleep apnea in a patient complaining of insomnia.

Drug-Dependency Insomnia

As suggested earlier, the widespread chronic use of drugs for the symptomatic treatment of the complaint of insomnia has led to drug-dependency insomnia (9). The diagnosis is confirmed when successful withdrawal of sleep medication alleviates the complaint. A chronic, objectively verified sleep disturbance can be induced exclusively by sleeping pills in an individual whose sleep is otherwise completely normal. However, removal of a drug may reveal a second cause of insomnia, which first initiated the use of sleeping pills and the ultimate development of drug dependency.

Circadian Rhythm Disturbances

A variety of studies have shown conclusively that there is a twenty-four-hour rhythm for sleep, with a peak tendency to sleep occurring once daily. This rhythm parallels body temperature and is inversely related to performance. Sleep disturbance consistently occurs when subjects are expected to reverse their normal sleep/wake cycle. Furthermore, they have symptoms of fatigue and sleepiness during the newly scheduled hours of wakefulness. Though this is a very new area of investigation, it is clear that attempts to sleep at other than the "natural" time could lead to sleep problems. A familiar example of this phenomenon is the well-known "jet lag" syndrome.

The most clearly documented problem in cycle abnormalities is phase lag syndrome, in which a patient typically complains of a long history of inability to fall asleep. He is either taking or has often taken short-acting sleeping pills in an attempt to induce sleep at a normal bedtime. The patient does not feel sleepy at a conventional bedtime and describes long hours of lying in bed worrying and coping with anxiety. However, the patient also states that once asleep, he generally has no problem sleeping; instead, he finds it difficult to get up in the morning at a conventional time and maintain alertness and performance in the early hours of the day. Characteristically, he can "sleep in" on weekends or on vacation. A theoretical discussion of the potential sleep problems associated with pathology in this area may be found elsewhere (10).

Insomnia Complaint as a Nonspecific Symptom

The complaint of insomnia is associated with many other psychiatric and medical conditions. Neurotic depression and chronic anxiety with a characterologic disturbance may account for 20 percent and 10 percent, respectively, of patients with insomnia. In all of these cases, the insomnia must be regarded as a symptom, unless it is documented by polysomnography; and, in all such cases, causal relationships must remain uncertain. Pharmacological intervention depends upon the associated condition. Behavior modification, biofeedback and electro-sleep, and sleep hygiene counseling are important in many cases.

EXCESSIVE DAYTIME SLEEPINESS

Patients with excessive daytime sleepiness, or hypersomnia, typically complain of inappropriate sleep episodes during the day, which cannot be explained by sleep loss at night. Such episodes tend to begin at a specific time in life, mitigating against a constitutional requirement for more sleep than the patient habitually obtains. The inappropriateness of sleep frequently can be verified by observers, but the objective definition of excessive sleepiness is a little more complex. In some cases, the sleepiness is so continuous and pervasive that the patient loses his frame of reference, stating that he is fully alert even when he is patently sleepy to an observer.

The existence of excessive daytime sleepiness seems to be relatively easy to validate in questionable cases, using repeated testing of sleep latency. In normal volunteers, sleep latency has been reliably related to subjective sleepiness prior to the test (Fig. 14-3). If allowed to go to bed every two hours, subjects who are pathologically sleepy will invariably fall asleep in less than five minutes after the lights are turned out and often will doze in less than one minute. Normal subjects generally show much longer sleep latencies and are still awake after twenty minutes. A physician can be certain of the pathology when the patient falls asleep in highly inappropriate situations, such as when talking with a salesman, being scolded by a teacher, having intercourse, or riding a bicycle. Often hypersomnia appears to come on insidiously, with an increase in the tendency to fall asleep in soporific situations. Some care must be taken to be sure that nocturnal sleep is not, in fact, disturbed. The physician should also be aware that profound sleepiness is associated with performance and memory impairment. Thus an automatic behavior syndrome which has been associated with excessive daytime sleepiness may be mistaken for the fugue states of psychomotor epilepsy (11).

Because the area is still in a highly formative state, it is not surprising that there is great variation in reports of prevalence and in the description of hypersomnia syndromes. There is also a great deal of mythology. For example, in a recent survey, practicing physicians were asked

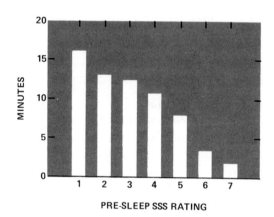

FIGURE 14-3. Relation of Subjective Sleepiness to Subsequent Electroencephalographic Sleep Latency

Abscissa: Stanford Sleepiness Scale (SSS) ratings from most awake (1 = feeling active and vital, alert, wide awake) to most sleepy (7 = almost in reveries, sleep onset soon, losing struggle to remain awake); ordinate: mean sleep latency. SSS rating 5 indicates unequivocal sleepiness, while sleep latencies under 10 minutes would suggest sleepiness.

to name the most common cause of hypersomnia. The three most frequently named disorders were hypothyroidism, hypoglycemia, and encephalitis. In contrast, a study of patients complaining of excessive daytime sleepiness revealed that 80 percent of them had either the narcolepsy syndrome or upper airway sleep apnea (12).

SPECIFIC CAUSES

The Narcolepsy Syndrome

The narcoleptic tetrad consists of sleep attacks, extreme muscular weakness (cataplexy), sleep paralysis, and hypnagogic or sleep-onset hallucinations (12). Severe narcoleptics may experience these attacks while standing, running, or driving. Narcolepsy is characterized by sleep disturbances, such as hypersomnia, disturbed nocturnal sleep, and pathological manifestations of REM sleep. The abnormalities in REM sleep include the appearance of sleep-onset REM periods and of dissociated REM-sleep inhibitory processes—cataplexy, and sleep paralysis. The diagnosis is relatively easy to make, if the patient has clear-cut cataplexy; if he does not, repeated observation and polysomnograms may be necessary to establish the cause of sleep attacks.

Upper Airway Sleep Apnea

During sleep, respiratory problems in the upper airway appear to be extremely common. Even normally, sleep onset is associated with an increase in upper airway resistance, as documented by the widespread occurrence of snoring. The problem is thought to result from a loss of tone in the muscles of the tongue, throat, and larynx. When this loss of tone is pathological, a complete functional obstruction of the upper airway can occur during sleep. In most cases, the patient has normal respiration when awake. There is no abnormality in respiratory drive, which is increased during apneic periods. Typically, the complaint of profound daytime sleepiness is related to excessive snoring, abnormal movement during sleep, morning headaches, loss of memory, and chronic hypertension. It is of major importance to differentiate sleep apnea from narcolepsy and other hypersomnia problems, because the treatment of choice for the upper airway sleep apnea is clearly surgical. Dramatic improvements have been seen in all signs and symptoms following chronic tracheostomy (13).

SPECIFIC PHARMACOLOGICAL TREATMENT
OF SLEEP DISORDERS

Unfortunately, the pharmacological approach to sleep disorders is hampered by the rather formative stage of our understanding of sleep biochemistry (14,15). In addition, many chemicals can affect sleep and wakefulness in multiple, often unknown ways. As a result, the treatment of specific sleep disorders syndromes has developed by trial and error and by serendipity.

INSOMNIA

Nocturnal Myoclonus

At the present time, there is no specific pharmacological treatment for nocturnal myoclonus. Symptomatic relief has been obtained with diazepam (Valium), 5–20 mg before bedtime, with a repeat dose upon undesired awakening. Interestingly, chronic use of chlorimipramine in narcoleptics has been associated with the development of this distressing leg movement syndrome.

Restless Legs Syndrome

Since the restless leg syndrome has been known for a relatively long time, a number of treatments have been proposed, including quinine, vitamin E, and barbiturates. Considerable relief can be obtained with carbamazepine (Tegretol). Patients on this medication must be followed very carefully, because of occasional bone marrow depression. Oxycodone (Percodan), one tablet before bedtime, is also useful; but the patient must be cautioned and supported, to avoid the danger of pharmacological addiction.

Central Sleep Apnea Syndrome

The physician should ask every patient complaining of insomnia whether or not he snores. In heavy snorers, symptomatic treatment should be avoided, since most currently available hypnotics are respiratory depressants; that effect, added to a central sleep apnea syndrome, could be fatal. The complaint and the incidence of apneas has been reduced with chlorimipramine, but effectiveness is lost with chronic administration (16).

Circadian Phase Lag Syndrome

As yet, no drug has been found which favorably shifts circadian rhythms. Therefore, pharmacological treatment of the phase lag is undesirable. As a major complicating problem in treating this syndrome, many patients are addicted to sleeping pills. This addiction must be treated first.

Symptomatic Treatment of Drug-Dependent Insomnia

Treatment of drug-dependency insomnia can often be surprisingly difficult for three reasons: 1) the patient strongly believes in the necessity of the drug and in the fact that he has insomnia, 2) the actual drug ingestion often involves multiple drugs and very inconsistent schedules of self-administration, and 3) the most effective program of withdrawal involves a very demanding interaction between physician and patient and the use of behavior-change contracts. Most hypnotic compounds cannot be withdrawn suddenly without serious consequences. Withdrawal programs for opiates, sedative-hypnotics, and alcohol are described in Chapter 23. Although these procedures can be used for treating drug-dependency insomnia, they often do not help the patient to reassess his beliefs about his sleeping problem. A program which may be more successful in these patients involves slow, stepwise withdrawal of the drug, aided by polygraphic monitoring of sleep, when necessary.

The first step of withdrawal is education of the patient. The true status of chronic hypnotic ingestion must be carefully explained. The patient must understand that inability to sleep upon cessation of sleep medication results from drug dependency, not insomnia. He must understand that he cannot always accurately assess his own sleep parameters and that he will sleep just as much and just as well at lower levels of medication, at which his normal sleep tendencies will eventually reassert themselves.

Step two is stabilization of the patient. The physician should assume complete control of the patient's medication, and all other involved physicians must stop writing prescriptions. Prescriptions should be issued to the patient on no more than a weekly basis; some pharmacists will even agree to a daily issue of sleeping medications. Furthermore, once the dose is set, the patient should be instructed to take the entire dose at the specified time. Even relatively high doses can usually be taken as a single dose. Many patients take a capsule or two and wait for something to happen; when nothing does, they may continue taking sleep medication throughout the night. Others will start taking medication early in the day, partly in anticipation of sleep and partly to counteract withdrawal symptomatology that they begin to experience either late in the previous sleep period or during the day.

The third step is actual withdrawal. If several drugs are being used, they should be withdrawn one drug at a time. As a drug is being withdrawn, the dose should be reduced by one unit each week. For example, if a patient were taking 1 g of sodium pentobarbital (Nembutal), on the first week he would take 900 mg and on the second week 800 mg. As the dose approaches zero, this schedule can be slowed, if needed. At each step, the patient will generally experience a slight worsening of subjective sleep parameters, with subsequent improvement. If possible, the withdrawal should be preceded by polygraphic monitoring; then, if the patient experiences doubt and skepticism about his sleep duration, he can be re-recorded and confronted with objective data that he is sleeping better with fewer drugs.

The final step is the complete withdrawal. There is some question whether placebos should be administered; some physicians find them to be beneficial (cf. Chapter 31). After complete withdrawal, there can be a very gradual improvement of symptoms over a four- to six-week period. Therefore, the patient should be cautioned to expect only gradual improvement over that time. It is possible that the patient will still have a sleep disturbance, and further study and treatment may well be necessary. In about 20 percent of insomniac complainers, drug withdrawal alone relieves the problem, verifying the diagnosis of drug dependency insomnia. In addition, about 50 percent of insomniacs have drug-induced insomnia as at least part of their problem.

EXCESSIVE DAYTIME SLEEPINESS

The Narcolepsy Syndrome

The narcoleptic has two problems: sleepiness and REM-sleep manifestations such as cataplexy, sleep paralysis, and hypnagogic hallucinations. These are affected by different drug treatments.

There are many difficulties with treating narcoleptic sleepiness. Tolerance to central stimulants almost invariably develops. In chronic users, sudden withdrawal from dextroamphetamine (Dexedrine) or methylphenidate (Ritalin) can lead to hypersomnia and serious depression (Chapter 21). In a narcoleptic patient who complains of excessive daytime sleepiness, some effort should be made to evaluate the actual intensity and the frequency of overwhelming sleep urges. The lowest effective dose of a stimulant medication should be prescribed. For example, methylphenidate, 5–20 mg, three to four times a day, can be used; the dose should be adjusted to minimize side effects. Often the narcoleptic patient has considerable difficulty in evaluating his subjective state of alertness. He is subject to automatic behaviors and may state that he is alert, only to fall asleep a few seconds later. There is some question, therefore, about the overall effectiveness of stimulants. As tolerance develops, patients should be withdrawn or given a "drug holiday." A few weeks after complete withdrawal, the compound can be reintroduced at a much lower dose. Tolerance is a continuing problem, since the illness is lifelong and the treatment is inadequate.

Abundant evidence suggests that cataplexy is a dissociated manifestation of the motor inhibitory process associated with REM sleep (2). Most drugs that are effective in treating cataplexy, e.g., the tricyclic antidepressants (tricyclics) and the monoamine oxidase (MAO) inhibitors, also are potent suppressors of REM sleep. Imipramine (Tofranil) is the drug of choice in treating cataplexy; 25–50 mg, one to three times a day is the dosage range. Tolerance may develop over time. The most troublesome long-term side effects of imipramine are the anticholinergic side effects, e.g., dry mouth and blurred vision (Chapter 11). In some males, there is considerable difficulty with sexual performance. Chlorimipramine is significantly more effective than imipramine and may work when imipramine has lost its effectiveness, even after withdrawal and reintroduction. High doses of amphetamine do not always block cataplexy, nor does methylphenidate. MAO inhibitors have been effective but should be used only as a last resort, because of the troublesome side effects (17).

USE OF SLEEP MEDICATIONS

As mentioned earlier, for about 20 percent of insomniac complainers, drug withdrawal alone relieves the problem, verifying a diagnosis of drug-dependency insomnia. In addition, about 50 percent of insomniacs have drug-induced insomnia as at least part of their problem. For this reason, chronic prescription of sleeping pills without careful investigation of the etiology of the complaint is unjustified and dangerous. If short-term symptomatic relief seems urgently desirable, a very definite course of hypnotic medication might be prescribed. Several rules should be followed:

- Only effective hypnotics should be used, and the period of use should be consistent with the demonstrated effectiveness of the drug. Thus, flurazepam (Dalmane) can be prescribed for twenty-eight consecutive nights, while secobarbital (Seconal) should be given for two to three days at most (9).
- Hypnotics should not be prescribed to heavy snorers without prior polysomnography, since snoring is a frequent sign of a sleep apnea syndrome.
- The dose of the hypnotic should never be escalated. If the hypnotic is ineffective in the therapeutic dose range, the patient probably does not have true insomnia.
- Drug accumulation should be avoided, to prevent daytime sedation. Drug doses should be kept at the minimum effective level. In addition, with chronic medication, it may be appropriate to schedule "drug holidays" (9). Whether these holidays lengthen the period of drug effectiveness is still unclear.

FUTURE DIRECTIONS

One of the exciting aspects of current sleep research is the effort to relate specific sleep disorders with abnormalities in brain function. As exemplified by our increased understanding of the "restless leg" syndrome and of the upper airway sleep apnea syndrome, careful physiological measures of sleep parameters have been of great value. However, there are still many instances in which such studies have not uncovered the etiology of the sleep disturbance. Recently, investigators have begun to examine central neuroregulator activity in sleep disorders, as reflected by measurable metabolites in the cerebrospinal fluid.

Although these studies are still relatively novel, they have already begun to yield interesting results. For example, a nonwakefulness syndrome has recently been associated with abnormally low cerebrospinal concentrations of homovanillic acid, a metabolite of dopamine (18). Another study identified hypersomniacs who had abnormally high cerebrospinal concentrations of 5-hydroxyindoleacetic acid (5-HIAA), the major metabolite of 5-hydroxytryptamine (serotonin) (19). Identification of normal mechanisms and of specific abnormalities in patients with various problems may greatly enhance our ability to devise appropriate pharmacological treatments for the disorders.

REFERENCES

1. Pollak, C. P., McGregor, P., and Weitzman, E. D. The effects of flurazepam on daytime sleep after acute sleep-wake cycle reversal. *Sleep Res.* 4:112, 1975.
2. Zarcone, V. Narcolepsy. *N. Engl. J. Med.* 288:1156–1165, 1973.
3. Guilleminault, C., Dement, W. C., and Passouant, P., *eds. Narcolepsy.* New York: Spectrum Publications, 1976.
4. Carskadon, M. A., Dement, W. C., Mitler, M. M., Guilleminault, C., Zarcone, V. P., and Spiegel, R. Self-reports versus sleep laboratory findings in 122 drug-free subjects with complaints of chronic insomnia. *Am. J. Psychiatry, 133:*1382–1388, 1976.
5. Guilleminault, C., Raynal, D., Weitzman, E., Dement, W. Sleep-related periodic myoclonus in patients complaining of insomnia. *Trans. Am. Neurol. Assoc. 100:*19-22, 1975.
6. Ekbom, K. A. Restless legs. *Acta Med. Scand., Suppl. 158:*1–123, 1945.
7. Guilleminault, C., Eldreidge, F. L., and Dement, W. C. Insomnia with sleep apnea: a new syndrome. *Science 181:*856–858, 1973.
8. Kales, A. and Kales, J. D. Sleep disorders: recent findings in the diagnosis and treatment of disturbed sleep. *N. Engl. J. Med. 290:*487–499, 1974.
9. Kales, A., Bixler, E. O., Tan, T., Scharf, M. B., and Kales, J. D. Chronic hypnotic-drug use. *J. Am. Med. Assoc. 227:*513–517, 1974.
10. Dement, W. C., Guilleminault, C., and Zarcone, V. The pathologies of sleep: a case series approach. *In: The Nervous System, Vol. 2: The Clinical Neurosciences.* D. B. Tower, *ed.,* New York: Raven Press, 1975, pp. 501–518.
11. Guilleminault, C., Billiard, M., Montplaisir, J., and Dement, W. C. Altered states of consciousness in disorders of daytime sleepiness. *J. Neurol. Sci. 26:*377–393, 1975.
12. Guilleminault, C. and Dement, W. C. 235 cases of excessive daytime sleepiness: diagnosis and tentative classification. *J. Neurol. Sci.,* 31:13–27, 1977.
13. Guilleminault, C., Tilkian, A., and Dement, W. C. The sleep apnea syndromes. *Ann. Rev. Med. 27:*465–484, 1976.
14. Jouvet, M. The role of monoamines and acetylcholine-containing neurons in the regulation of the sleep-waking cycle. *Ergeb. Physiol. 64:* 166–307, 1972.
15. Holman, R. B., Elliott, G. R., and Barchas, J. D. Neuroregulators and sleep mechanisms. *Ann. Rev. Med. 26:*499–520, 1975.
16. Kumashiro, H., Sato, M., Hirata, J., Baba, O., and Otsuki, S. Sleep apnea and sleep regulating mechanisms. *Folia Psychiatry Neurol. Jpn.* 25:41–49, 1971.
17. Wyatt, R. J., Fram, D. H., Buchbinder, R., and Snyder, F. Treatment of intractable narcolepsy with a monoamine oxidase inhibitor. *N. Engl. J. Med. 285:*987–991, 1971.
18. Mouret, J., Renaud, B., Quenin, P., Michel, D., and Schott, B. Monoamines et régulation de la vigilance. Apport et interpretation bio-

chemique des données polygraphiques. *In: Les Médiateurs Chimiques.* P. Girard and R. Couteaux, *eds.*, Paris: Masson, 1972, pp. 139–155.

19. Guilleminault, C. and Dement, W. C.   Pathologies of excessive sleep. *In: Advances in Sleep Research, Vol. 1.* E. Weitzman, *ed.*, New York: Spectrum Publications, 1974, pp. 345–390.

15 | Pharmacological Treatment of Aggressive Disturbances

BURR EICHELMAN

INTRODUCTION

This chapter is concerned with pharmacological treatment of individuals who are prone to displays of violence which are frequently beyond their control and are irrelevant in the context of the larger society. The psychiatrist dealing with such aggressive behavior continually must keep in mind that he is dealing with a symptom rather than a disease. Aggression may be defined as behavior leading to "the damage or destruction of some goal entity" (1). If the patient perceives his aggressive tendencies to be deleterious, he may approach the physician for aid in controlling the behavior in accordance with the usual voluntary patient-physician relationship. Alternatively, the society may consider an individual's behavior to be dangerous or antisocial and request that the psychiatrist intervene to control it. Psychiatrists should carefully scrutinize such interventions to evaluate whether they are acting as the agent of the patient or of society, whether they are functioning as physicians or as executors of the law, and whether their evaluation and treatment of the patient helps to reveal the underlying etiology of the violent behavior.

There are many interpersonal means for intervening with the potentially violent patient (2). Essentially, these methods focus upon teaching the patient to recognize with whom he is angry and to express his anger verbally rather than physically. Therapists need to have empathy with the patient, while setting firm limits and conveying an understanding of the potential consequences of the violent behavior. Initially, therapists often concentrate upon teaching the patient to introspect, to role-play, and to fantasize the contemplated violent event and its consequences. Such training may help to decrease the impulsiveness of certain violence-prone individuals. In addition, therapy can focus upon the development of other coping strategies. Patients may learn how to be verbally aggressive or how to bolster self-esteem without resorting to violence, perhaps through reachable achievements in vocation, sports, or interpersonal relationships. Therapy may also involve changing the milieu of the violent individual, particularly if a part of this environment includes potential victims who appear to taunt and dare the patient and who may even provide the weapon. Finally, therapy must remove the potential weapons from both the violence-prone individual and his victims.

Most states offer legal means for the involuntary detention of a patient who is imminently dangerous to others. The therapist should not reject this option automatically, if detention is in the interest of the patient and of his potential victim. Irretrievable loss of life outweighs a *transient* trespass on civil liberties. Further, following the Tarasoff case in California, it appears that the courts may mandate the therapist to warn the potential victim of an imminently dangerous or threatening individual, overriding elements of confidentiality.

The sources of aggressive behavior are multiple. We will focus here on some of the biological areas which have reference to psychopharmacology. Other biological aspects have been reviewed in a comprehensive report prepared by the National Institute of Neurological Diseases and Stroke (3), while other reviews consider various aspects of the aggressive behavior (4). Animal models, which may be profoundly limited when applied to the human, suggest that aggressive behavior has strong genetic predispositions (5) and neurochemical controls (6). However, there is no compelling evidence of genetic factors in human aggressive behavior. Animal aggression can be markedly altered by brain lesions and by drugs which alter brain neurotransmitter activity. Environmental stress also appears to function in the induction of animal aggression (7). Lastly, social learning theory underscores the power of reinforcement and modeling as a causal element in nonhuman and human aggressive behavior (8). The symptomatic violent behavior which the clinical psychiatrist witnesses may involve aspects of all of these potential influences. Consequently, intervention for this kind of behavioral problem must also become multifaceted. As already indicated, psychopharmacological treatment is only one part of clinical intervention.

BIOLOGICAL ASPECTS OF AGGRESSION

Although many of the current clinical interventions for violent behavior in humans have been developed empirically, new research with animal models of aggression may shed additional light on the functioning of neuronal systems associated with aggression. Models of animal aggression have been categorized in several ways. Moyer (1) has divided aggressive behavior into the following seven classes: predatory, intermale, fear-induced, irritable, territorial, maternal, and instrumental. Reis (9) has attempted to merge these groupings into two—predatory and affective aggression.

Predatory aggression is illustrated by mouse-killing (muricide) behavior in the rat or rat-killing in the cat. This behavior is often stereotyped, characterized by quiet biting in the cervical region of the prey and killing by cervical dislocation. In rats, certain members of the species persistently show this behavior, while others never exhibit it. The behavior can be induced in rats by facilitation of central brain cholinergic activity or by interference with brain levels of 5-hydroxytryptamine (9). Cholinergic implants by cannula into the hypothalamus or thalamus can induce this behavior. Treatment of rats with p-chlorophenylalanine (PCPA), a tryptophan hydroxylase inhibitor, lowers brain content of 5-hydroxytryptamine (Chapter 3) and also induces muricide. In combination, these findings suggest that a brain cholinergic system appears to induce this behavior, while a brain serotonergic system appears to inhibit it. These two systems may also be modulated by other neurotransmitters, such as norepinephrine.

Affective aggression is illustrated by rage behavior in the cat (9). Rage can be induced by electrical stimulation of the hypothalamus or amygdala or by cerebral transection. This behavior is enhanced by drugs which appear to facilitate the adrenergic systems of the brain, such as L-DOPA or protriptyline, and suppressed by drugs which block them, like haloperidol (Chapter 2). Neurochemical analyses of brain metabolites suggest that norepinephrine metabolites increase during this behavior, while brain norepinephrine itself decreases. This is compatible with the theory that enhanced noradrenergic activity is involved in the elicitation of affective aggression in the cat.

Central adrenergic metabolism also seems to play an important role in shock-induced aggression in the rat. Shock-induced aggression is instigated by placing two rats together in a gridded box and subjecting them to electric footshock. Under these conditions, they will attack each other. This behavior is facilitated by drugs and environmental stresses which seem to increase brain catecholamine metabolism or turnover (10), including drugs like antidepressants, rubidium, methylxanthines, and stresses such as rapid eye movement (REM) sleep deprivation or immobilization. It is inhibited by drugs such as lithium, which appear to decrease central catecholaminergic activity (Chapters 2 and 12).

There is a large literature on animal aggression, well beyond the scope of this chapter (6,9). However, the preclinical research in the neurochemistry of aggression suggests that we should begin to catalogue human aggressive behaviors more carefully, since various forms of inappropriate aggressive behaviors may have different neurochemical correlates and, potentially, different means for neurochemical intervention. Thus, it is important to study appropriate research patients for neurochemical correlates of their aggressive behavior. This might lead to a more directed and successful approach to the treatment of those forms of human aggressive behavior in which aggression is not a direct response to social conditions.

PHARMACOLOGICAL TREATMENTS OF HUMAN AGGRESSIVE BEHAVIOR

In reviewing possible pharmacological treatment paradigms for patients manifesting violent behavior, the reader should keep clearly in mind that the medications mentioned are usually approved only for treating the suspected underlying etiology of the aggressive behavior, rather than for treating aggression per se (Table 15-1). Thus, phenytoin (Dilantin) can be used if the physician believes there is an underlying, but as yet undocumented, seizure disorder; or a phenothiazine may be used when the physician suspects the aggression to be secondary to schizophrenia. Without a suspected underlying etiology, it is possible to overstep the accepted usage of an agent and enter into

TABLE 15-1.
TYPES OF HUMAN AGGRESSION

Origin of Violence	Drugs of Choice
Schizophrenic psychosis	Antipsychotics
Acute brain syndromes	Benzodiazepines Antipsychotics
Chronic brain syndromes	Antipsychotics Antihistamines
Mental retardation	Antipsychotics Anticonvulsants Benzodiazepines Lithium
Seizures and dyscontrol syndromes	Anticonvulsants
Mania	Lithium
Depression	Tricyclic Antidepressants Lithium
Sexual violence	Antipsychotics Antiandrogens

experimental treatment. This properly should be carried out only under approved protocols and investigational drug status.

Excellent references for a more comprehensive documentation of material given below are papers presented at the American Psychiatric Association's Meeting in 1973 (11–16). The philosophy of this chapter and of those papers is *to treat the underlying disorder if it is known or suspected.* Thus, if a patient is psychotic, with a diagnosis of acute schizophrenia, and is violent as a consequence of delusions or hallucinations secondary to his psychosis, antipsychotics should be used to treat the schizophrenia (Chapter 9). In cases of catatonic excitement, intramuscular doses of 5 mg of haloperidol (Haldol), repeated as often as every thirty minutes, may be necessary to reduce the agitation and violent behavior.

Acute organic brain syndromes or undiagnosed aberrant behavior should be treated with as little medication as possible (cf. Chapter 24). If medication is indicated, benzodiazepines should be used. When acute management is imperative, intravenous diazepam (Valium) can be given at a rate of up to 5 mg per minute to a total dose of 20–30 mg, just as it is administered for seizures. Antipsychotics may also be used.

Pericyazine (Aolept) has been suggested for treating psychomotor agitation in post-traumatic acute brain syndromes (12).

In chronic organic brain syndromes from senile dementia or arterio-sclerotic vascular disease, which can lead to violent behavior, antipsychotics are used. Haloperidol, 2 mg one to two times daily, can be effective. Thioridazine (Mellaril) and thiothixene (Navane) have also been recommended (12). In addition, the antihistamine diphenhydramine (Benadryl), 50 mg one to four times daily, can be useful.

In one recent report, mentally retarded, violent patients have been treated with phenothiazines, phenytoin, and lithium (12). A new benzodiazepine, SCH 12,679, was also suggested as potentially useful for treating aggressive behavior in retarded children. This same study recommends chlorpromazine (Thorazine) or haloperidol for the treatment of violent behavior associated with alcohol or narcotic withdrawal. However, since seizure thresholds are lowered during alcohol withdrawal, chlordiazepoxide (Librium), 100 mg every two to four hours, may be more appropriate. The treatment of violence associated with alcohol intoxication or withdrawal is discussed in Chapter 23.

Seizure disorders and seizure-like behavior such as the episodic dyscontrol syndrome (15) first require a thorough neurological evaluation, including repeated electroencephalograms (EEGs) with nasopharyngeal leads to rule out temporal lobe epilepsy. Even if no epileptogenic focus is found, such patients may well merit a trial course of anticonvulsant medication (15). Phenytoin or pimidone (Mysoline), may be used for patients with the episodic dyscontrol syndrome and additional seizure history. For those without a seizure history, chlordiazepoxide can be used, starting at 10 mg four times daily and increasing to 200 mg per day or until side effects develop.

Animal studies with lithium (14) and the clinical use of lithium in mania (Chapter 12) suggest that this agent might successfully inhibit certain types of violent behavior associated with disturbances of affect. Lithium has been used successfully in suppressing aggressive behavior in violent prison populations (14,17). This effect awaits further confirmation through double-blind studies. Lithium has also been reported to stabilize the mood swings associated with aggression in "emotionally unstable character disordered" girls (18).

Traditionally, patients whose violent behavior was thought to stem from an underlying depression have been treated with tricyclic antidepressants. Pharmacological treatment for this population of patients should now be subjected to closer controlled evaluation, since lithium also has antidepressant qualities (19), lithium appears to attenuate some types of human aggressive behavior (14), and tricyclic antidepressants exacerbate affective aggression in animal models (6).

The benzodiazepines, often used in the treatment of anxiety states (Chapter 13), have also been tried in the treatment of aggressive behavior (13). However, the efficacy of these agents appears to be inconsistent (20). In addition, there is no good characterization of an "anxious-aggressive" population that might be particularly targeted for receiving benzodiazepines. Furthermore, there are reports that benzodiazepines can enhance aggressive behavior in some clinical populations (13). It is still unclear whether this last effect stems directly from a neurochemical action or secondarily from a lowering of anxiety levels. Pragmatically, benzodiazepines should be reserved for patients complaining of irritability and violent behavior. When these drugs are prescribed, the behavior of the patients must be monitored, so that the medication can be withdrawn swiftly if the violent behavior appears to be increasing.

A final category of patients is designated as sexually violent. Whether the neurochemistry or learning contingencies for these individuals will prove different from "normals" or from other violent populations is a question for future clinical research. Empirically, many of these patients are treated with antipsychotics. Preliminary data suggest that antiandrogen agents like medroxyprogesterone acetate (Provera) may be beneficial for some members of this subgroup of patients (16).

CONCLUSION

Both the diagnosis and the pharmacological and behavioral treatment of disorders involving aggression and violence are in their infancy. Considerable preclinical work with animal models of agonistic and violent behavior is still needed (21–23). Human studies will require careful consideration of ethical and moral issues, particularly in terms of identifying those individuals who are appropriate for psychopharmacological therapy. For specific patients who may endanger themselves and others and who do not appear to have control over their violent behavior, psychopharmacological agents may be appropriate and helpful. Success with such agents usually will rest upon our ability to treat the underlying condition. Drug treatment of aggressive behavior highlights serious ethical issues of research on mental disorders; it would be inappropriate for research and treatment to be misused and misdirected as a means of social control. This topic is discussed further in Chapter 34.

REFERENCES

1. Moyer, K. E. Kinds of aggression and their physiological basis. *Commun. Behav. Biol. (Part A)* 2:65–87, 1968.
2. Lion, J. *Evaluation and Management of the Violent Patient.* Springfield: Thomas, 1972.
3. Goldstein, M., Woodhall, B., Huber, W., Purpura, D., Barchas, J., Flynn, J., and Walter, R. *(eds.)* Brain research and violent behavior. *Arch. Neurol.* 30:1–35, 1974.
4. Barchas, P. Approaches to aggression as a social behavior. *In: Interpersonal Behavior in Small Groups.* R. Ofshee, *ed.,* Englewood Cliffs: Prentice-Hall, 1973, pp. 388–401.
5. Orenberg, E. K., Renson, J., Elliott, G. R., Barchas, J. D., and Kessler, S. Genetic determination of aggressive behavior and brain cyclic AMP. *Psychopharmacol. Commun.* 1:99–107, 1975.
6. Eichelman, B. The catecholamines and aggressive behavior. *Neurosci. Res.* 5:109–129, 1973.
7. Lamprecht, F., Eichelman, B., Thoa, N. B., Williams, R. B., and Kopin, I. J. Rat fighting behavior: serum dopamine-beta-hydroxylase and hypothalamic tyrosine hydroxylase. *Science* 177:1214–1215, 1972.
8. Bandura, A. Social learning theory of aggression. *In: Control of Aggression: Implications from Basic Research.* J. F. Knutson, *ed.,* Chicago: Aldine, 1971, pp. 201–250.
9. Reis, D. J. Central neurotransmitters in aggression. *Res. Publ. Assoc. Res. Nerv. Ment. Dis.* 52:119–148, 1974.
10. Eichelman, B. Catecholamines and aggressive behavior. *In: Neuroregulators and Psychiatric Disorders.* E. Usdin, D. A. Hamburg, and J. D. Barchas, *eds.,* New York: Oxford University Press, 1977, pp. 146–150.
11. Lion, J. Conceptual issues in the use of drugs for the treatment of aggression in man. *J. Nerv. Ment. Dis.* 160:76–82, 1975.
12. Itil, T. M. and Wadud, A. Treatment of human aggression with major tranquilizers, antidepressants, and newer psychotropic drugs. *J. Nerv. Ment. Dis.* 160:83–99, 1975.
13. Azcarate, C. L. Minor tranquilizers in the treatment of aggression. *J. Nerv. Ment. Dis.* 160:100–107, 1975.
14. Sheard, M. H. Lithium in the treatment of aggression. *J. Nerv. Ment. Dis.* 160:108–118, 1975.
15. Monroe, R. R. Anticonvulsants in the treatment of aggression. *J. Nerv. Ment. Dis.* 160:119–126, 1975.
16. Blumer, D. and Migeon, C. Hormones and hormonal agents in the treatment of aggression. *J. Nerv. Ment. Dis.* 160:127–137, 1975.
17. Tupin, J. P., Smith, D. B., Classon, T. L., Kim, L. I., Nugent, A., and Groupe, A. Long term use of lithium in aggressive prisoners. *Compr. Psychiatry* 14:311–317, 1973.
18. Rifkin, A., Quitkin, F., Carrillo, C., Blumberg, A. G., and Klein, D. Lithium carbonate in emotionally unstable character disorders. *Arch. Gen. Psychiatry* 27:519–523, 1972.
19. Mendels, J. Lithium and depression. *In: Lithium: Its Role in Psychi-*

atric Research and Treatment. S. Gershon and B. Shopsin, *eds.,* New York: Plenum Press, 1973.

20. Garattini, S., Mussini, E., and Randall, L. O. (*eds.*) *The Benzodiazepines.* New York: Raven Press, 1973.

21. Stolk, J. M., Conner, R. L., Levine, S., and Barchas, J. D. Brain norepinephrine metabolism and shock-induced fighting behavior in rats: differential effects of shock and fighting on the neurochemical response to a common footshock stimulus. *J. Pharmacol. Exp. Ther. 190:*193–209, 1974.

22. Ciaranello, R. D., Lipsky, A., and Axelrod, J. Association between fighting behavior and catecholamine biosynthetic enzymes in two sublines of an inbred mouse strain. *Proc. Nat. Acad. Sci (U.S.A.) 71:*3006–3008, 1974.

23. Hamburg, D. A. Psychobiological studies of aggresive behavior. *Nature 230:*19–23, 1971.

16 | Hypnotic Agents in Psychiatric Evaluations

BURR EICHELMAN, FLOYD M. ESTESS,
and THOMAS A. GONDA

INTRODUCTION

Psychiatrists have capitalized upon the ability of several drugs to enhance aspects of interpersonal dialogue by incorporating their use into some interview methods. In the past several decades, classes of drugs which are used as acute facilitators of the psychiatric interview have been narrowed to include primarily the short-acting barbiturates. This chapter briefly reviews the history of the use of these drugs in the psychiatric interview and describes techniques for conducting such a session.

HISTORY AND CURRENT USE

Prior to the widespread use of phenothiazines, psychiatrists noted that barbiturates could have a normalizing effect on some schizophrenic patients. Catatonic patients in either excited or retarded states would often temporarily relate in nonpsychotic ways during treatment with intravenous barbiturates (1,2). Severely schizophrenic patients who were resistive, mute, and unwilling to eat, drink, or give essential information frequently became tractable and facilitative under the influence of a barbiturate. "Narcoanalysis" was developed as a diagnostic and therapeutic tool for neurotic disorders (3) and reached its pinnacle during World War II in the diagnosis and treatment of war neuroses, as reported in the classic monograph of Grinker and Spiegel (4). Barbiturates were also employed to differentiate schizophrenia from organic brain syndromes. This differential diagnosis relied upon observations that patients with an organic brain syndrome often worsen or become paradoxically agitated on barbiturates, while schizophrenic patients frequently behave less psychotically.

Stimulants have also been used as facilitators of the psychiatric interview, either alone or in conjunction with short-acting barbiturates. Methamphetamine has been used in the interview process with schizophrenic patients (2,5). Similar reports for methylphenidate also have reached the literature, with particular emphasis upon the usefulness of this drug in increasing the rate of speech in interviews (6).

Currently, short-acting barbiturates have three major uses in the psychiatric interview. First, sodium amobarbital (Amytal) can be used as a diagnostic tool to determine the degree of suicidal ideation and depressive affect which may be present in fugue or "accident-prone" patients whose illness appears to involve a major element of dissociation and denial. Second, Amytal interviews are useful in the search for a precipitating event of hysterical conversion reactions. Finally, sodium methohexital (Brevital), in concert with the procedures described by Brady (7), can act as an ancillary facilitator of relaxation during the development of a desensitization hierarchy for phobias. Until recently, concurrent use of sodium amobarbital and methylphenidate has been indicated in patients who become more relaxed with sodium amobarbital but whose speaking rate is laboriously retarded. With these patients, sodium amobarbital appears to allow relaxation and reduce editing, denial, and dissociation during the interview, while methylphenidate increases both the tempo and pressure of speech and the expression of affect (8).

TECHNIQUES FOR AMYTAL INTERVIEW

The physician should begin the Amytal interview by carefully explaining the procedure to the patient and obtaining a written informed consent from him. During this discussion, the physician should verify that barbiturates are not contraindicated for the patient. Contraindications include pharyngitis or post-intubation status, a previous history of laryngospasm with barbiturates, liver failure or hepatitis, porphyria, and recent treatment with heavily sedating drugs.

Interviews should be conducted in a setting in which appropriate resuscitation equipment is immediately available should laryngospasm occur. This complication is rare but potentially life-threatening. The patient should abstain from all food and liquids for the morning, to avoid the risks of aspiration. The Amytal solution should be prepared in advance and consists of 1 g of sodium amobarbital in 20 ml of sterile water.

For the interview, the patient reclines in a softly lighted room. Depending upon the expectations for the interview and its potential for later use in therapy, the session may be recorded on audio- or video-tape, with the patient's consent. A butterfly intravenous line, with a stopcock, is established. Then, induction is achieved by injecting the sodium amobarbital at a rate of approximately 2 ml per minute, while the patient counts backward from a hundred. Generally, by the time a count of 50 to 40 has been reached, the patient's speech is slurred and errors in the reversed counting are being committed. At this time, the injection is temporarily stopped, and the intravenous line is irrigated with saline. The interview commences and need not deviate in format from an interview in the waking state. However, it is usually directed toward specific goals, such as determining the level of suicidal risk or ascertaining the precipitant for a fugue or conversion symptom which has not been consciously presented in prior interviews. During the course of the interview, the patient's degree of relaxation will lighten, requiring additional administration of sodium amobarbital. No more than 1 g of sodium amobarbital should be used, but this is more than sufficient for a two-hour interview. Following the interview, the intra-venous line is removed, and the patient is allowed to rest or to fall asleep. He should be observed regularly for any signs of deepening sedation. Generally, the patient is kept under observation for several hours after he awakens from the interview; he can then be released, preferably to friends or family who can stay with him for several more hours. Patients are often amnesic in recalling part or even most of the interview.

For a patient extremely slow in speech or for one who previously had difficulty in self-expression, either in a nondrug interview or in an Amy-tal interview, methylphenidate has been added to the interview medica-tion. The initial induction procedure is identical to that for Amytal alone. The intravenous line is then flushed with saline to remove the barbitu-rate, which otherwise will precipitate methylphenidate. Generally, a total dose of 15 mg is sufficient, with doses in the literature ranging from 10–50 mg (9,10). However, intravenous methylphenidate is no longer available, except as an investigational drug.

The Brevital interview described by Brady is part of a technique of systematic desensitization (7). Systematic desensitization is an attempt to decrease a patient's anxiety by progressively exposing him to a feared situation, while his anxiety has been inhibited. Progressive muscle relaxation is the most common method for inhibiting anxiety during systematic desensitization. However, sodium methohexital can also produce potent and reliable anxiety-inhibition for the brief periods necessary for desensitization. Brady utilizes 1.0–1.5 ml (10–15 mg) of sodium methohexital, given intravenously over two to three minutes. The therapist can give up to an additional 4 ml over the next twenty to thirty minutes. Following the desensitization session, the patient is alert in ten to fifteen minutes.

CASE HISTORY

The following case history illustrates the initial use of the Amytal interview for diagnostic purposes. The results of this interview encouraged a subsequent successful hypnotherapeutic intervention in a patient with recurrent fugues:

J.H. was a twenty-four-year-old single white woman with a chief complaint of blackout spells. She had been referred to the University from the Community Mental Health Center. She reported a nine-month history of blackout spells characterized by periods of absence of awareness for seemingly purposeful activities. On one occasion she reportedly opened her car door into oncoming traffic, not having been aware of how she got there. On another, while totally unaware of her actions, she left her apartment at night, drove twenty miles to the beach, parked her car, and began wading into the ocean, at which time she regained awareness.

The patient worked as a telephone operator. She was in a relationship with a single man who was prepared to marry her when she had lost sufficient weight; if she couldn't reduce, he was going to leave her. No other acute situational stress was uncovered during the initial history. Although somewhat cheerful, J.H. was very concerned about her obesity. She denied any current suicidal ideation, although she acknowledged that she had nearly succeeded in a suicide attempt three years previously, following the termination of an affair. Since this behavior was compatible with the presence of dissociative episodes, it seemed appropriate to conduct an Amytal interview, to reveal the triggering mechanisms for them and to see whether they included an unconscious suicide plan.

The Amytal interview was performed and videotaped with the patient's written consent. During this interview, J.H. presented many previously repressed, affect-laden areas of history. She related how fearful she was of her parents' increasing disability and approaching deaths. But she also told how her mother had beaten her and locked her into closets as a young child and had had her committed to a foster home as an adolescent. J.H. related that she had been raped by her cousins as a preadolescent. She described her desperate feelings of abandonment at the end of her affair three years ago and her wish that she had succeeded with the suicide. During this interview her demeanor was one of intense distress and pain. She trembled and shook, crying deeply. The following day she had no recollection of the content or affect presented in the interview.

On the basis of the findings during the Amytal interview and in the presence of a completely negative neurological evaluation, she was treated for dissociative reaction accompanied by marked depression with uncovering psychotherapy facilitated by hypnosis. She is fugue-free, has lost over forty pounds, is engaged, and is gainfully employed.

SUMMARY

Short-acting barbiturates, used either alone or in combination with methylphenidate, can facilitate evaluative psychiatric interviews, particularly for patients with dissociative or conversion symptoms. These techniques have also been employed to differentiate organic brain syndromes from schizophrenias and other psychiatric disorders. In addition, short-acting barbiturates can be utilized as an ancillary aid in desensitization therapy. The reader is referred to the references for further information about these latter uses of hypnotic agents in psychiatric practice.

REFERENCES

1. Bleckwenn, W. J. Production of sleep and rest in psychotic cases. *Arch. Neurol. Psychiatry* 24:365–372, 1930.
2. Pennes, H. H. Clinical reactions of schizophrenics to sodium Amytal, Pervitin hydrochloride, mescaline sulfate, and d-lysergic acid diethyl-amide (LSD-25). *J. Nerv. Ment. Dis.* 119:95–112, 1954.
3. Horsley, J. S. Narcoanalysis. *J. Ment. Sci.* 82:416–422, 1936.
4. Grinker, R. R. and Spiegel, J. P. *War Neuroses.* New York: McGraw-Hill, 1945.
5. Hope, J. M., Callaway, E., and Sands, S. L. Intravenous Pervitin and the psychopathology of schizophrenia. *Dis. Nerv. Sys.* 12:67–72, 1951.
6. Guile, L. A. Intravenous methylphenidate—a pilot study. *Med. J. Aust.* 2:93–97, 1963.
7. Brady, J. P. Systematic desensitization. *In: Behavior Modification: Principles and Clinical Applications,* W. Stewart Agras, *ed.,* Boston: Little, Brown, 1972, pp. 127–150.
8. Yalom, I. D. Plantar warts: a case study. *J. Nerv. Ment. Dis.* 138:163–171, 1964.
9. Freed, H. The use of Ritalin intravenously as a diagnostic adjuvant in psychiatry. *Am. J. Psychiatry* 114:944, 1958.
10. Witton, K. Directive psychotherapy with parenteral Ritalin in advanced schizophrenia. *Dis. Nerv. Sys.* 21:683–685, 1960.

17 | Side Effects of and Adverse Reactions to Psychotropic Medications

ROBERT L. SACK

INTRODUCTION

To some extent, side effects are a matter of definition. For example, the sedative effects of some of the major tranquilizers may be a useful property when dealing with a highly excited patient but an adverse effect when treating a patient who must remain alert in order to maintain an occupation. Likewise, the anticholinergic activity of the tricyclic antidepressants (tricyclics) may cause unwanted urinary retention in the elderly and yet be a useful property when treating children with urinary incontinence (enuresis). Since psychotropic drugs within each major class are very similar in action and efficacy on target symptoms, the selection of a particular drug often involves consideration of certain side effects. Thus, thioridazine (Mellaril) and trifluoperazine (Stelazine) have similar antipsychotic efficacy, so that the relative sedative side effects of the two drugs may determine the choice of treatment for a particular patient.

Many of the side effects and toxic reactions described below have been mentioned in previous chapters in association with particular drugs. However, instead of cataloging toxic and side effects as they pertain to each drug or class of drugs, this chapter will focus on particular organ systems as they are affected by psychotropic drugs (Table 17-1). Effects on organ systems are especially relevant in dealing with patients who have a concurrent medical problem, since questions often arise as to what interactions can be expected between a particular drug and a diseased organ. For additional information about the complex area of drug side effects, the reader may refer to several excellent and more detailed reviews (1–6). Problems of overdose and addiction with psychoactive drugs are discussed in the chapters on each agent and in Chapters 23 and 24.

TABLE 17-1.

ADVERSE EFFECTS OF PSYCHOTROPIC DRUGS ON ORGAN SYSTEMS

SYSTEM	EFFECTS	DRUGS
Autonomic	Anticholinergic Dry mouth and skin Urinary retention Poor visual accommo- dation	Antipsychotics, Tricyclics
	Excessive perspiration	Phenothiazines, Tricyclics, Benzodiazepines
Cardiac	ECG abnormalities and arrhythmias	Phenothiazines (esp. thioridazine), Tricyclics
Cardiovascular	Hypotension	Phenothiazines, Tricyclics, MAO inhibitors
	Hypertension	MAO inhibitors + Adrenergic stimulators (e.g., tyramine, amphetamines, epinephrine, norepinephrine, and L-DOPA)
Dermatological	Skin rash Photosensitivity	All drugs Phenothiazines (esp. chlorproma- zine)
	Pigmentation	Phenothiazines (esp. chlorproma- zine)
Endocrinological	Amenorrhea Galactorrhea and gynecomastia	Antipsychotics Antipsychotics
Gastrointestinal	Nausea and vomiting Constipation Paralytic ileus	Antipsychotics Phenothiazines and Tricyclics Phenothiazines + Tricyclics + Antiparkinsonian agents
	Increased body weight	Antipsychotics, Tricyclics
Hematological	Leukopenia and agranulocytosis Leukocyctosis	Antipsychotics Lithium
Hepatic	Induction of metabolic enzymes	Barbiturates, Haloperidol (possibly)
	Toxic reactions Cholestatis Hepatotoxicity	Phenothiazines (esp. chlorproma- zine), Tricyclics MAO inhibitors
Neurological	Extrapyramidal reactions Parkinsonian syndrome Acute dystonias Akathisia	Antipsychotics
	Tardive Dyskinesia	Antipsychotics
Ophthalmological	Lens Pigmentation	Phenothiazines (esp. chlorproma- zine and thioridazine)
	Pigmentary Retinopathy	Thioridazine

AUTONOMIC EFFECTS

Both the antipsychotics and the tricyclics are potent anticholinergics and frequently produce symptoms of dry mouth and skin, urinary retention, and poor visual accommodation (7). Dry mouth usually diminishes with time. Some patients counteract the effect with hard candy. Unfortunately, this sometimes leads to monilial infestations in the mouth; therefore, it is better to use a sugarless breath-freshener if the dry mouth is bothersome. Dry skin from the anticholinergic suppression of sweating is not noticed by most patients. However, in hot weather, hyperthermic reactions and deaths have occurred in patients taking phenothiazines, in part because of an inability to dissipate heat.

Urinary retention is a frequent problem with phenothiazines or tricyclics, especially in older males with prostatic hypertrophy. It is probably much more common than reported by patients. If the patient cannot void, he may require catheterization, which can precipitate a urinary-tract infection. Bethanecol chloride (Urecholine) is sometimes useful for acute retention (Chapter 11). Dosage of the psychotropic drug should be reduced when this side effect occurs; once the urinary function has improved, a higher dose may often be resumed without further problems.

Difficulties with visual accommodation are a common anticholinergic effect of the tricyclics and phenothiazines, resulting from relaxation of the ciliary muscle of the eye. This problem usually disappears after the first week. Patients who have to read can use inexpensive, ready-made reading glasses until the blurred vision passes.

Excessive perspiration (hyperhydrosis) has been reported with tricyclics, phenothiazines, and benzodiazepines. A particularly dramatic form of hyperhydrosis sometimes occurs, involving only the upper half of the body and face. Changing to another drug is recommended if the problem persists. The mechanism of this hyperhydrosis is unknown.

CARDIAC EFFECTS

The phenothiazines, particularly thioridazine, and the tricyclics regularly cause electrocardiographic (ECG) changes. Most frequent abnormalities are prolongation of the P-R interval, lowering of the S-T segment, and flattening of the T-wave. The significance of these changes has been a source of controversy, but generally they are considered to be benign. However, it is well known that, in toxic doses, tricyclics can cause severe disturbances in cardiac rhythm (8). Furthermore, in one group of patients with pre-existing cardiac disease, there were sudden deaths in 13 of 119 patients treated with amitriptyline, as compared to 3 in a comparable control group (9). The high incidence was not found with patients on imipramine or in noncardiac patients. There have been reports of sudden death in otherwise healthy young adults taking phenothiazines or tricyclics in which cardiac disturbances have been proposed as the mechanism of death. However, this hypothesis is without direct verification.

Obviously, caution should be exercised in treating patients with known cardiac abnormalities. The greatest concern is hypotension, which can compromise cardiac perfusion. Patients with known rhythm abnormalities should be treated cautiously, with frequent ECG monitoring. Since most patients with cardiac disease are elderly and since older patients often respond to less than the usual dose of psychotropic drugs, lower doses should be employed in this age group (Chapter 28). Of the antipsychotics, haloperidol (Haldol) probably has the fewest cardiovascular side effects. In questionable cases, a cardiology consultation should be obtained. The benzodiazepines are quite safe in patients with heart disease.

CARDIOVASCULAR EFFECTS

The phenothiazines, the tricyclics, and the monoamine oxidase (MAO) inhibitors all routinely cause some problems with postural hypotension in otherwise healthy patients. Ordinarily, postural hypotension is more bothersome than dangerous. However, in patients with arteriosclerotic vascular disease or peripheral neuropathy, blood pressure may drop to dangerous levels. Risks include a cerebrovascular occlusion, myocardial infarct, and injury from falling during a fainting episode.

The mechanism of postural hypotension is probably different for the drugs mentioned. The phenothiazines have a strong α-adrenergic blocking effect which probably accounts for their blood-pressure-reducing activity. The MAO inhibitors may induce formation of a false transmitter substance at the sympathetic nerve junction, resulting in decreased sympathetic tone (Chapter 11).

The usual treatment of postural hypotension is simply to warn the patient not to assume an upright position suddenly. It may be desirable to give the drug only at night, to reduce the chances of syncope. If the problem is more acute, the patient should be placed at bed rest, with the head below the pelvis, until the crisis has passed. Since postural hypotension can result from volume depletion, any dehydration should be corrected. If the hypotension is severe and pressor agents are required, *epinephrine should be avoided,* since the β-receptor vasodilating properties of the drug in the presence of phenothiazine-induced α-blockade may aggravate the problem. Severe hypotension can be treated with *norepinephrine* in doses sufficient to overcome phenothiazine blockade. Of the antipsychotic drugs, haloperidol may have the least hypotensive effects and is the drug of choice in problematical situations.

The most notorious elevations in blood pressure are the hypertensive crises occurring with MAO inhibitors. Episodes occur when a patient taking one of these drugs is given an adrenergic agonist or ingests a food high in tyramine content. Symptoms include headache, palpitations, nausea, vomiting, flushing, photophobia, and fever. The mechanism for these reactions is thought to be an exaggerated effect of exogenous adrenergic agonists on blood pressure when MAO is inhibited. Ordinarily MAO in the gut and liver metabolizes tyramine from food before it is absorbed into the systemic circulation; when the enzyme is inhibited, tyramine enters the circulation and acts on sympathetic neurons to rapidly raise blood pressure. Foods that can produce this reaction include nonprocessed cheese, herring, canned figs, chocolate, yeasts, red wine (especially Chianti), chicken livers, fava beans, beer, and meat extracts. Medicines which can cause a hypertensive crisis are amphetamines, epinephrine, norepinephrine, L-DOPA, certain cold remedies, nasal decongestants, and anorexiants. Patients should be warned to avoid preparations of local anesthetics which contain epinephrine.

Although the tricyclics potentiate amines and have been reported to be incompatible with the MAO inhibitors in some cases, the combination has been used extensively by some clinicians with no serious problems. This combination may prove to be justified in certain serious cases of depression (Chapter 11). If the combination is to be used, it may be better to start with the tricyclics and then add the MAO inhibitor cautiously.

DERMATOLOGICAL EFFECTS

Skin reactions to psychotropic drugs are common but usually are not serious. From 5 to 10 percent of patients taking chlorpromazine experience an allergic skin rash. Interruption of the drug is usually required, but treatment may be resumed once the rash has subsided. Because many patients are on more than one drug, the specific offender may never be identified. It seems quite clear that phenothiazine drug rashes do not signal impending anaphylactoid reactions; therefore, drug therapy need not be stopped altogether. Photosensitivity reactions are characteristic of phenothiazines, with an incidence of about 3 percent. The counteractive measure is to advise vulnerable patients to use a sun-screen lotion when they expect to be in direct sunlight for a protracted period of time. The thioxanthine antipsychotics have a very low incidence of photosensitivity and are preferred for vulnerable patients. Skin pigmentation may also occur with phenothiazines, particularly with chlorpromazine and thioridazine. Skin pigmentation should alert the physician to possible pigmentation in the eye as well.

ENDOCRINOLOGICAL EFFECTS

Amenorrhea is reported to be a common side effect of psychotropic drugs, particularly phenothiazines. The incidence is uncertain, since menstrual irregularities are common in untreated patients as well. The effect should not cause alarm but may be reversed by decreasing the dosage or introducing intermittent dosage regimens. It is, of course, important to rule out other possibilities for amenorrhea, including pregnancy.

Infrequently, galactorrhea and gynecomastia are side effects of psychotropic drugs, especially with the antipsychotics. The mechanism appears to involve blockade of dopaminergic neurons, resulting in decreased release of prolactin inhibitory factor. This permits increased prolactin secretion by the pituitary, which stimulates the mammary glands. Usually the problem can be corrected by lowering the dose or by changing to a different antipsychotic agent.

GASTROINTESTINAL EFFECTS

Paradoxically, although the antipsychotics are used in the treatment of nausea and vomiting, they can also induce these disturbances. The mechanism is unknown but may result from anticholinergic effects of decreased motility and relaxation of the stomach. Constipation is a much more common side effect of phenothiazines and tricyclics. In more severe cases, it may lead to impaction and paradoxical diarrhea. Stool softeners are a useful counteractive measure. Some cases of paralytic ileus have been attributed to the combination of phenothiazines, tricyclic antidepressants, and antiparkinsonian drugs. All three of these drugs have potent anticholinergic activity; in combination the effects are synergistic. It is unnecessary, and sometimes dangerous, to add antiparkinsonian agents to a phenothiazine-tricyclic regimen: the anticholinergic effects of this latter combination are usually quite sufficient to prevent extrapyramidal symptoms.

Increases in body weight often accompany treatment with the tricyclics and the antipsychotics. With depressed patients, this is usually a desirable effect, since it reflects the reversal of anorexia and correlates with clinical improvement. With other patients, an increase in body weight may be quite undesirable. There is no specific counteractive measure, except for the obvious one of dieting.

HEMATOLOGICAL EFFECTS

Agranulocytosis is the most common and significant blood dyscrasia caused by psychotropic drugs. In fact, in terms of the absolute number of cases, antipsychotics may currently be the most important drugs causing agranulocytosis (10). The exact incidence is unknown but is probably about 0.1 percent. Older individuals are more susceptible, as are women and Caucasians. There is a continuing dispute as to whether the reaction is dose related. Nearly all of the antipsychotics and tricyclics have been reported to cause this complication, although haloperidol may not.

When it occurs, agranulocytosis usually appears within the first eight weeks of treatment. The white count drops precipitously over two to five days. Because of the rapid decline in the white count, routine monitoring is probably not helpful, although some cases have been discovered before the development of symptoms. The patient typically complains of fever, pharyngeal soreness and ulcerations, adenopathy, and sometimes an infection which fails to heal. Some patients may develop a leukopenia without developing agranulocytosis; however, if the total leukocyte count falls below 3500, the drug should be stopped.

The basic principle of treatment is to stop the drug and treat any infection vigorously. In most patients with agranulocytosis, recovery will take place within two weeks, although fatalities from agranulocytosis do occur. Reverse isolation may be needed to protect the patient from infection.

Lithium carbonate can produce a leukocytosis which may reach levels suggestive of infection. The leukocytosis is apparently benign and is only of importance in that it may confuse the diagnosis when a source of infection is suspected (Chapter 12).

HEPATIC EFFECTS

As a rule, most drugs are metabolized in the liver to products which are biologically less active and more water soluble, so that excretion by the kidney can take place. The exceptions to this rule are useful to keep in mind when treating patients with marginal liver function. For example, one may choose a drug like paraldehyde, which, in part, is excreted by the lungs, or phenobarbital, which is excreted, to a large extent, by the kidneys. Some drugs are excreted by the bile, but ordinarily reabsorption takes place in the intestinal tract and ultimately the drug is excreted in the kidney. In cases of biliary obstruction, excretion of these drugs is greatly reduced.

The enzyme systems concerned with the biotransformation of drugs are located in the microsomal endoplasmic reticulum. Treatment of a patient with certain drugs may stimulate the activities of these enzymes, resulting in increasing tolerance to the drug or to other drugs metabolized by the same system. The best-known example of this effect is the stimulation of liver microsomal enzymes by repeated administration of barbiturates (Chapter 19). This can result in decreased blood levels of barbiturates and of other metabolic competitors, including warfarin anticoagulants, meprobamate, estrogens, and phenytoin. Of particular concern is the dangerously erratic control of anticoagulation in patients treated with barbiturates. There is some evidence that haloperidol may stimulate liver microsomal enzymes as well. As knowledge of drug interactions expands, other examples of enzyme induction probably will be discovered.

Toxic effects on the liver have been reported for phenothiazines, tricyclics, and MAO inhibitors. Chlorpromazine-induced jaundice was of much greater concern in the earlier years of its use and now has practically disappeared. The cause of this decline is unknown. Transient abnormalities in liver-function tests are not uncommon in the course of phenothiazine therapy, but they ordinarily do not herald the onset of a toxic reaction. Several of the first MAO inhibitors, such as iproniazid and pheniprazine, have been withdrawn from the market because of liver toxicity. The liver toxicity differs from the self-limited cholestatic jaundice of chlorpromazine; rather, the reaction is a fulminating hepatocellular necrosis which is indistinguishable from viral hepatitis. The hydrazine MAO inhibitors cause liver toxicity more frequently than do the nonhydrazines.

In view of the above toxic effects, there is often concern about giving antipsychotic and antidepressant drugs to a patient with pre-existing liver disease. However, there is no evidence that pre-existing liver disease predisposes patients to these reactions. Consequently, the patient's risk for the development of a toxic hepatitis is no greater than that for the general population. If a reaction were to occur, the effect would be cumulative; still, hepatotoxic reactions are now so rare that this risk is small.

NEUROLOGIC EFFECTS

All of the antipsychotic drugs currently marketed in the United States can cause extrapyramidal reactions. Clozapine and lenperone, which are not yet released, rarely, if ever, cause them. The commonly used antipsychotic drugs differ significantly in their tendency to induce these side effects: piperazine phenothiazines and butyrophenones are the most common offenders, while thioridazine is the least. The occurrence of extrapyramidal reactions is also related to individual differences in susceptibility. The three general types of extrapyramidal reactions have the following manifestations:

Parkinsonian Syndrome—"pill-rolling" tremor, slow movements, cogwheel rigidity, drooling, masklike face, and slow mental activity.

Acute Dystonias—severe rolling of eyes (oculogyric crises), and spasms of the tongue and face, of the neck (torticollis), and, occasionally, of the spine and extremities (opisthotonos).

Akathisia—restlessness, with particular difficulties in sitting still; patient typically shifts his weight from foot to foot and paces about.

Akathisia is the most easily missed of the extrapyramidal reactions, since it may resemble psychotic excitement or agitated depression; sometimes a repetitious, alternating rhythm of the movements will suggest the diagnosis. Acute dystonic reactions are more frequent among young males, while parkinsonian reactions and akathisia are more frequent among the middle-aged.

There is general agreement that antipsychotic drugs produce these effects through receptor blockade of dopaminergic motor tracts. At least two explanations have been offered about the different incidences of extrapyramidal reactions for various antipsychotic drugs. First, these drugs have different anticholinergic potencies, which may determine the ability to act as their own antiparkinsonian agents. Second, they may be differentially active on specific dopaminergic tracts, so that drugs with the least tendency to produce extrapyramidal reactions are those which have least activity on the dopaminergic motor tracts.

In principle, all extrapyramidal reactions can be treated either by reducing the dose of antipsychotic drug or by balancing dopaminergic blockade with an anticholinergic drug. Some of the reactions will disappear with increasing doses of the antipsychotic drug, because of the concomitant increase in anticholinergic effects. With the parkinsonian syndrome, the addition of an oral antiparkinsonian drug will usually bring dramatic relief. Acute dystonic reactions can be treated with intramuscular or intravenous injections of antiparkinsonian agents for more rapid onset of action (Chapter 7). Akathisia is the most refractory reaction to treat with anticholinergics and often requires substitution of another preparation.

Opinions differ as to whether antiparkinsonian drugs should be administered prophylactically or only upon development of the extrapyramidal reactions. Since about 15 percent of patients receiving antipsychotic drugs develop these reactions and since they can be a frightening experience for a patient, an argument can be made for the prophylactic use of antiparkinsonian drugs. On the other hand, extrapyramidal reactions are never fatal in themselves, while co-administration of antiparkinson drugs increases the intensity of anticholinergic side effects. Once instituted, an antiparkinsonian agent need not be given indefinitely. Only about 25 percent of the patients receiving antiparkinsonian agents for previous extrapyramidal reactions will have any further symptoms if the drug is withdrawn.

Tardive dyskinesia, the other major and extremely important neurological side effect of the antipsychotics, is discussed in Chapter 9.

OPHTHALMOLOGICAL EFFECTS

Pigmentary changes in the eye were not appreciated as a problem with phenothiazine treatment until a number of patients had been on high doses for a considerable length of time (11). It is now recognized that these problems can occur rather early in high-dose treatment. There are apparently two distinct syndromes. The first is typically associated with chlorpromazine treatment and consists of a deposit of light, dusty pigment on the anterior portion of the lens. This eventually develops into a stellate, cataract-like formation. In severe cases, pigmentation may be noted in the anterior lens, posterior cornea, anterior cornea, conjunctiva, skin, and, finally, retina. Pigmentation in the skin is invariably associated with changes in the eye and calls for a thorough ocular examination. Ordinarily, these deposits do not affect visual acuity, although they can in severe cases. Composition of this pigment is still unknown; it may be melanin or some metabolite of chlorpromazine. A number of treatments have resulted in some improvement, but substitution of a different phenothiazine seems to be the simplest approach. These deposits are definitely dose related. Patients on high doses of chlorpromazine or thioridazine, the most frequently reported offenders, should receive a slit-lamp examination periodically.

Pigmentary retinopathy is a more serious complication associated with high-dose thioridazine therapy. It occurs in vulnerable patients after doses of over 1.2 g per day for four to eight weeks. There are clumps of pigment on the retina and retinal edema. The patient complains of a brownish discoloration of vision and may notice a marked slowing of dark adaptation. In severe cases, a significant decrease in visual acuity, or even blindness, may result. However, visual acuity usually returns to normal once the drug is discontinued. Apparently, doses of thioridazine less than 800 mg per day are safe.

CONCLUSION

Rapid recognition and prompt treatment of unwanted side effects is an important part of clinical practice. In general, an open discussion with the patient of potential side effects enhances trust rather than arouses apprehension. For example, unless the patient is forewarned, unexpected blurred vision from psychotropic medication may seem to confirm delusions of bodily deterioration in a psychotically depressed individual. Furthermore, some side effects can be alleviated by counteractive measures which will result in greater patient compliance with treatment. This is particularly important when relapse is likely if the patient fails to take his medication. Since many patients will not relate side-effect symptoms to the medication they are taking, it is important to make frequent inquiries.

Side effects can also have important theoretical implications. In some cases, an analysis of side effects has helped to elucidate the major action of a drug. For example, the close connection between antipsychotic efficacy and the production of extrapyramidal side effects contributed significantly to the development of the hypothesis that dopamine receptor blockade is the major mechanism of action of these drugs (Chapter 8). Thus, attention to side effects is sometimes relevant to scientific progress as well as to good clinical practice.

REFERENCES

1. Shader, R. I. and DiMascio, A., eds., *Psychotropic Drug Side Effects*. Baltimore: Williams and Wilkins, 1970.
2. Kline, N. S. and Angst, J. Side effects of psychotropic drugs. *Psychiatr. Ann.* 5:8–39, 1975.
3. Mielke, D. Adverse reactions associated with mood altering drugs. *Psychiatr. Ann.* 5:71–89, 1975.
4. Davis, J. M., Bartlett, E., and Termini, B. A. Overdosage of psychotherapeutic drugs—a review. *Dis. Nerv. Syst.* 29:157–164, 1968.
5. Hollister, L. E. Toxicology of psychotherapeutic drugs. *In: Principles of Psychopharmacology*. W. G. Clark and J. del Guidice, *eds.*, New York: Academic Press, 1970, pp. 537–546.
6. Kline, N. S., Alexander, S., and Chamberlain, A. *Manual of Overdoses with Psychotropic Drugs*. Oxadell, N.J.: Medical Economics, 1974.
7. Hsu, J. J. and Yap, A. T. Autonomic reactions in relation to psychotropic drugs. *Dis. Nerv. Syst.* 28:304–310, 1976.
8. Jefferson, J. W. A review of the cardiovascular effects and toxicity of tricyclic antidepressants. *Psychosom. Med.* 37:160–179, 1975.
9. Couel, D. C., Crooks, J., Dingwall-Fordyce, I., Scott, A. M., and Weir, R. D. A method of monitoring drugs for adverse reactions. II. Amitriptyline and cardiac disease. *Eur. J. Clin. Pharmacol.* 3:51–55, 1970.
10. Huguley, C. M., Jr. Drug-induced blood dyscrasias. *In: Disease-a-Month*. H. F. Dowling, *ed.*, Chicago: Year Book Medical Publishers, 1963.
11. Siddall, J. R. The ocular toxic findings with prolonged and high dosage chlorpromazine intake. *Arch. Ophthal.* 74:460–464, 1965.

III | Psychopharmacology of Drug Abuse

The drugs of abuse are of intense interest from both theoretical and clinical standpoints. The powerful effects of these generally small molecules raise important questions about the mechanisms by which they act. For example, it is astounding that the complex human organism can become addicted to a two-carbon compound, ethanol. Yet addiction does occur—and with high psychological, social, and economic costs. The first five chapters focus upon our current understanding of the biochemistry of major addicting and nonaddicting drugs of abuse, including opiates, sedative hypnotics, alcohol, central nervous system stimulants, and hallucinogens.

Chapters 23 and 24 contain a detailed discussion of the problems of diagnosing and treating drug abuse. While Part II concentrated upon the positive uses of psychopharmacological agents in treating psychiatric disorders, these two chapters examine the negative effects of abusing psychoactive drugs. Thus, alcohol abuse may affect more than ten percent of the population and is probably the most serious public health problem confronting the middle aged. Drug overdose and withdrawal constitute a growing emergency-room problem that requires insightful but speedy intervention. The long-term treatment and rehabilitation of alcoholics and other drug abusers continues to be a perplexing problem for both physicians and society.

291

18 | Opiates:
Biological Mechanisms

HUDA AKIL

INTRODUCTION

The opiates are probably unequaled in their power to bewilder both the user and the observer. They induce effects ranging from pain reduction and pleasure to the misery of "cold turkey" withdrawal. To the clinician, they represent a valuable tool for pain relief, even though their utility is marred by the rapid development of tolerance and by the serious potential for addiction. To the pharmacologist and neuroscientist, they have opened avenues of investigation into drug receptor interactions, pain systems, and feedback mechanisms. Their action appears to involve the complex interfaces of sensory, autonomic, motivational, and emotional systems. Thus, difficulties in uncovering the basic mechanisms underlying the acute and chronic effects of opiates have been immense. And yet, in the last few years, dramatic advances have been made in our understanding of opiate-related phenomena, rendering narcotic research one of the fastest advancing fields in the neurosciences.

HISTORY

No one knows when opium was first discovered, but there are records of its use by Sumerians nearly six thousand years ago. Techniques for collecting opium from the seed boll of the poppy *Papaver somniferum* were detailed by the Assyrians and are essentially unchanged today. Greek physicians used opium as a medicant, as did Galen. By the ninth century, opium was also known in China, where it was introduced by the Arabs.

During the nineteenth century, opium use was widespread. Both in the United States and in England, grocery stores, general stores, and mail-order catalogues advertised opium preparations as "pain killers," "cough mixtures," "women's friends," and "consumption cures." Factory workers used laudanum, an alcoholic solution of opium, to quiet crying babies. Even a popular drink called "Godfrey's Cordial" contained opium, along with molasses and sassafras flavoring (1). In 1805, Saturner, a pharmacist in Hanover, Germany, reported the isolation of a pure alkaloid base from opium. He named it "morphine," after the Greek god of sleep, Morpheus. Diacetylmorphine, or heroin, was not produced until 1874. Preparations containing either of these two substances became increasingly popular during the last part of that century.

While opium use was legal in the 1800's, many considered it to be disreputable, if not immoral. Crusades against opium use led first to laws banning "opium dens." where opium was smoked, and then to increased tariffs on opium imports. Further pressures resulted from the 1906 Pure Food and Drug Act, which required that medicines state their contents on the label, if they contained drugs such as the opiates. This was followed, in 1914, by the Harrison Narcotic Act, which restricted legal distribution of opiates to physicians. Opiates are still of major importance in medicine, since they are potent analgesics. In addition, however, illegal users of opiates currently may number more than 500,000 in the United States alone, despite strict laws against non-medicinal sale and use (1).

STRUCTURE-ACTIVITY RELATIONSHIPS

Figure 18-1 shows a schematic illustration of the three-dimensional configuration of morphine. This T-shaped molecule has two broad, hydrophobic surfaces which are at right angles and a methylated nitrogen which is usually charged at physiological pH. This charged nitrogen is essential for activity and lies in one of the hydrophobic planes. The hydroxyl group at carbon 3 on the other plane is also essential. On the other hand, neither the hydroxyl group at carbon 6 nor the ester linkage is needed for activity, as demonstrated by the activity of levorphanol (Fig. 18-2).

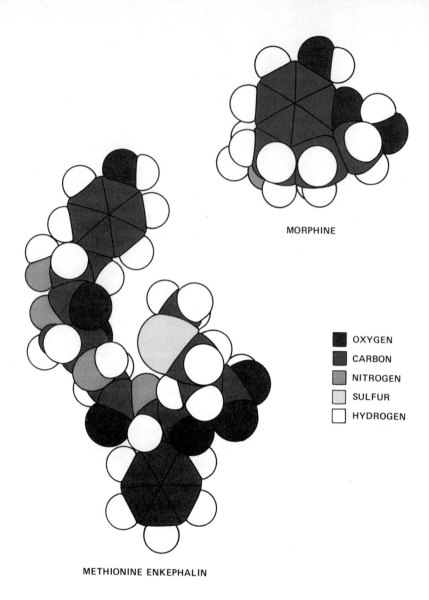

MORPHINE

OXYGEN
CARBON
NITROGEN
SULFUR
HYDROGEN

METHIONINE ENKEPHALIN

FIGURE 18-1. Three-Dimensional Illustrations of Morphine and Methionine Enkephalin

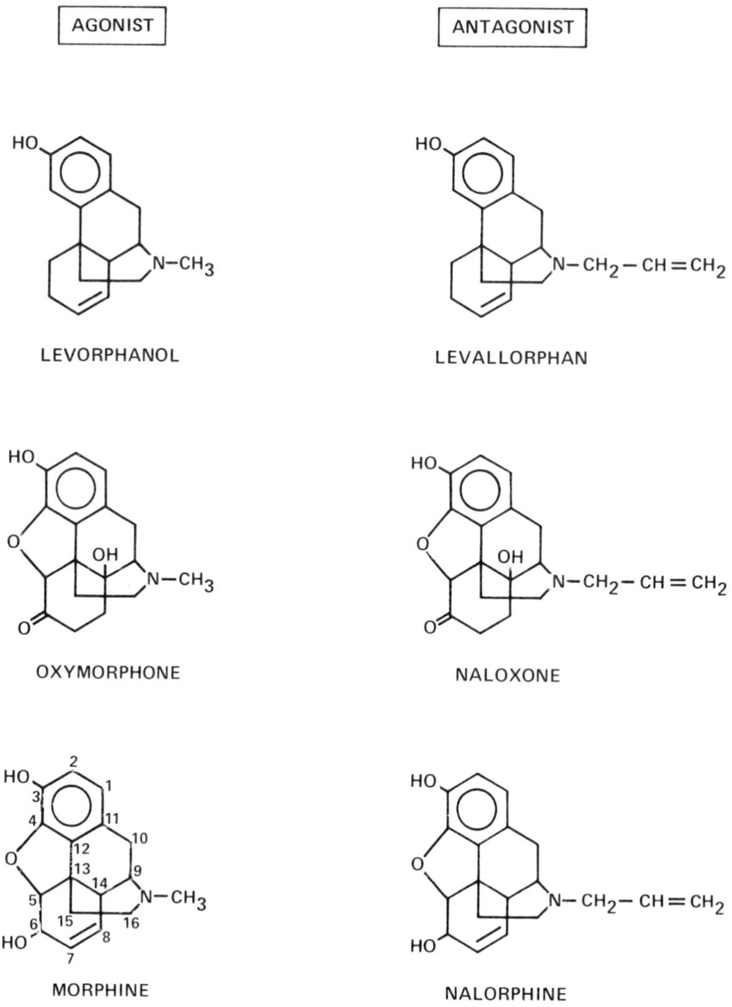

AGONIST   ANTAGONIST

LEVORPHANOL   LEVALLORPHAN

OXYMORPHONE   NALOXONE

MORPHINE   NALORPHINE

FIGURE 18-2. Several Opiate Agonist-Antagonist Pairs

Note that the pairs differ only in the presence or absence of an allyl group on the nitrogen.

Most natural and synthetic opiates exhibit the same T-shaped configuration. Even with methadone, which looks strikingly different, steric forces produce a configuration which closely resembles that of other opiates (2). Most opiates exist in two forms, differing only by being mirror images of one another. These forms can be distinguished by their ability to rotate polarized light to the left (levorotary) or right (dextrorotary). Typically, pharmacological activity resides only in the levo isomers of opiates, while the dextro isomers are usually devoid of analgesic activity.

Relatively minor substitutions in the opiate molecule can lead to the production of opiate antagonists, which are not only poor agonists but actually prevent or reverse the effects of agonists. These drugs usually differ from their corresponding agonists by having allyl, cyclopropyl, methyl, or propyl substituents on the nitrogen. Figure 18-2 depicts some agonist-antagonist pairs which involve the substitution of an allyl function for the nitrogen methyl group.

OPIATE RECEPTORS

The strict structural requirements of opiates, their high potency, their stereospecificity, and the existence of agonists and antagonists all favored the proposal that narcotics exert their action by binding to specific opiate receptors (3). In 1973, three separate groups—headed by E. Simon at New York Medical Center, L. Terrenius in Uppsala, Sweden, and S. Snyder at Johns Hopkins—demonstrated specific opiate binding in the nervous system. Employing a paradigm suggested by A. Goldstein (4), they showed that opiate binding is saturable and stereospecific and occurs at low concentrations of ligand. The binding sites are selective, exhibiting little or no binding of nonopiate agents. In addition, the affinity of a given opiate for the receptor correlates well with its activity in bioassay systems and with its clinical potency.

Both Snyder and Simon demonstrated a differential distribution of the opiate binding sites within the mammalian brain. Generally, regions associated with pain transmission are rich in opiate receptors. These areas include the dorsal horn of the spinal cord and the gray core surrounding the 4th ventricle, the aqueduct of Sylvius, and the 3rd ventricle. In rat and monkey, these same midbrain and medial thalamic sites are also very sensitive to morphine. Furthermore, morphine infusion in the midbrain periaqueductal gray sites brings about tolerance and abstinence symptoms upon withdrawal (5,6). Two receptor-rich areas which do not appear to be closely related to pain transmission are the striatum and the amygdala. These latter structures are thought to mediate opiate motor effects and emotional concomitants, respectively.

Snyder and Simon also described what is commonly known as the "sodium effect" on opiate receptors. In the *in vitro* binding procedure, even low concentrations of sodium induce dramatic alterations in the receptor affinities: antagonist binding increases, while that of agonists decreases. This and other evidence led Snyder (7) to propose that the opiate receptor exists in two conformations: an antagonist form, which binds sodium, and an agonist form, which does not. The exact mechanisms regulating interconversion between configurations and the physiological consequences of such changes remain unknown.

BEHAVIORAL AND NEUROCHEMICAL EFFECTS

Opiates bring about important mood changes, sleepiness, mental clouding, and autonomic signs like pupillary constriction and respiratory depression. The spectrum of these effects varies dramatically between species and even among individuals within a species. For example, morphine produces drowsiness in man and in several other species; in others, it creates a stimulated state known, in the cat, as "morphine mania." The mood changes in man are equally unpredictable. While some describe a peculiar state of well-being and euphoria during opiate use, other subjects feel only negative effects such as nausea. Although many of these opiate effects are intriguing, those of primary interest are analgesia, tolerance, and dependence.

ANALGESIA

Narcotics are the most potent analgesic agents known. They markedly reduce pain responsiveness in animals and appear to decrease both sensory and emotional components of pain in man. The mechanisms by which the opiates produce this effect are unknown, and a complete review of this topic lies outside the scope of this psychopharmacology text. However, since pain is the basis of a great deal of emotional learning, a better understanding of its inhibition might be one key to the study of mood and emotional disturbances. Thus, several features of opiate analgesia are of potential relevance to our understanding of other important opiate effects, including euphoria, tolerance, and dependence.

As described earlier, the brain contains specific regions which are rich in opiate receptors; these same areas are also sensitive to microinjections of opiates. Such data suggest that there may be a neuronal system involved in opiate-induced analgesia. This system appears to interact with other brain neuroregulators, since disruption of serotonergic activity can block opiate analgesia. Very recently, investigators have also shown that this system can be activated by electrical stimulation. This has already proven to be a useful clinical tool with human patients who have intractable pain: a few minutes of stimulation can provide several hours of pain relief and appear to avoid many of the side effects of narcotics (8). Stimulation-produced analgesia shares several characteristics of opiates, being partially reversed by naloxone (9) and exhibiting partial tolerance and cross-tolerance with opiates (10). These findings provide physiological evidence of an endogenous opiate-like system with an anatomical distribution paralleling that of the opiate receptors. Thus, both opiates and electrical stimulation could activate the same pain inhibitory system, with morphine binding to the receptors and electrical stimulation releasing an endogenous opiate-like factor. The recent discovery of such a factor is described later in this chapter.

TOLERANCE AND DEPENDENCE

The physical and psychological effects of opiate addiction and withdrawal are described in Chapter 23. As indicated in that chapter, tolerance to opiates develops with chronic use of the drug; the abstinence syndrome also has a characteristic timecourse. Thus, both effects appear to involve some relatively slow physiological change. Although the underlying mechanisms of these phenomena are unknown, there are several interesting hypotheses about biological processes which might be involved.

Any reasonable hypothesis must explain important empirical facts about opiate addiction. For example, tolerance and physical dependence appear to be inextricably linked. That is, a tolerant individual will enter withdrawal if the drug is withheld, but when withdrawal is complete, tolerance to all opiates disappears. Furthermore, decreased sensitivity to agonists is accompanied by an increased sensitivity to antagonists, so that, in tolerant individuals, very small doses of the latter reverse agonist effects and precipitate withdrawal. Theories of tolerance and dependence cannot invoke major changes of narcotic concentrations in blood or brain, since the rate of absorption or metabolism are not dramatically altered in addicted animals and cannot account for the magnitude of tolerance and dependence.

Many theories of opiate addiction start with the concepts of specific opiate receptors and drug-receptor interactions. While some focus upon the opiate receptors themselves, others concentrate upon central pathways which might be influenced by these receptors. Several of the theories revolve around the concept of physiological adaptation. The body frequently responds to a disturbance in homeostasis by initiating counteracting processes. If these processes are successful, increasingly higher doses of the disruptive agent are needed to obtain a response, i.e., tolerance develops. Withdrawal of the disruptive agent leaves the compensating forces unopposed, disrupting homeostasis in the opposite direction and leading to symptoms opposite to those occurring with acute administration. As the body recovers from this second disturbance, homeostasis is restored.

The denervation supersensitivity hypothesis offers a good example of an application of these concepts to opiate tolerance and dependence (11). Anatomical or pharmacological denervation can lead to increased sensitivity of the denervated receptor to its ligand, a neurotransmitter. By binding to the opiate receptor, morphine might produce a sustained decrease in neuronal firing. This functional denervation could lead to sensitization of the postsynaptic receptors in the terminal fields of that neuron. As the receptors become more responsive to smaller concentrations of the neurotransmitter, more morphine will be required to effectively block transmission. Upon morphine withdrawal, supersensitivity becomes apparent and is manifested as abstinence. This interesting hypothesis will be difficult to test until the connection between the opiate system and other neuroregulators is established.

Goldstein *et al.* (2) have suggested that tolerance may reflect an increase in the absolute number of opiate receptors, so that higher concentrations of drug are needed to maintain the same number of unoccupied receptors. When the drug is withdrawn, the expanded receptor pool would be uncovered, producing effects which are opposite to those initially caused by receptor occupancy with narcotics. This hypothesis has not been supported by opiate binding studies, which have failed to detect any changes in number of opiate receptors in tolerant animals. Takemori (12) suggested a variant of this idea, proposing that qualitatively different receptors may develop during tolerance. Again, however, opiate binding studies show no obvious changes in binding affinity *in vitro*.

Snyder (7) has argued that *in vivo* conformational changes of the receptor may be the crucial factor, based upon the existence of the two conformational forms of the opiate receptor, which were mentioned earlier. Since tolerance and dependence involve decreased sensitivity to agonists and increased susceptibility to antagonists, Snyder proposed that these processes are associated with a change in the opiate receptor which favors the antagonist form at the expense of the agonist form. This attractive theory places the change at the receptor and takes into consideration the paradoxical increase in sensitivity to antagonists. Currently, it is difficult to test, since available procedures are not well suited for studying the dynamic interconversion of the receptor between conformational states.

The most recent hypotheses of tolerance and dependence focus upon the regulatory mechanism of the endogenous opiate peptides. Unlike the above proposals, these emphasize possible changes on the presynaptic side of opiate-sensitive synapse. An example of such theories will be described in the next section of this chapter.

ENDOGENOUS OPIATES

The existence of specific opiate receptors, as demonstrated both by pharmacological and by binding studies, suggested that endogenous opiate-like factors might be the natural ligands to these receptors. If such a system existed in the brain, one might expect opiate antagonists to produce physiological and behavioral changes. And yet, opiate antagonists have little or no effects on their own. The possibility remained, however, that the endogenous opiate system was relatively "silent" under normal conditions and that it needed to be activated before an antagonist effect could be uncovered, as might occur with stimulation-produced analgesia. The convergence of physiological evidence with the pharmacological evidence rendered the existence of endogenous opiates increasingly likely.

In 1974, Hughes and Kosterlitz reported the existence of a substance in brain which produced opiate-like effects on the vas deferens bioassay for narcotics. These effects were reversible by the antagonist naloxone. The Aberdeen group subsequently purified this substance (13), characterized it as a peptide, and identified its sequence (14). The activity was found to reside in two pentapeptides which were termed "enkephalins" and which differed by one terminal residue:

Methionine-enkephalin (see Fig. 18-1)—
 H · Tyrosine · Glycine · Glycine · Phenylalanine · Methionine · OH
Leucine-enkephalin
 H · Tyrosine · Glycine · Glycine · Phenylalanine · Leucine · OH

Subsequently, the enkephalins were identified by Snyder's group, employing the radioreceptor assay (15). Both groups reported that the enkephalins are unevenly distributed in the brain and that their distribution parallels that of opiate receptors. Detailed information about pathways must await extensive immunocytochemical mapping.

Hughes *et al.* (14) noted that the sequence of methionine-enkephalin occurs in the C-fragment of β-lipotropin, a pituitary peptide thought to be the β-MSH prohormone. Other investigators reported that various fragments of β-lipotropin did, in fact, possess opiate-like activity (16). These fragments all began with the five amino acid residues which constitute methionine-enkephalin (β-LPH 61–65). By consensus, the entire class of endogenous factors with morphine-like activity are called "endorphins," while "enkephalins" denotes the two specific pentapeptides identified by Hughes and his co-workers.

The exact relationship between the pituitary endorphins and the enkephalins is still unknown. Furthermore, there is recent evidence that large endorphins may also exist in brain (17). These endorphins appear to differ structurally from the pituitary peptides, although their exact sequence is still unknown. It is generally hypothesized that larger endorphins may be active neuromodulators in their own right and may also constitute the precursors of the enkephalins.

A number of recent pharmacological studies have shown that both enkephalins and endorphins produce naloxone-reversible analgesia when microinjected into opiate-sensitive sites and sustain the development of opiate-like tolerance, cross-tolerance, and physical dependence in rats and mice (6,18). While enkephalin and the β-lipotropin fragments are equipotent in bio- and binding assays, enkephalins are rapidly degraded *in vivo*. Therefore, their pharmacological effects are far more transient than are those of the pituitary endorphins, which produce powerful and long-term analgesia, even with intravenous administration.

If the endorphins are the natural ligands for the opiate receptors, it is reasonable to expect that they exhibit significant changes if the receptor is repeatedly bombarded with an exogenous drug such as morphine. Enkephalin levels increase as tolerance develops and decrease with naloxone-precipitated withdrawal (19). This suggests that continuous morphine administration may lead to a decrease in firing of enkephalin-containing neurons—reflected as increased content. Precipitated withdrawal leads to the opposite effects, i.e., compensatory increases in firing and release, leading to decreased levels. Whether these compensatory changes in opiate peptides are of a large enough magnitude to account for tolerance and withdrawal remains to be determined.

CONCLUSION

What began as an investigation into the potent effects of a few plant alkaloids has led to the discovery of a whole neuronal system in mammalian brains. Furthermore, it is a system for which scientists are in the enviable position of having a wide spectrum of agonists and antagonists, a receptor assay, and several bioassays. Rapid progress is already being made in establishing how much of the opiate effects involve interactions with this system. However, that is but a portion of the future task, for we still know little about the normal function of this fascinating new system.

The endorphins may be at the crossroad of several neuronal mechanisms. They may have evolved from rather primitive systems involved in pain and stress modulation to become critical in drives, emotions, and mood states, and in their interfaces with sensory and hormonal mechanisms. While it may be tempting to think of the endorphins as the "pleasure substrate," it is probably more realistic to conceive of them as critical in the fine tuning of sensory phenomena with affect. It is, therefore, conceivable that such a system would be disrupted in human psychiatric disorders. Preliminary work already supports this possibility. Thus, acute and chronic stress lead to dramatic change in pain sensitivity and in levels of endogenous opiate peptides (20). In addition, cerebrospinal fluid concentrations of endorphins have been reported to be high in schizophrenics, decreasing with clinical improvement (21). In manic-depressives, rhythmic changes were seen which also paralleled clinical status. The same authors have further reported that the opiate antagonist naloxone blocks auditory hallucinations in schizophrenics, a finding which we have confirmed in some patients. These results must be verified, but further work in this field could prove tremendously rewarding.

REFERENCES

1. Becher, E. M. *Licit and Illicit Drugs.* Boston: Little, Brown, 1972.
2. Goldstein, A., Aronow, L., and Kalman, S. M. *Principles of Drug Action: The Basis of Pharmacology,* 2nd ed. New York: John Wiley & Sons, 1974.
3. Snyder, S. H. and Pert, C. B. Membrane receptor. *In: Opiate Receptor Mechanisms.* S. H. Snyder and S. Matthysse, *eds.,* Cambridge: MIT Press, 1975, pp. 26–34.
4. Goldstein, A., Lowney, L. J., and Pal, B. K. Stereospecific and nonspecific interactions of the morphine congener levorphanol in subcellular fractions of mouse brain. *Proc. Nat. Acad. Sci., U.S.A. 68*:1742–1747, 1971.
5. Pert, A. and Yaksh, T. Sites of morphine induced analgesia in the primate brain: relation to pain pathways. *Brain Res. 80*:135–140, 1974.
6. Wei, E. and Loh, H. Chronic intracerebral infusion of morphine and peptides with osmotic minipumps, and the development of physical dependence. *In: Opiates and Endogenous Opioid Peptides.* H. W. Kosterlitz, *ed.,* Amsterdam: North-Holland Publishing Co., 1976, pp. 303–310.
7. Snyder, S. H. A model of opiate receptor function with implications for a theory of addiction. *In: Opiate Receptor Mechanisms.* S. H. Snyder and S. Matthysse, *eds.,* Cambridge: MIT Press, 1975, pp. 137–141.
8. Richardson, D. E. and Akil, H. Stimulation-produced analgesia: chronic produced analgesia by naloxone, a narcotic antagonist. *Science 191:* 961–962, 1976.
9. Akil, H., Mayer, D. J., and Liebeskind, J. C. Antagonism of stimulation-self-administration in periventricular sites in intractable pain patients. *J. Neurosurg.,* in press.
10. Mayer, D. J. and Hayes, R. Stimulation-produced analgesia: development of tolerance and cross-tolerance to morphine. *Science 188*:941–943, 1975.
11. Jaffe, J. H. and Sharpless, S. K. Pharmacological denervation supersensitivity in the central nervous system: a theory of physical dependence. *Res. Publ. Assoc. Res. Nerv. Ment. Dis. 46*:226–246, 1968.
12. Takemori, A. E. The effects of morphine, other opioids and their derivatives on the metabolism of the cerebral cortex. *Res. Publ. Assoc. Res. Nerv. Ment. Dis. 46*:53–73, 1968.
13. Hughes, J. Isolation of an endogenous compound from the brain with pharmacological properties similar to morphine. *Brain Res. 88*:295–308, 1975.
14. Hughes, J., Smith, T. W., Kosterlitz, H. W., Fothergill, L. A., Morgan, B. A., and Morris, H. R. Identification of two related pentapeptides from the brain with potent opiate agonist activity. *Nature 258*:577–579, 1975.
15. Simantov, R. and Snyder, S. H. Isolation and structure identification of a morphine-like peptide "enkephalin" in bovine brain. *Life Sci. 18:* 781–788, 1976.
16. Li, H. L. and Chung, D. Isolation and structure of an untriakontapep-

tide with opiate activity from camel pituitary glands. *Proc. Nat. Acad. Sci., U.S.A. 73*:1145–1148, 1976.

17. Ross, M., Su, T-P., Cox, B. M., and Goldstein, A. Brain endorphins. *In: Opiates and Endogenous Opioid Peptides.* H. W. Kosterlitz, *ed.,* Amsterdam: North-Holland Publishing Co., 1976, pp. 35–40.

18. Beluzzi, J. D., Grant, N., Garsky, V., Sarantakis, D., Wise, C. D., and Stein, L. Analgesia induced *in vivo* by central administration of enkephalin in rat. *Nature 260*:625–626, 1976.

19. Simantov, R. and Snyder, S. H. Elevated levels of enkephalin in morphine-dependent rats. *Nature 262*:505–507, 1976.

20. Akil, H., Madden, J., IV, Patrick, R. L., and Barchas, J. D. Stress-induced increase in endogenous opiate peptides: concurrent analgesia and its partial reversal by naloxone. *In: Opiates and Endogenous Opioid Peptides.* H. W. Kosterlitz, *ed.,* Amsterdam: North-Holland Publishing Co., 1976, pp. 63–70.

21. Whalström, A., Johansson, L., and Terenius, L. Characterization of endorphines (endogenous morphine-like factors) in human CSF and brain extracts. *In: Opiates and Endogenous Opioid Peptides.* H. W. Kosterlitz, *ed.,* Amsterdam: North-Holland Publishing Co., 1976, pp. 49–56.

19 | Sedative Hypnotics: Biological Mechanisms

JOACHIM RAESE

INTRODUCTION

This chapter explores some of the pharmacological properties of the sedative-hypnotic barbiturates and benzodiazepines. Since the turn of the century, sedative hypnotics have been among the drugs most heavily prescribed by the medical profession. Their appropriate use in the treatment of anxiety and of sleep disorders is discussed in Chapter 13 and 14, respectively. Unfortunately, these substances have also proven to possess a tremendous potential for abuse, as described in Chapter 23. Partly because of their widespread availability, that abuse is an increasingly important problem for the medical profession. Thus, it is potentially of profound clinical importance to uncover some of the mechanisms by which these substances exert their effects.

The sedative hypnotics are also of strong interest to basic scientists. These substances seem to be able to selectively modulate such basic behaviors as arousal and stress response. An understanding of their actions might help elucidate the neurochemical and neurophysiological control of these behaviors. While we are far from obtaining final answers as to which of the many effects of these drugs are most important, there have been some exciting developments in recent years.

BARBITURATES

HISTORY

Barbiturates are derivatives of barbituric acid (malonylurea) (Fig. 19-1), which may have gotten its name because it was first synthesized

306

from uric acid by Von Baeyer on St. Barbara's day. Barbital, which was developed by the great organic chemist Fischer in collaboration with Von Mering, was the first barbiturate used in clinical medicine. Barbital's trade name, Veronal, probably derives from the fact that Von Mering was in Verona when he learned of barbital's synthesis in a telegram from Fischer. Subsequently, barbital was shown to facilitate sleep and to have some antianxiety effects when used during the daytime (1).

Soon after its introduction in 1903, barbital became extremely popular in clinical medicine. The next important barbiturate was phenobarbital, introduced in 1912. In addition to its use as a sedative, phenobarbital has become one of the most important pharmacological treatments for epilepsy. The systematic search for shorter acting barbiturates led to pentobarbital and secobarbital in 1930. These two medications are still widely used to induce sleep and are also the most widely abused barbiturates. The development of amobarbital in 1923 led to the use of "amytal interview" as a diagnostic and therapeutic instrument in psychiatry (Chapter 16), while the synthesis of thiopental in 1935 produced a short-lived agent useful for intravenous anesthesia.

STRUCTURE-ACTIVITY RELATIONSHIPS

Barbituric acid, the parent compound of the barbiturates, is not a central depressant. Sedative activity requires the introduction of two alkyl groups at position 5 (Fig. 19-1B,D). In general, longer alkyl sidechains yield compounds which are both shorter acting and more potent. Compounds with sidechains exceeding 6–7 carbon atoms lose their hypnotic activity and become convulsants. In contrast, introduction of aryl or reactive alkyl sidechains imparts anticonvulsant activity (Fig. 19-1C) (2).

For the barbiturates, duration of action is inversely related to lipid solubility. The lipid-soluble, short-acting thiobarbiturates are formed by replacing the oxygen at position 2 with a sulfur atom (Fig. 19-1B). These compounds tend to be more toxic than their oxybarbiturate analogues, but several are safe for clinical use. Lipid solubility is also enhanced by a methyl substitution on one of the nitrogens (Fig. 19-1C). Interestingly, alkylation of both nitrogens yields drugs which have convulsant activity (2).

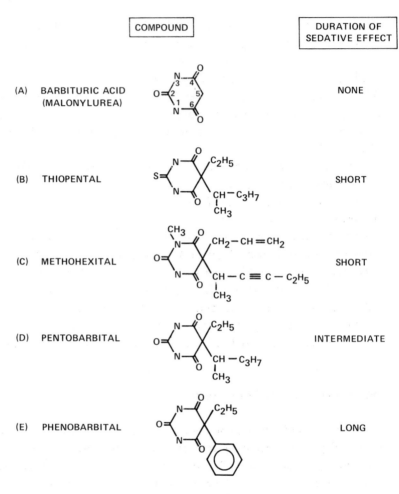

FIGURE 19-1. Structure-Activity Relationships Among Barbiturates

METABOLISM

Metabolic degradation of barbiturates primarily involves liver microsomal enzyme systems. Oxidation of the larger of the two side-chains at position 5 is the major pathway; the resulting polar metabolites are generally inactive and are excreted in the urine. N-Dealkylation can be important for compounds with a nitrogen methyl group. For example, the action of mephobarbital is greatly prolonged by the formation and accumulation of its N-demethyl metabolite, phenobarbital. There is also a small, but measurable, exchange of oxygen for sulfur in thiobarbiturates, to form the analogous oxybarbiturates (3).

Since barbiturate metabolism is so highly dependent upon liver enzymes, changes in liver function can markedly alter the rate at which these compounds are inactivated. Thus, conditions such as hepatitis and obstructive jaundice may significantly prolong the sedative effects of these drugs. Similarly, prolongation can arise from competition of several compounds for the same metabolic enzymes. Furthermore, barbiturates induce the metabolic capacity of these enzymes; over several days, metabolic activity may increase by two- to threefold. Clinically, these changes can be of particular importance with patients who are also receiving metabolic competitors like warfarin or digitoxin, for which careful control of plasma concentrations is essential (2).

BEHAVIORAL AND NEUROCHEMICAL EFFECTS

Both in man and in animals, the main effects of barbiturates are sedation and sleep induction. As mentioned earlier, phenobarbital has selective anticonvulsant properties. The sedative and anticonvulsant actions appear to be independent, since nonsedative doses of phenobarbital are effective in the treatment of epilepsy and the sedative effects of the drug can be completely antagonized by amphetamine, with no loss of anticonvulsant potency. Another important effect of the barbiturates is addiction. Tolerance develops fairly rapidly and cannot be adequately explained by increases in degradative activity. The clinical implications of addiction are discussed in Chapter 23.

The central systems involved in the sedative effects of the barbiturates are unknown. Much attention has been given to the reticular activating system as a possible site of action. As described in Chapter 4, this brain region has extensive interconnections with auditory, visual, olfactory, and somatic systems and is thought to play a central role in arousal mechanisms. Many studies have shown that the reticular activating system is extremely sensitive to the depressant effects of the barbiturates (4).

Barbiturates appear to act by depressing neuronal transmission. At pharmacologically effective concentrations, they selectively block chemical transmission across the synapse, without affecting electrical transmission along the axon. At higher concentrations, however, they have local anesthetic actions, increasing the sodium conductance of the axons and thereby producing a depolarization block of nerve impulse conduction. Depression of neuronal activity has been demonstrated at various levels of organization, such as the neuromuscular junction, autonomic ganglia, monosynaptic spinal reflexes, and various brain regions. The synaptic depression appears to result from decreased responsiveness of both pre- and postsynaptic mechanisms.

Presynaptically, the barbiturates may interfere with the normal link between depolarization and calcium uptake. Thus, pentobarbital inhibits the depolarization-induced uptake of calcium into neuronal synaptosomes (5). Without calcium uptake, the transmitter release is blocked, thereby preventing normal transmission. Barbiturates may act through GABAergic presynaptic terminals. These usually inhibitory synapses, which are described in Chapter 3, appear to produce a refractory depolarization which prevents transmission. Barbiturates appear to produce a similar depolarization in dorsal root ganglia primary afferents, the first synapses of sensory pathways; this effect is blocked by γ-aminobutyric acid (GABA) antagonists such as picrotoxin and bicuculline (6).

Barbiturates also block the postsynaptic response to transmitter release. This effect seems to be specific, both for brain region and for transmitter. In the cerebral cortex, the drugs reportedly block postsynaptic response in excitatory but not in inhibitory noradrenergic synapses, with no effect on cholinergic or serotonergic synapses (7), while in the brainstem, they appear to block the postsynaptic response to acetylcholine (8). Richards (9) concluded that barbiturates generally inhibit the postsynaptic response at excitatory synapses and have variable effects at inhibitory ones. The molecular and ionic mechanisms of these selective inhibitions remain to be determined.

To date, studies have failed to connect specific transmitters to specific behavioral effects of the barbiturates. Barbiturates decrease the stress-induced acceleration of norepinephrine turnover, reduce dopamine turnover in the neostriatum and limbic forebrain, and decrease turnover of 5-hydroxytryptamine in the cerebral cortex (10). However, it is still uncertain whether these changes have a causal role in the sedative and hypnotic effects of these drugs or represent a secondary effect of some other action, possibly upon the GABA system.

BENZODIAZEPINES

The benzodiazepines have been available clinically for less than 20 years; yet, they have become the most frequently prescribed drugs in medicine. Their impact upon the treatment of anxiety states has been immense, and a description of their development and history is given in Chapter 13, the chapter on antianxiety medications. The following material describes some of the important metabolic and biochemical information which investigators have obtained about these fascinating compounds.

METABOLISM

Most of the clinically useful benzodiazepines are structurally similar. Several of the more commonly used compounds are illustrated in Figure 19-2. A substituent at position 7 is essential for biological activity; the 7-chloro derivatives are most common. A carbonyl at position 2 enhances activity and is generally present. Most of the newest products also take advantage of the increased activity resulting from a halogen at the 2' position, as seen with flurazepam. These general features are important in considering the metabolic fate of the benzodiazepines. Since the 7 and 2' positions of the molecule are essentially inert to the major degradative pathways, many of the metabolites retain substantial pharmacological activity.

The major metabolic pathways for the 1,4-benzodiazepines have been reviewed recently (11). Those compounds with an alkyl function at position 1—e.g., flurazepam—undergo N-dealkylation, resulting in compounds which retain their biological activity. Those like chlordiazepoxide and flurazepam, which contain aliphatic nitrogens, also undergo N-dealkylation at those positions. Benzodiazepines which do not originally have a carbonyl at position 2 often obtain one by undergoing oxidation to form the analogous lactam. Finally, the lactams are readily hydroxylated at position 3. Subsequent glucuronide conjugation at this position leads to rapid urinary excretion of these metabo-

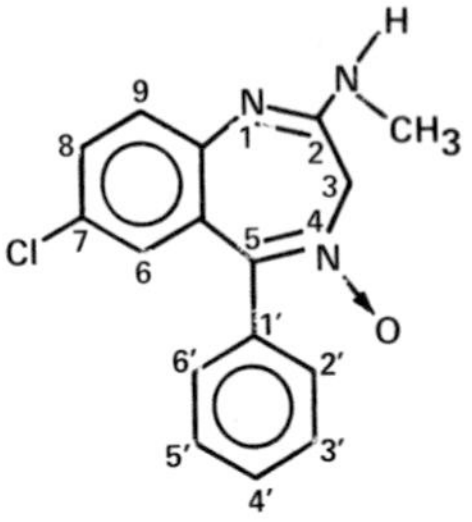

CHLORDIAZEPOXIDE

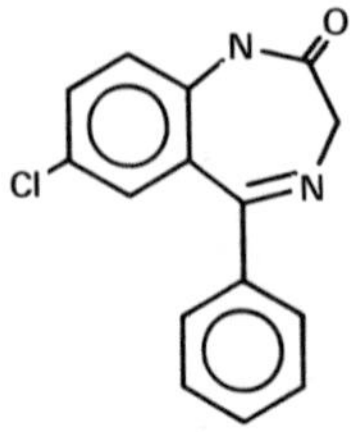

DIAZEPAM

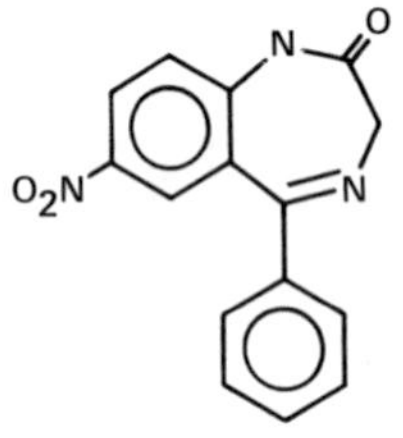

NITRAZEPAM

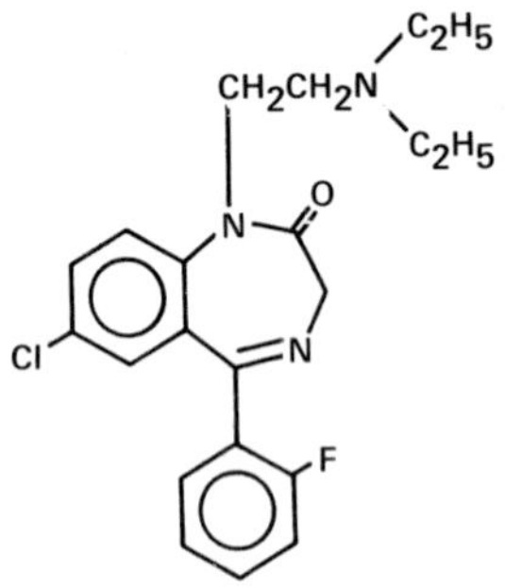

FLURAZEPAM

FIGURE 19-2. Several Common Benzodiazepines

lites. Many of the above reactions involve the liver microsomal enzymes, and changes in the activity of this enzymatic system will alter the rate of their metabolism. However, unlike the barbiturates, the benzodiazepines do not induce this system themselves.

Behavioral and Neurochemical Effects

The benzodiazepines share with the barbiturates anticonvulsant, sedative, and hypnotic effects. In addition, however, they possess the remarkable ability to reduce anxiety and aggression (12). Although the addictive potential of these substances is somewhat less than that for the barbiturates, the benzodiazepines have become common drugs of abuse. The toxicity and abstinence syndromes associated with these drugs are described in Chapter 23.

Until recently, attempts to elucidate the mechanisms by which the benzodiazepines exert their effects met with limited success. Like the barbiturates, benzodiazepines were shown to decrease turnover rates of both dopamine and 5-hydroxytryptamine in specific brain regions and to block stress-induced acceleration of norepinephrine turnover (10). However, the cause of this reduction in turnover remained unclear, since the drugs were shown to affect neither uptake mechanism nor degradative and metabolic enzymes of these neuroregulators and had no direct effects on pre- or postsynaptic sites.

A rapidly increasing body of evidence suggests that GABAergic systems have an important role in the effects of the benzodiazepines. Initially, this connection was made through the anticonvulsant properties of these drugs. Although there is no clearly demonstrable relationship between drug-induced seizures and central GABA levels, ample evidence suggests that interference with GABA transmission can induce convulsions. The benzodiazepines are particularly potent antagonists of seizures produced by compounds such as isoniazid, which blocks GABA synthesis, or picrotoxin and pentylenetetrazol, which are GABA receptor blockers (13). In addition, the benzodiazepines prolong presynaptic inhibition in the primary afferent of the spinal cord, as do the barbiturates. Again, this effect appears to involve GABAergic neurons; in accord with that conclusion, GABA blocking agents prevent this action of the benzodiazepines (14).

The recent demonstration of extensive connections between dopaminergic and GABAergic systems in the midbrain (15) suggests a straightforward way in which the benzodiazepines might produce a decrease in dopamine turnover. Thus, with GABA acting as an inhibitory transmitter in the dopaminergic nigrostriatal pathway, facilitation of GABA transmission should produce a decrease in dopamine turnover (Fig. 19-3). In support of such a model, bicuculline reduces the inhibitory effect of chlordiazepoxide on striatal dopamine turnover (16). Similar mechanisms might be involved in the effects on norepinephrine and 5-hydroxytryptamine.

Although the precise neurochemical pathways are far from clear, there is some evidence that the antianxiety effects of the benzodiazepines may involve serotonergic systems (12). Thus, p-chlorophenylalanine, which blocks the synthesis of 5-hydroxytryptamine, also alters the suppressive effects of chlordiazepoxide in animal models of anxiety, while the presumed 5-hydroxytryptamine antagonists cinanserin and methysergide both reduce anxiety in these models and add to the

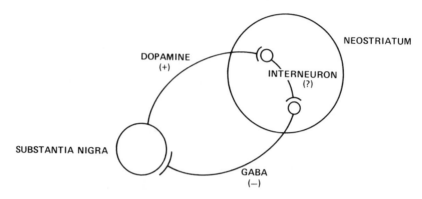

FIGURE 19-3. Schematic Representation of Possible GABA Involvement in the Dopaminergic Striatonigral Pathway

effects of the benzodiazepines. In addition, the benzodiazepines reduce the turnover of 5-hydroxytryptamine in some brain regions, with no change in total content (17). These studies suggest that at least in part the antianxiety effects may result from the reduction of serotonergic activity. Stein (18) has proposed that 5-hydroxytryptamine is involved in a "punishment" system and that a reduction in the activity of that system diminishes the "anxiety" of potentially harmful situations. Both the practical and the theoretical implications of that hypothesis will require further research.

SUMMARY

The recent progress in developing an understanding of the biochemical actions of the benzodiazepines and barbiturates offers a classical example of the continuing need for basic research. Most of the data has become available only in the last three to four years. Much of the research thrust derives from our expanding knowledge of the GABAergic system and from the development of new technologies to permit scientists to study that system. Many questions remain unanswered. In view of the tremendous importance of the benzodiazepines both in psychiatry and in general medicine, those questions must be answered and should ultimately provide better treatment. Undoubtedly, complete answers will require not only a fuller investigation of known systems in the brain but also the exploration of systems and regulatory mechanisms about which we still know little.

REFERENCES

1. Maynert, E. W. Sedatives and hypnotics. II: Bartiburates. *In: Drill's Pharmacology in Medicine*. J. R. DiPalma, ed., New York: McGraw-Hill, 1965, pp. 188–209.
2. Harvey, S. C. Hypnotics and sedatives. The barbiturates. *In: The Pharmacological Basis of Therapeutics*, 5th ed. L. S. Goodman and A. Gilman, eds., New York: Macmillan Co., 1975, pp. 102–123.
3. Parke, D. V. Biochemistry of the barbiturates. *In: Acute Barbiturate Poisoning*. H. Matthew, ed., Amsterdam: Excerpta Medica, 1971, pp. 7–53.
4. Killam, K. Drug action on the brainstem reticular formation. *Pharmacol. Rev.* 14:175–224, 1962.
5. Blaustein, M. P. and Ector, A. C. Barbiturate inhibition of calcium uptake by depolarized nerve terminals *in vitro*. *Mol. Pharmacol.* 11:369–378, 1975.
6. Nicoll, R. A. Presynaptic action of barbiturates in the frog spinal cord. *Proc. Nat. Acad. Sci., U.S.A.* 72:1460–1463, 1975.
7. Johnsson, E. S., Roberts, M. H. T., and Straughn, D. W. The response of cortical neurones to monoamines under different anesthetic conditions. *J. Physiol. (Lond.)* 203:261–280, 1969.
8. Bradley, P. B. and Dray, A. Modification of the responses of brainstem neurons to transmitter substances by anaesthetic agents. *Br. J. Pharmacol.* 48:212–224, 1973.
9. Richards, C. D. On the mechanism of barbiturate anesthesia. *J. Physiol. (Lond.)* 227:749–767, 1972.
10. Lidbrink, P., Corrodi, H., Fuxe, K., and Olson, L. The effects of benzodiazepines, meprobamate, and barbiturates on central monoamine neurons. *In: The Benzodiazepines*. S. Garattini, E. Mussini, and L. O. Randall, eds., New York: Raven Press, 1973, pp. 203–223.
11. Randall, L. O., Schallek, W., Sternbach, L. H., and Ning, R. Y. Chemistry and pharmacology of the 1,4-benzodiazepines. *In: Psychopharmacological Agents*, Vol. III. M. Gordon, ed., New York: Academic Press, 1974, pp. 175–281.
12. Cook, L. and Sepinwall, J. Behavioral analysis of the effects and mechanisms of action of benzodiazepines. *Adv. Biochem. Psychopharmacol.* 14:1–28, 1975.
13. Costa, E., Guidotti, A., Mao, C. C., and Suria, A. New concepts on the mechanism of action of benzodiazepines. *Life Sci.* 17:167–186, 1975.
14. Suria, A. and Costa, E. Action of diazepam, dibutyryl cGMP, and GABA on presynaptic nerve terminals in bullfrog sympathetic ganglia. *Brain Res.* 87:102–106, 1975.
15. Hökfelt, T., Ljungdahl, Å., Fuxe, K., Johansson, O., Pérez de la Mora, M., and Agnati, L. Some attempts to explore possible central GABAergic mechanisms with special reference to control of dopamine neurons. *In: Neuroregulators and Psychiatric Disorders*. E. Usdin, D. A. Hamburg, and J. D. Barchas, eds., New York: Oxford University Press, 1977, pp. 358–372.
16. Fuxe, K., Agnati, L. F., Bolme, P., Hökfelt, T., Lidbrink, P., Ljungdahl, Å., Pérez de la Mora, M., and Ögren, S.-O. The possible involve-

ment of GABA mechanisms in the action of benzodiazepines on central catecholamine neurons. *Adv. Biochem. Psychopharmacol. 14:* 45–61, 1975.

17. Dominic, J. A., Sinha, A. K., and Barchas, J. D. Effect of benzodiazepine compounds on brain amine metabolism. *Eur. J. Pharmacol. 32:* 124–127, 1975.

18. Stein, L., Wise, C. D., and Berger, B. D. Antianxiety action of benzodiazepines: decrease in activity of serotonin neurons in the punishment system. *In: The Benzodiazepines.* S. Garattini, E. Mussini, and L. O. Randall, *eds.,* New York: Raven Press, 1973, pp. 299–326.

20 | Alcohol: Biological Mechanisms

R. BRUCE HOLMAN

INTRODUCTION

Man has been aware of the pharmacological properties of the various alcohols for many centuries. Alkyl alcohols are monohydroxy derivatives of hydrocarbon chains, having a general formula of R-OH. Table 20-1 lists formulas and names of some of the more common alcohols. These compounds are widely used in making flavor essences and perfumes or as solvents for paints, varnishes, resins, and cellulose esters. All alcohols produce dose-dependent toxic responses in humans which range from irritation of the eyes and mucous membranes, headache, dizziness, flushing, and vomiting to mental depression, anesthesia, coma, and death. Of the alcohols, only ethanol is sufficiently nontoxic to permit regular human consumption. For that reason, the terms "alcohol" and "ethanol" will be used interchangeably in this chapter.

The history of ethanol is such an integral part of our society that it need hardly be reviewed here. This drug is unique among addicting agents in being legally sanctioned. Alcoholism is the major drug addiction problem in America. Not surprisingly, alcohol has been the focus of a considerable body of research aimed at determining its mechanisms of action. As can be seen in the following pages, that work is far from complete.

METABOLISM

Alcohol is rapidly absorbed and distributed throughout the general body water, but it is not stored in tissues. Although some unchanged ethanol can be detected in urine and expired air, most is oxidized by

TABLE 20-1.
COMMON ALCOHOLS

Formula	General Nomenclature	
CH_3OH	Methyl Alcohol	Methanol
CH_3CH_2OH	Ethyl Alcohol	Ethanol
$CH_3CH_2CH_2OH$	n-Propyl Alcohol	1-Propanol
$CH_3CH(OH)CH_3$	Isopropyl Alcohol	2-Propanol
$CH_3CH_2CH_2CH_2OH$	n-Butyl Alcohol	1-Butanol
$CH_3CH_2CH(OH)CH_3$	sec-Butyl Alcohol	2-Butanol
$(CH_3)_2CHCH_2OH$	Isobutyl Alcohol	2-Methyl-1-Propanol
$(CH_3)_3COH$	tert-Butyl Alcohol	2-Methyl-2-Propanol

the enzyme alcohol dehydrogenase to acetaldehyde and then further metabolized to acetic acid by aldehyde dehydrogenase (Fig. 20-1). This metabolic pathway has been reviewed by others (1,2) and will be discussed only briefly.

ALCOHOL DEHYDROGENASE

The conversion of ethanol to acetaldehyde is catalyzed by alcohol dehydrogenase. This enzyme is found in many organs of the body, but its greatest concentration is in the liver, the primary site of alcohol metabolism. Although recent studies have demonstrated the presence of alcohol dehydrogenase in the brain (3), the activity levels are sufficiently low to suggest that this is not a major metabolic site. Alcohol

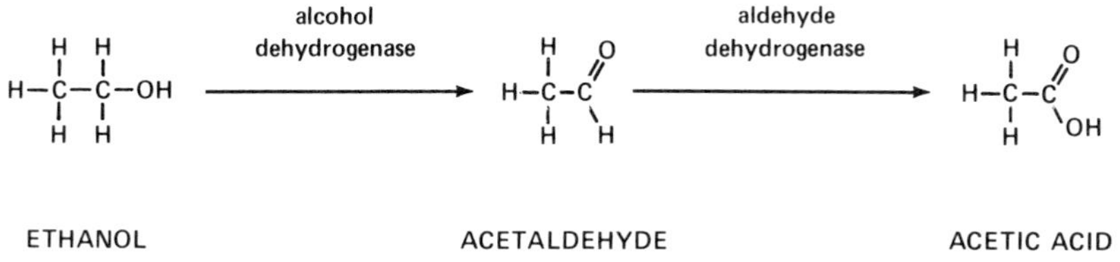

FIGURE 20-1: Major Metabolic Pathway for Ethanol

dehydrogenase requires nicotinic acid dinucleotide (NAD) as a cofactor. Enzyme activity is not highly substrate-specific, and the enzyme will oxidize a wide variety of alcohols. The rate of metabolism is fairly constant and apparently is not enhanced either by increased doses of ethanol or by any known pharmacological agent. Alcohol dehydrogenase can be inhibited by drugs such as pyrazole, resulting in prolonged maintenance of elevated blood alcohol concentrations.

OTHER OXIDATIVE SYSTEMS

Although alcohol dehydrogenase is the primary route of alcohol metabolism, two other systems may also play important roles. A second ethanol oxidizing system in the liver appears to become increasingly important as an oxidative pathway during chronic administration of ethanol (4). In addition, a small percentage of alcohol can be metabolized by a catalase system. Ethanol is the antidote of choice for methanol poisoning, since it will competitively inhibit methanol metabolism.

ALDEHYDE DEHYDROGENASE

Acetaldehyde is a normal constituent of body fluids; however, concentrations rise significantly after ethanol consumption. The oxidation of acetaldehyde to acetic acid is catalyzed by aldehyde dehydrogenase, a nonspecific, NAD-dependent dehydrogenase which acts on a number of aldehyde substrates. Although this enzyme is present in numerous body tissues, including brain, the liver again appears to be the major site of action. Thus, 80 percent of the acetic acid formed from ethanol can be recovered in the hepatic venous drainage (1,2). Since blood acetaldehyde content increases after ethanol administration, its synthesis must exceed its metabolism. This makes it a potentially important agent in alcoholic states. Acetaldehyde itself enhances the activity of aldehyde dehydrogenase and competes with other endogenous aldehydes. Although no other known drugs will induce this system, several are potent inhibitors of aldehyde metabolism including propranolol, p-chloromercuribenzoate, and disulfiram (1,2).

PHYSIOLOGICAL AND NEUROCHEMICAL EFFECTS

Administered acutely, increasing doses of ethanol produce behavioral effects ranging from calming and sedation to loss of motor coordination, disturbed thought processes, unconsciousness, and, ultimately, death. Ethanol is an addictive drug and as with other addictive agents, chronic abuse leads to tolerance, physical dependence, and withdrawal (Chapter 23). Even simple misuse of ethanol can profoundly impair an individual's ability to function in our society.

Several important changes in body function occur as sequelae of alcohol use and abuse in humans. Unfortunately, it has proven extremely difficult to determine which of these changes are directly related to the physiological and behavioral effects of ethanol. Controversies abound. Even the apparently straightforward matter of the relative biological importance of ethanol and acetaldehyde continues to be a center of controversy. Despite these difficulties, some progress has been made in establishing important peripheral and central effects of these two compounds.

PERIPHERAL EFFECTS OF ALCOHOL

Ethanol is primarily metabolized in the liver; it is not surprising, then, that ethanol consumption impairs several important hepatic metabolic systems. These effects appear to result not from ethanol itself but from the requirements for its metabolism. Ethanol oxidation utilizes 75–100 percent of the oxygen which is normally available to the liver for other oxidative reactions (5). The diversion of other cofactors, such as NAD, to this single metabolic process may also disturb normal liver function. In addition, the overproduction of acetic acid disrupts such crucial energy processes as the Krebs cycle and free fatty acid oxidation. These disruptive effects, coupled with increased release of free fatty acids from adipose tissue, may contribute to the alcoholic cirrhotic liver condition (5). Furthermore, ethanol decreases metabolism of carbohydrates, which may also contribute to the fatty liver problem of chronic alcoholics. Decreased carbohydrate metabolism increases the presence of glycerol phosphate and, thus, indirectly increases formation of triglycerides. Of more immediate clinical concern, the reduction in carbohydrate metabolism can also result in lowered glucose production (5). Normal, well-fed adults are able to maintain sufficient blood glucose levels following alcohol consumption. However, hypoglycemia does occur following alcohol administration in children and fasting adults. As emphasized in Chapter 23, severe hypoglycemia can be an important complicating factor in both acute toxicity and withdrawal syndromes.

PERIPHERAL EFFECTS OF ACETALDEHYDE

Acetaldehyde metabolism results in substantial diversion of liver cofactors such as oxygen and NAD from other metabolic reactions. The toxic consequences to hepatic cells are similar to those caused by alcohol (6). Although acetaldehyde does not block carbohydrate metabolism, it does disrupt the degradative pathway of glucose, resulting in hyperglycemia. Acetaldehyde is also a competitive inhibitor of other reactions in which aldehyde dehydrogenase participates. This has major implications for the metabolism of the biogenic amines. For example, 5-hydroxytryptamine is normally metabolized via 5-hydroxyindoleacetaldehyde to either 5-hydroxytryptophol or 5-hydroxyindoleacetic acid (Chapter 3). During alcohol and acetaldehyde metabolism, there is a decrease in the formation of acid metabolites, with a concomitant increase in 5-hydroxytryptophol. Similar shifts to more neutral products occur for the catecholamines.

CENTRAL EFFECTS OF ALCOHOL

Since very little alcohol is actually oxidized in cerebral tissue, the direct inhibitory effects on normal metabolic processes are not as marked as they are in the liver (6). *In vitro*, alcohol can decrease the respiratory activity of cerebral tissue, but only at large, nonphysiological doses. This suggests that the behavioral effects of alcohol stem primarily from actions of this drug upon neuronal function. Since information processing in the brain is dependent on transmission between neurons and neuronal networks, investigators have concentrated largely upon alterations in neurotransmitter function which might occur during ethanol consumption, intoxication, and withdrawal.

Early studies of the effect of ethanol on brain function looked for changes in neurotransmitter content. Most studies have focused on the indole- and catecholamines, although some information is also available on acetylcholine and γ-aminobutyric acid (GABA). Such investigations have yielded inconsistent and conflicting results, partly because experimental procedures vary markedly among studies. Most investigators agree that acute administration of alcohol does not alter the cerebral content of 5-hydroxytryptamine, dopamine, or norepinephrine but increases both acetylcholine and GABA concentrations. Chronic treatment produces a decrease in cerebral norepinephrine, with variable effects on 5-hydroxytryptamine and dopamine.

However, there is evidence suggesting that some of these systems are involved in the effects of ethanol. Drugs which interrupt noradrenergic transmission, such as reserpine, increase the severity of alcohol withdrawal, while those which raise cerebral GABA levels, such as aminooxyacetic acid, reduce withdrawal convulsions. It is not known whether these agents are blocking a primary or secondary pharmacological effect of alcohol. For example, the role of the noradrenergic system might involve response to the nonspecific stress of chronic ethanol injections. Similarly, GABA may diminish withdrawal seizures through a general anticonvulsant action, with no specific association to ethanol (7). Fortunately, studies of transmitter turnover are beginning to provide a better picture of the dynamic changes induced in the brain by ethanol.

Recent studies indicate that alcohol has a marked effect on neurotransmitter turnover. Acute alcohol administration increases synthesis, release, and metabolism of norepinephrine, with no measurable change in transmitter content. During chronic alcohol administration and during withdrawal, norepinephrine metabolism stays high (8). Dopamine synthesis and metabolism also increase with acute alcohol consumption, but turnover decreases during withdrawal. The effects of ethanol on the serotonergic system are much less clear. The variability of the results suggest that effects on this system may differ significantly between species and with drug dose.

Although progress is being made in establishing the effects of ethanol on brain neuroregulators, much less is known about the specific mechanisms of those effects. While global effects of ethanol on transmitter metabolism exist, extensive *in vitro* and *in vivo* studies have failed to reveal actions upon either the synthetic or the degradative pathways for these neuroregulators which entirely explain these effects. This suggests that the observed changes are only secondary to other processes.

CENTRAL EFFECTS OF ACETALDEHYDE

Acetaldehyde formation is a major consequence of peripheral ethanol metabolism; acetaldehyde may also mediate many of the important central effects of alcohol. One basis for such an hypothesis is the interaction between alcohol and disulfiram (Antabuse). Disulfiram blocks the oxidation of acetaldehyde. When given to human subjects who have consumed ethanol, it produces violent and unpleasant physical symptoms. These symptoms are so profound that chronic disulfiram administration is used as a means of deterring ethanol consumption in alcoholics (Chapter 23).

Although acetaldehyde might reasonably be expected to have direct effects upon neuronal systems, most recent investigations have concentrated upon the possible production of abnormal substances from reactions involving acetaldehyde and biogenic amines. As previously mentioned, acetaldehyde competitively inhibits aldehyde dehydrogenase in the periphery, thus preventing normal oxidation of the biogenic amine aldehydes. One of the abnormal metabolites which theoretically might accumulate under these conditions is the aldehyde derivative of dopamine, 3,4-dihydroxyphenylacetaldehyde. This reactive product could, in turn, react with a second dopamine molecule to form tetrahydropapaveroline (Fig. 20-2) (9). Tetrahydropapaveroline is structurally similar to morphine, a fact which has excited speculation about a common basis for such mutual properties of ethanol and morphine as addiction. Tetrahydropapaveroline has been detected in the urine of patients with Parkinson's disease receiving L-DOPA, and concentrations were increased following ethanol consumption. As yet, however, tetrahydropapaveroline has not been detected in brains of animals or humans either before or after alcohol consumption (10). Nor is much information available about the effects of this compound on alcohol-related behaviors. Without such data, the relevance of this compound to the actions of acetaldehyde must remain speculative.

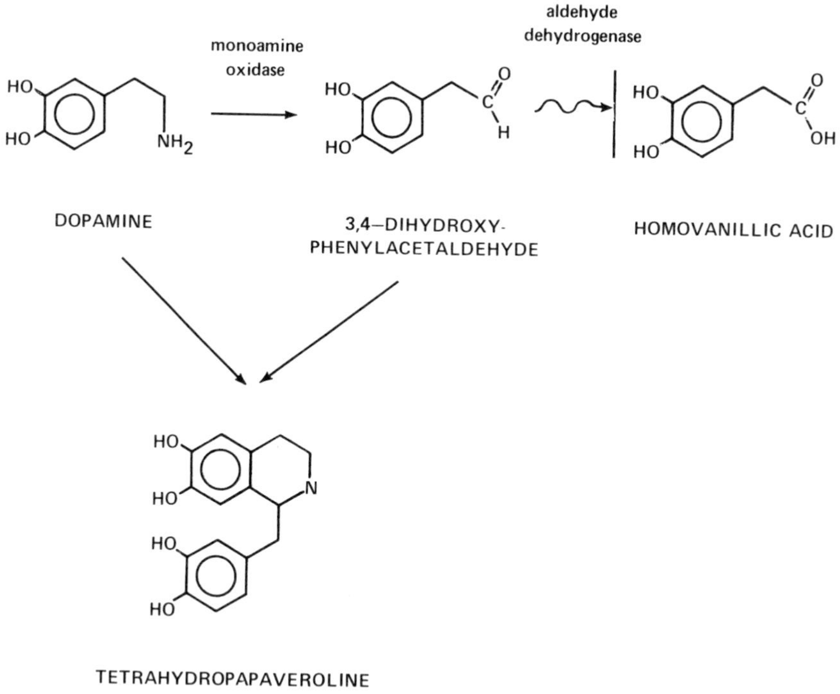

FIGURE 20-2: Proposed Mechanism for Formation of Tetrahydropapa-veroline

Another product of potential biological interest results from direct Pictet-Spengler condensation of biogenic amines with acetaldehyde (Fig. 20-3). The general class of compounds formed from catecholamines are known as tetrahydroisoquinolines, of which salsolinol, the dopamine metabolite, has received the most attention. Salsolinol is also present in the urine of Parkinson patients receiving L-DOPA therapy and ethanol (10). Recently, salsolinol has been detected in rat brain after administration of ethanol plus blockers of biogenic amine and of acetaldehyde metabolism (11). As yet, its presence in brain has not been demonstrated following the consumption of ethanol alone. *In vitro* studies have shown that salsolinol can be taken up and stored by catecholaminergic neurons, releasing catecholamines and acting as a false transmitter. Salsolinol also inhibits catecholamine metabolism and reuptake mechanisms (12). These capacities to modulate various specific aspects of catecholaminergic transmission suggest a mode by which salsolinol and other tetrahydroisoquinolines might affect alcohol-related behaviors. For example, administration of tetrahydroisoquino-lines to mice withdrawing from alcohol increased the intensity of the withdrawal (13).

Indoleamines can react with aldehydes to form tryptolines (tetra-hydro-β-carbolines) (14). For example, 5-hydroxytryptamine can condense with acetaldehyde to form 5-hydroxymethtryptoline (Fig. 20-3). Methtryptolines have been tentatively identified in the urine of rats receiving ethanol and inhibitors of biogenic amine and acetalde-hyde metabolism. Although methtryptolines have not yet been isolated

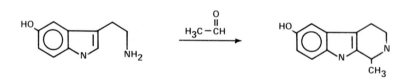

DOPAMINE

SALSOLINOL
(1−METHYL−6,7−DIHYDROXY−
1,2,3,4−TETRAHYDROISOQUINOLINE)

NOREPINEPHRINE

1−METHYL−4,6,7−TRIHYDROXY−
1,2,3,4−TETRAHYDROISOQUINOLINE

5−HYDROXYTRYPTAMINE

5−HYDROXYMETHTRYPTOLINE
(6−HYDROXY−1−METHYL−
1,2,3,4−TETRAHYDRO−β−CARBOLINE)

FIGURE 20-3: Condensation Products of Biogenic Amines and Acetalde-hyde

from brain, they have been shown to have potent pharmacological and behavioral effects which appear to be mediated via inhibition of serotonergic reuptake mechanisms. In tests on alcohol consumption in rats, 5-methoxymethtryptoline reduced the selection of ethanol versus water in a forced-choice drinking paradigm (15).

Studies of condensation products such as the tetrahydroisoquinolines and the tryptolines have begun only recently. Remarkably little is known about the general behavioral effects of these drugs, and even less is known about their specific action on alcohol-related behaviors. Furthermore, methods for their detection and quantitation are at the limit of current technology, so that careful studies of these substances in brain tissue are only now becoming feasible. Nonetheless, the information which is already available suggests that these compounds deserve further attention as possible links between ethanol and its effects on the brain.

NEURONAL MEMBRANES AND ALCOHOL

In trying to understand how alcohol can have its profound influence upon brain function, investigators have explored rather complex mechanisms. Quite recently, several investigators have suggested that the effect might be much more direct and much simpler than presently thought. For example, recent theories about anesthetic agents invoke alterations in neuronal membrane characteristics to explain the effects of these drugs (16,17). A similar disruption of membrane architecture by ethanol might underlie some of its biological actions, such as addiction, tolerance, and withdrawal. Perhaps, in the presence of alcohol, the neuronal membrane must adapt to a new "environment" by changing its lipid composition. Tolerance, then, could reflect the need for more drug to overcome some aspects of this adaptation, while withdrawal would occur when removal of the drug caused a return of the membrane to its predrug state. *In vitro*, ethanol specifically inhibits passive and active ionic movement by disrupting the environment in the synaptic plasma membrane. This disruption may represent a change in the arrangement of lipid molecules of the membrane. In addition, alcohol reduces the calcium concentrations of specific brain regions of the rat (18). Calcium is known to be involved in many neuronal processes, including neurotransmitter release (Chapter 2). Once again, only further study will determine if such speculation is relevant to the *in vivo* situation and how such changes relate to neurochemical and behavioral observations.

REFERENCES

1. Lundquist, F. The metabolism of alcohol. *In: Biological Basis of Alcoholism.* Y. Israel and J. Mardonnes, *eds.,* New York: Wiley-Interscience, 1971, pp. 1–52.
2. von Wartburg, J. P. The metabolism of alcohol in normals and alcoholics: enzymes. *In: The Biology of Alcoholism: Vol. 1: Biochemistry.* B. Kissin and H. Begleiter, *eds.,* New York: Plenum Press, 1971, pp. 63–102.
3. Tabakoff, B. and Gulpke, C. C. Alcohol and aldehyde metabolism in brain. *Adv. Exp. Med. Biol.* 56:141–164, 1975.
4. Lieber, C. S., Hasumura, Y., Teschke, R., Matsuzaki, S., and Korsten, M. The effect of chronic ethanol consumption on acetaldehyde metabolism. *In: The Role of Acetaldehyde in the Actions of Ethanol.* K. O. Lindros and C. J. P. Eriksson, *eds.,* Helsinki: The Finnish Foundation for Alcohol Studies, 1975, pp. 83–104.
5. Majchrowicz, E. Metabolic correlates of ethanol, acetaldehyde, acetate and methanol in humans and animals. *Adv. Exp. Med. Biol.* 56:111–140, 1975.
6. Truitt, E. B., Jr., and Walsh, M. J. The role of acetaldehyde in the actions of ethanol. *In: The Biology of Alcoholism, Vol. 1: Biochemistry.* B. Kissin and H. Begleiter, *eds.,* New York: Plenum Press, 1971, pp. 161–195.
7. Goldstein, D. B. Physical dependence on alcohol in mice. *Fed. Proc. 34:* 1953–1961, 1975.
8. Karoum, F., Wyatt, R. J., and Majchrowicz, E. Brain concentrations of biogenic amine metabolites in acutely treated and ethanol-dependent rats. *Br. J. Pharmacol.* 56:403–411, 1976.
9. Alivisatos, S. G. A. and Arora, R. C. Formation of aberrant neurotransmitters and its implication for alcohol addiction and intoxication. *Adv. Exp. Med. Biol.* 5:255–289, 1975.
10. Sandler, M., Carter, S. B., Hunter, K. R., and Stern, G. M. Tetrahydroisoquinoline alkaloids: *in vivo* metabolites of L-DOPA in man. *Nature* 241:439–443, 1973.
11. Collins, M. A. and Bigdeli, M. G. Tetrahydroisoquinolines *in vivo.* I. Rat brain formation of salsolinol, a condensation product of dopamine and acetaldehyde, under certain conditions during ethanol intoxication. *Life Sci.* 16:585–602, 1975.
12. Cohen, G. Some neuropharmacological properties of tetrahydroisoquinolines derived from the condensation of aldehydes with catecholamines. *In: The Role of Acetaldehyde in the Actions of Ethanol.* K. O. Lindros and C. J. P. Eriksson, *eds.,* Helsinki: The Finnish Foundation for Alcohol Studies, 1975, pp. 187–195.
13. Blum, K., Eubanks, J. D., Wallace, J. E., Schwertner, H., and Morgan, W. W. Possible role of tetrahydroisoquinoline alkaloids in postalcohol intoxication states. *Ann. N. Y. Acad. Sci.* 273:234–246, 1976.
14. Holman, R. B., Elliott, G. R., Seagraves, E., DoAmaral, J. R., Vernikos-Danellis, J., Kellar, K. J., and Barchas, J. D. Tryptolines: their potential role in the effects of ethanol. *In: The Role of Acetaldehyde in the Actions of Ethanol.* K. O. Lindros and C. J. P. Eriksson, *eds.,*

Helsinki: The Finnish Foundation for Alcohol Studies, 1975, pp. 207–216.

15. Geller, I. and Purdy, R. Alteration of ethanol preference in rats; effects of β-carbolines. *Adv. Exp. Med. Biol. 59*:295–301, 1975.

16. Grenell, R. G. The binding of alcohol to brain membranes. *Adv. Exp. Med. Biol. 59*:11–22, 1975.

17. Bangham, A. D. Alcohol, anaesthetics and membranes. *In: Central Nervous System and Behavioral Pharmacology.* M. Airaksinen, *eds.,* New York: Pergamon Press, 1976, pp. 33–39.

18. Ross, D. H. Selective action of alcohols on cerebral calcium levels. *Ann. N. Y. Acad. Sci. 273*:280–294, 1976.

21 | Amphetamine and Cocaine: Biological Mechanisms

ROBERT L. PATRICK

INTRODUCTION

Cocaine and amphetamine are potent psychomotor stimulants which are of great interest because of their biochemical actions and behavioral effects. Despite their dissimilar chemical structures, these two compounds have remarkably similar pharmacological properties. Both can produce general hyperactivity in a variety of animal species, including man. At higher doses, they induce stereotypies in animals—sniffing, biting, and gnawing in rats and mice and picking and self-grooming in nonhuman primates. In humans they also produce behaviors characterized by meticulous and repetitious arrangement of objects, which may be analogous to the animal stereotypies. Interestingly, both amphetamines and cocaine were introduced in medicine because they temporarily alleviate fatigue and enhance mental and physical performance. Unfortunately, both have proven to have serious abuse potential, as discussed in Chapter 23. This chapter provides a brief history of cocaine and amphetamine and a description of our current understanding of the biochemical mechanisms by which they exert their profound effects on behavior.

COCAINE

HISTORY

Cocaine use has a long and varied history. When the Spanish conquered the Inca Empire, they discovered that the Andesan Indians of South America chewed the leaves of the plant now known as *Eryth-*

roxylon coca. These leaves produced mild euphoria, alertness, a feeling of increased energy, and decreased appetite. Although chewing of coca leaves was never widespread in Europe or America, small amounts of coca extracts were added to various "medicinal" drinks. For example, one American drink was introduced by J. S. Pemberton in Atlanta in 1886. Pemberton, who combined extracts of the cola nut and of coca leaves, called the product "Coca-Cola." However, by the early 1900's, Coca-Cola was being made from decocainized coca leaves (1).

Cocaine, the principal active agent in coca leaves, was first isolated in the mid-eighteenth century (Fig. 21-1). In 1884, Aschenbrandt gave pure cocaine to Bavarian soldiers and reported that it decreased fatigue. This report was read by a young and poor neurologist in Vienna named Sigmund Freud. He tried cocaine himself with pleasant results and subsequently gave it to his colleague von Fleischl-Marzow, who was addicted to morphine because of painful neuromata. Fleischl took increasing doses of cocaine and, within a year, was taking doses far above those that Freud occasionally used. Fleischl then apparently developed cocaine psychosis, a syndrome which resembles acute paranoid schizophrenia. This incident prompted Freud to completely abandon his support for the therapeutic use of cocaine.

Today the legal use of cocaine is restricted to the production of local anesthesia. Since cocaine is still obtained as a plant product from coca leaves by a relatively expensive process, its illegal use is far less extensive than that of the more readily available amphetamines. However, cocaine abuse is a continuing and growing problem. The euphoria it produces is a transient but powerful reinforcer, encouraging repeated administrations and often resulting in cocaine psychosis.

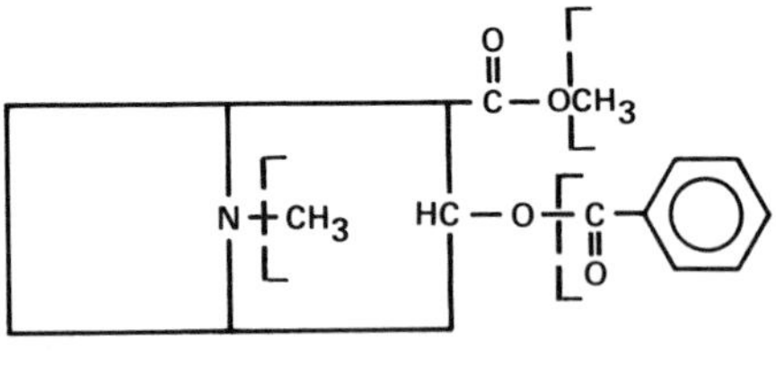

FIGURE 21-1. Cocaine
    Brackets indicate groups which are enzymatically cleaved during metabolism.

Metabolism

Cocaine appears to be metabolized primarily by serum esterases, although it can also lose the methyl group from the nitrogen. The major cleavage sites are indicated in Figure 21-1, and all possible metabolic combinations can be found (2). When given intravenously, cocaine is cleared rapidly from both brain and plasma, with a half-life of about twenty minutes (2). In contrast, the common practice of applying cocaine to nasal mucosa produces peak concentrations at about one hour, with measurable amounts remaining at six hours. This difference is attributable, at least in part, to the continued presence of cocaine on the nasal mucosa for as long as three hours (3).

Behavioral and Neurochemical Effects

Studies on the behavioral effects of cocaine have been reviewed by Kosman and Unna (4). Cocaine increases general locomotor activity, enhances physical and mental endurance, and decreases appetite. Tolerance does not develop to cocaine's excitatory effects. In fact, chronic administration usually results in an apparent sensitization to them. Physiological addiction does not appear to occur with cocaine, and abrupt withdrawal in either man or animals does not lead to an abstinence syndrome. Psychological addiction, however, can be a serious problem.

Cocaine is thought to exert most of its behavioral and psychological effects through central catecholaminergic systems (5). Thus, cocaine no longer increases locomotor activity in mice after catecholaminergic pathways have been chemically lesioned (6). In addition, cocaine is a potent inhibitor of neuronal uptake mechanisms for norepinephrine, dopamine, and 5-hydroxytryptamine. In contrast to some other types of uptake inhibitors, such as amphetamine, cocaine does not exhibit much potency as a stimulator of release in these systems (7). Cocaine also differs from the tricyclic antidepressants, another class of uptake inhibitors, since the former but not the latter strongly inhibits striatal dopamine uptake (8). Such differences in specific potencies in different brain regions may be a crucial key for understanding why cocaine itself is not a good antidepressant (Chapter 10).

Except at high concentrations, cocaine has no direct effect on dopamine synthesis *in vitro;* however, it is extremely effective in blocking the feedback inhibition of dopamine synthesis normally produced by the addition of dopamine. Presumably, cocaine exerts this effect by preventing the entry of exogenous dopamine into the nerve endings (9). Cocaine does inhibit 5-hydroxytryptamine synthesis; it appears to be an inhibitor of the high affinity uptake mechanism of the amino-acid precursor, tryptophan (10). Cocaine is also an inhibitor of monoamine oxidase (MAO), one of the major metabolic enzymes for the biogenic amines (11).

The available evidence suggests that cocaine may markedly prolong the time that biogenic amines, particularly dopamine, spend in the synaptic cleft. This could lead to a functional overactivity of these systems. Unfortunately, the *in vivo* effects of cocaine on these systems, especially after chronic administration, have yet to be studied extensively. However, the striking similarities between the behavioral effects of cocaine and amphetamine suggest that they may share some common modes of action. As described in the next section of this chapter, there is good evidence that amphetamine acts primarily upon dopaminergic systems.

AMPHETAMINES

History

The discovery of the amphetamines has recently been told by Chauncey Leake (12). In the 1920's, K. K. Chen left Leake's laboratory to return to China, where he began a systematic investigation of the ancient Chinese drug codification. Chen noted repeated recommendations of the desert plant *ma huang* for asthma. Following this lead, Chen discovered that the plant was *Ephedra vulgaris.* The alkaloid ephedrine, which had been isolated from this plant about eighty years earlier, was rediscovered by Chen and Schmidt in 1925 (Fig. 21-2). It is still used in treating asthma.

Gordon Alles wanted to find a synthetic substitute for ephedrine. After synthesizing several related phenylalkylamines, he joined Leake

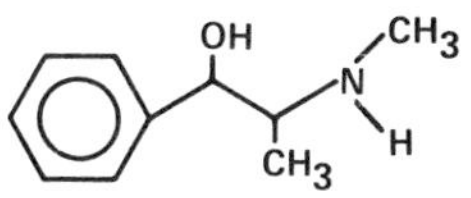

FIGURE 21-2. Ephedrine

to study their biological activity. These two investigators perfected careful techniques for evaluating the toxicity and activity of phenyl-alkylamines. The best compound of their first series was *d,l*-phenyliso-propylamine, or amphetamine. The carbonate of this racemic substance was volatile and could be used to treat asthma. After the optical isomers were isolated, dextroamphetamine, or dexedrine, was tried clinically. Investigators found that the drug increased alertness and wakefulness and improved physical and mental performance in people who were fatigued or bored. It also suppressed appetite.

Amphetamines were used extensively in World War II by both sides. After the war, Japan had huge supplies which were placed on the open market. This led to an epidemic of amphetamine abuse and yielded numerous cases of amphetamine psychosis. Other epidemics have followed, both in Sweden and in the United States. In fact, it is one of the ironies in the history of psychopharmacology that the Haight-Ashbury amphetamine epidemic took place less than a mile from the University of California San Francisco Medical Center, where Alles and Leake had first synthesized amphetamines more than forty years earlier.

METABOLISM

The structure and major metabolic pathways of amphetamine are indicated in Figure 21-3. As reviewed by Williams *et al.* (13), either aromatic or aliphatic hydroxylation can occur, yielding *p*-hydroxyamphetamine and norephedrine, respectively. Both of these metabolites are biologically active. Figure 21-3 also indicates the twenty-four-hour excretion pattern of amphetamine metabolites in normal humans. The major components are unmetabolized amphetamine and the deaminated product benzoic acid, while hydroxyl metabolites are present in much lower amounts. There are also suggestions that N-hydroxylation may occur, although this has yet to be confirmed *in vivo*. Excretion patterns vary both with species and with individuals. In addition, they are affected by a variety of factors. For example, chronic users excrete more unmetabolized amphetamine, norephedrine, and 4-hydroxynorephedrine than do normal controls. Similarly, conditions which produce an acidic urine greatly enhance excretion, with a marked shift toward unmetabolized amphetamine. This enhanced excretion can be a valuable clinical tool (Chapter 24).

Behavioral and Neurochemical Effects

The behavioral effects of amphetamine resemble those of cocaine: general locomotor activity is increased, physical and mental fatigue is

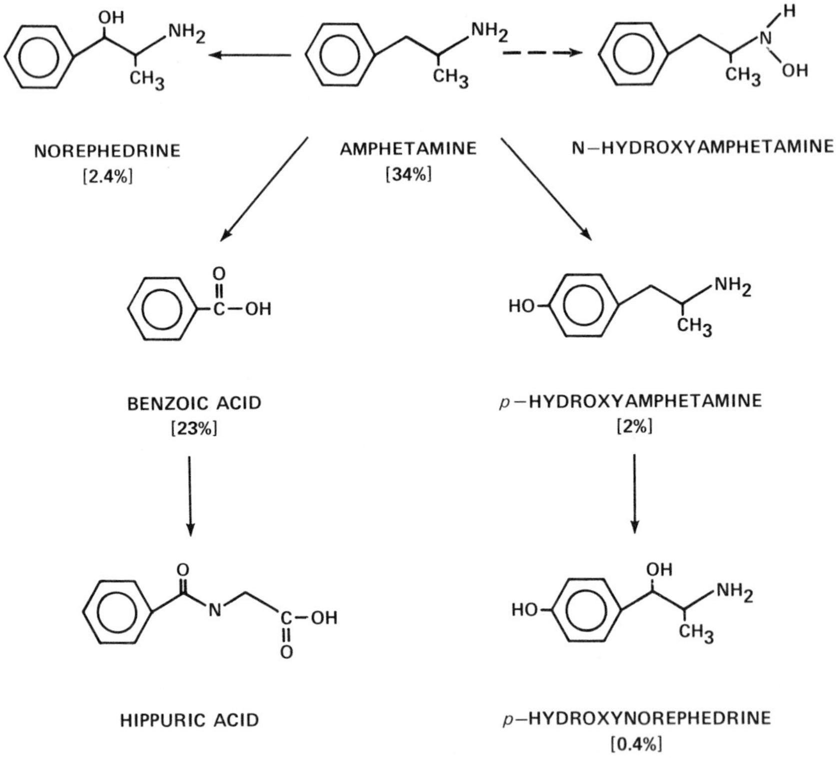

FIGURE 21-3. Metabolic Pathway for Amphetamine in Humans
Bracketed figures under a metabolite indicate urinary excretion in normal human subjects as a percent of the amphetamine dose (from Williams *et al.* [13]). Dashed line indicates possible metabolic pathway not confirmed *in vivo*.

reduced, and appetite is decreased (4). Evidence is not definitive, but tolerance probably develops for some but not all of the effects. Thus, the anorexic effect declines with time, particularly in man. In contrast, chronic administration actually sensitizes animals to amphetamine-induced hyperactivity and stereotypy (14). As with cocaine, amphetamine does not produce a physiological addiction, although abrupt withdrawal can lead to a suppression of activity in animals and to a possible depression in man (9).

Amphetamine exhibits a wide range of pharmacological activity; however, the most important actions are thought to involve the biogenic amines, particularly the catecholamines. Amphetamine inhibits MAO, blocks neuronal uptake mechanisms for the catecholamines and 5-hydroxytryptamine, and causes a release of catecholamines from nerve endings. It may also act directly on noradrenergic receptors (5). Amphetamine contains an asymmetric carbon, so that it exists in two forms which differ only in their spatial arrangement. It is of both theoretical and practical interest that the relative potencies of these optical isomers depends upon the action being studied (15). As described in Chapter 8, such differences are controversial and have been of particular interest in attempts to uncover the neurochemical basis of amphetamine psychosis.

Even though the exact mechanisms are unknown, amphetamine's net effect appears to be an increase in catecholaminergic activity and, perhaps, in serotonergic activity. It also has an interesting and specific effect on striatal dopamine, producing a rapid decrease in synthesis (16). This effect is not found in either cerebral cortex or hypothalamus and can be blocked by pretreatment with an antipsychotic. A reduction also occurs in 5-hydroxytryptamine synthesis in the striatum (17). The ultimate importance of these decreases in synthetic rate will depend upon their generalizability to areas which may be related to the behavioral effects of the drug.

Although most of the behavioral effects of amphetamine have been related to its ability to increase the concentration of biogenic amines in the synaptic cleft by blocking inactivation and enhancing release, the relative importance of a particular amine appears to depend upon the behavior being studied. For example, depletion of the catecholamines or destruction of catecholaminergic pathways will block both stereotypies and hyperactivity (5,18). In contrast, selective depletion of norepinephrine alone reduces motor activity but does not prevent the appearance of stereotypy (5). Less is known about the role of serotonergic systems in amphetamine's effect; but there are suggestions that they, too, may play a role in some behavioral effects, such as in hyperactivity (19).

SUMMARY

The psychomotor stimulants, particularly amphetamine, have played a tremendously important role in the history of psychopharmacology. Their ability to reduce fatigue and to induce euphoria have been a continuing challenge to investigators who are interested in delineating the central mechanisms responsible for "mood," while widespread abuse is an important problem in clinical psychopharmacology. In addition, cocaine and amphetamine psychoses have had tremendous impact upon schizophrenia research, as already described in Chapter 8. It is exciting that much of the research reviewed in this chapter has been generated in the past five years. These studies have simultaneously helped to explain the actions of amphetamine and cocaine and to elucidate some of the functions of the catecholaminergic and serotonergic systems. Still, there are many unanswered questions. These systems must be explored more fully, to precisely define which pharmacological actions are most important for producing the behavioral effects. Furthermore, it will be important to examine other neuroregulators, to see what role they may play. Thus, these compounds continue to offer a rich and rewarding area for research.

REFERENCES

1. Brecher, E. M. Coca leaves and cocaine. *Consumer Reports: Licit and Illicit Drugs.* Boston: Little, Brown, 1972, pp. 269–277.
2. Misra, A. L., Nayak, P. K., Patel, M. N., Vadlamani, N. L., and Mulé, S. J. Identification of norcocaine as a metabolite of [³H]-cocaine in rat brain. *Experientia 30:*1312–1314, 1974.
3. Van Dyke, C., Barash, P. G., Jatlow, P., and Byck, R. Cocaine: plasma concentrations after intranasal application in man. *Science 191:*859–861, 1976.
4. Kosman, M. E. and Unna, K. R. Effects of administration of the amphetamines and other stimulants on behavior. *Clin. Pharmacol. Ther. 9:*240–254, 1968.
5. Caldwell, J. and Sever, P. S. The biochemical pharmacology of abused drugs. I. Amphetamines, cocaine, and LSD. *Clin. Pharmacol. Ther. 16:*625–638, 1974.
6. Ziegler, H., Del Basso, P., and Longo, V. G. Influence of 6-hydroxy-dopamine and of α-methyl-p-tyrosine on the effects of some centrally acting agents. *Physiol. Behav. 8:*391–396, 1972.
7. Heikkila, R. E., Orlansky, H., and Cohen, G. Studies on the distinction between uptake inhibition and release of [³H]dopamine in rat brain tissue slices. *Biochem. Pharmacol. 24:*847–852, 1975.
8. Shore, P. A. Transport and storage of biogenic amines. *Ann. Rev. Pharmacol. 12:*209–226, 1972.
9. Patrick, R. L., Snyder, T. E., and Barchas, J. D. Regulation of dopamine synthesis in rat brain striatal synaptosomes. *Mol. Pharmacol. 11:*621–631, 1975.
10. Knapp, S. and Mandell, A. J. Narcotic drugs: effects on the serotonin biosynthetic systems of the brain. *Science 177:*1209–1211, 1972.
11. Muschool, E. Effect of cocaine and related drugs on the uptake of noradrenaline by heart and spleen. *Br. J. Pharmacol. 16:*352–359, 1961.
12. Leake, C. D. The long road for a drug from idea to use. *In: Discoveries in Biological Psychiatry.* F. J. Ayd and B. Blackwell, *eds.,* Philadelphia: Lippincott Co., 1970, pp. 68–84.
13. Williams, R. T., Caldwell, J., and Dring, L. G. Comparative metabolism of some amphetamines in various species. *In: Frontiers of Catecholamine Research.* S. H. Snyder and E. Esdin, *eds.,* Oxford: Pergamon Press, 1973, pp. 927–932.
14. Segal, D. S. Behavioral and neurochemical correlates of repeated d-amphetamine administration. *In: Neurobiological Mechanisms of Adaptation and Behavior.* A. J. Mandell, *ed.,* New York: Raven Press, 1975, pp. 247–262.
15. Holmes, J. C. and Rutledge, C. O. Effects of the d- and l-isomers of amphetamine on uptake, release and catabolism of norepinephrine, dopamine and 5-hydroxytryptamine in several regions of rat brain. *Biochem. Pharmacol. 25:*447–451, 1976.
16. Harris, J. E., Baldessarini, R. J., and Roth, R. H. Amphetamine-induced inhibition of tyrosine hydroxylation in homogenates of rat corpus striatum. *Neuropharmacology 14:*457–471, 1975.
17. Knapp, S., Mandell, A. J., and Geyer, M. A. Effects of amphetamines

on regional tryptophan hydroxylase activity and synaptosomal conversion of tryptophan to 5-hydroxytryptamine in rat brain. *J. Pharmacol. Exp. Ther. 189*:676–689, 1974.

18. Randrup, A. and Munkvad, I.   Biochemical, anatomical, and psychological investigations of stereotyped behavior induced by amphetamines. *In: Amphetamines and Related Compounds.* E. Costa and S. Garattini, *eds.*, New York: Raven Press, 1970, pp. 695–713.

19. Breese, G. R., Cooper, B. R., and Mueller, R. A.   Evidence for involvement of 5-hydroxytryptamine in the action of amphetamine. *Br. J. Pharmacol. 52*:307–314, 1974.

22 | Hallucinogens and other Psychotomimetics: Biological Mechanisms

STANLEY J. WATSON

Hallucinogens are a diverse group of substances which share the ability to produce vivid sensory experiences that have no objectively verifiable basis. Agents fitting this general description are also called "psychotogens" and "psychotomimetics," to suggest that they mimic some of the symptoms of psychosis. Although several classes of drugs have the general ability to produce hallucinations, this chapter will focus on the agents in most common use. The main emphasis will be on LSD and agents with similar modes of action, such as psilocin, mescaline, and dimethyltryptamine. Only brief descriptions are given of phencyclidine, cannabis, the anticholinergics, and solvent hallucinogens.

LSD, PSILOCIN, DIMETHYLTRYPTAMINE, AND MESCALINE

History

The hallucinogens have both an ancient and a modern history. For centuries cultures have utilized plant extracts which contained natural hallucinogens, using them for religious ritual, for healing, and for predicting the future. For example, the early Spanish settlers in Mexico described the psychic effects of both the peyotl cactus and the teonanacatl mushroom. The modern era of the hallucinogens is confined almost entirely to this century. During that time scientists have made great strides in identifying these compounds and in elucidating some of the biochemical actions by which they exert their effects. Unfortunately, that same time period has witnessed a massive increase in the availability of such compounds and in their abuse.

The peyotl cactus was the first of the hallucinogenic plants to be scrutinized by the organic chemists. It was subsequently named *Anhalonium lewinii*, in honor of Lewin and Hefter, who isolated the active component, mescaline, in 1896. By 1919, Spath had identified mescaline as 3,4,5-trimethoxyphenylethylamine and synthesized it. During the late 1950's, Hofmann isolated the active principles of the "magic" mushroom, *Psilocybe mexicana*, and identified them as the indoleamines psilocybin and psilocin.

One of the major discoveries in this field was made by Hofmann. The work began in the 1930's with studies of ergot alkaloids, many of which were of interest to medicinal chemists because of their effects on smooth muscles. In the process of modifying the activity of these substances, Hofmann isolated the lysergic acid nucleus from the alkaloids and combined it with amines. One of these products was lysergic acid diethylamide-25 (LSD). On April 16, 1943, Hofmann accidentally ingested a small amount of this material. His description of the first LSD "trip" is as graphic as any that have followed (1).

The incredible effects that the hallucinogens have upon the mind are a continuing source of fascination and inspiration for scientist and philosopher alike. As described in Chapter 8, the discovery of such substances has had profound effects upon our theories about schizophrenia. Their role in medicine and in society remains undefined. As our understanding of the biological actions of hallucinogens improves, we may be able to more rationally evaluate the issues they raise.

BEHAVIORAL AND NEUROCHEMICAL EFFECTS

The primary behavioral effects of the hallucinogens is to produce intense visual hallucinations, mood changes, and complex sensory alterations. There are slight differences between agents, but these probably result from specific side effects and from contaminants in the preparation. Serotonergic systems have been implicated as the neurochemical basis for the hallucinogenic effects. A more recent hypothesis involving the possible effects of LSD on dopaminergic receptors will also be discussed. It is possible that both systems may be important, since the complex effects of hallucinogens could easily result from interactions with several neuroregulators.

Interactions with Serotonergic Systems

The line of evidence leading to the current connection between LSD action and 5-hydroxytryptamine is exemplary of careful scientific investigation combined with well-designed multidisciplinary research. For several years after LSD was first discovered there were few clues to its mode of action. Then, in 1953, Gaddum (2) reported that LSD inhibited some of the peripheral effects of 5-hydroxytryptamine and suggested that a similar action might account for the activity of LSD in the central nervous system. The proof for that thesis has been slowly but persistently developed by many investigators (cf. 3,4). One early landmark was the demonstration by Freedman (5) that LSD caused an increase in 5-hydroxytryptamine content and a decrease in its primary metabolite, 5-hydroxyindoleacetic acid. These data were seen as support for the inhibitory action of LSD on serotonergic cells.

With the development of techniques for visualizing serotonergic cells, axons, and terminals, investigators were able to study the specific anatomy of serotonergic systems in the brain. These pathways are discussed in Chapter 3. The serotonergic cells of the dorsal raphé have been particularly important in studies of the hallucinogens. Aghajanian and his co-workers (6) used both single-cell recording and microiontophoresis to uncover the specific effects of hallucinogens on this system (see Chapter 4).

While earlier data suggested an antagonism between LSD and 5-hydroxytryptamine, microiontophoretic studies showed that the two had similar effects on the raphé neurons (7). Thus, 5-hydroxytryptamine inhibited cell firing for short periods, and LSD produced a similar but longer-lasting inhibition. However, this effect of LSD did provide an electrophysiological explanation for the pharmacological evidence that LSD decreased serotonergic activity. Therefore, it was proposed that LSD acted in a competitive fashion with 5-hydroxytryptamine to inhibit serotonergic cells. In support of this hypothesis, depletion of 5-hydroxytryptamine was shown to prolong the action of LSD, presumably because the transmitter is no longer present to compete for a common receptor site.

Unfortunately, a problem for this hypothesis arose at the other end of the serotonergic system. Like the cell bodies, terminal endings of this system are also sensitive to both 5-hydroxytryptamine and LSD, with both producing postsynaptic inhibition (Fig. 22-1). If LSD acts

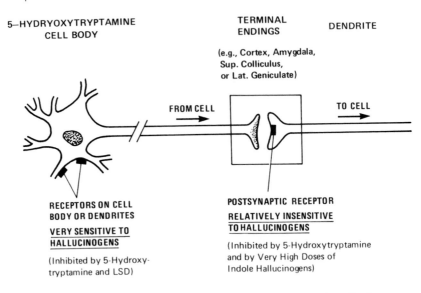

FIGURE 22-1. Schematic Representation of the Effect of Hallucinogens on Central Serotonergic Systems

Normally, an action potential propagates down the axon and releases 5-hydroxytryptamine, which activates the postsynaptic receptor and thus inhibits the postsynaptic dendrite and cell. The serotonergic cell may also inhibit itself or other nearby cells via short collaterals which release 5-hydroxytryptamine onto receptors of the serotonergic cell or its dendrites, thus preventing further firing. LSD appears to show preferential potency for the cell receptors, rather than for the postsynaptic receptors.

as an agonist at both sites, then it seemed logical that the net effect of systemic LSD should be to produce normal or even increased serotonergic activity, rather than antagonism of it. Further uncertainty about the relevance of these effects developed from the discovery that non-hallucinogenic analogues of LSD, like 2-bromo-LSD, were also active agonists at serotonergic postsynaptic receptors. Thus, there seemed to be no correlation between activity as a serotonergic agonist and potency as an hallucinogen.

Recently, a new insight has arisen from studies in which the serotonergic cell bodies and their terminal fields were examined separately. Aghajanian and Haigler (6) found that receptors on serotonergic raphé cells are far more sensitive to LSD inhibition than are the postsynaptic serotonergic receptors, even though receptors at both of these sites are equally sensitive to 5-hydroxytryptamine. Furthermore, 2-bromo-LSD is effective at the postsynaptic receptor but does not affect the cell body receptors. These results gave rise to the present theory that LSD exerts its primary effects by inhibiting serotonergic cells, rather than postsynaptic sites. Such inhibition should result in prolonged cessation of action of the serotonergic system, thereby freeing the systems which it normally inhibits. Many of the regions innervated by serotonergic systems are associated with the visual and limbic systems (Chapter 3) and could, therefore, account for most of the central effects of LSD.

In order to approach the question of whether other hallucinogens act by this same mechanism, it is important to know their clinical potencies and helpful to understand their structural similarities to LSD. Figure 22-2 emphasizes the structural similarities among 5-hydroxytryptamine and several hallucinogens and indicates their relative hallucinogenic potencies. If a common mechanism is to account for action of these drugs, their relative clinical potencies should resemble their relative pharmacological potencies. As shown, these agents exhibit the same rank order for inhibition of serotonergic cells as for hallucinogenic potency. Furthermore, as their hallucinogenic potentials decrease, so do their preferences for cell receptors over postsynaptic receptors.

Closely related to the above results are the data of Snyder and Richelson (8), who have carried out studies of several structural parameters of indole-containing molecules in relation to their hallucinogenic properties. They correlated clinical potency with the electron donating capacity of the highest occupied molecular orbital. The correlation was good for some but not all of the hallucinogens. The last line of Figure 22-2 shows the relative electron-donating capacity for these compounds. This structural parameter correlates well with both hallucinogenic and serotonergic inhibitory potencies.

The current thesis of the effect of indole hallucinogens on 5-hydroxytryptamine might be stated as follows: LSD acts to preferentially inhibit serotonergic cell firing and seems to spare postsynaptic serotonergic receptors. This preference is shared by other similar hallucinogens but in a limited fashion. Nonhallucinogenic analogues of LSD show no preference. These results suggest that there are two different steric conformations of serotonergic receptors, one of which has higher affinity for LSD than the other. In general, 5-hydroxytryptamine is an inhibitory transmitter; thus, when its activity is decreased, the next neuron in the

5–HYDROXYTRYPTAMINE

I STRUCTURAL FORMULA		II PSYCHOMIMETIC POTENCY (ARBITRARY DOSE UNITS)	III INHIBITION OF SEROT- ONERGIC CELL FIRING	IV ELECTRON DONATING CAPACITY (E_H)
	LSD	3,700	MOST	0.218
	PSILOCIN	31		0.460
	DIMETHYL-TRYPTAMINE	4		0.516
	MESCALINE	1	LEAST	0.536

chain is freed from inhibition and becomes more active. Since serotonergic systems appear to be intimately involved in the control of sensation, sleep, attention, and mood, it may be possible to explain the actions of LSD and other hallucinogens by their disinhibition of these critical systems.

The cause of the prolonged action of LSD and of the rapid development of tolerance may also entail interactions between LSD and serotonergic receptors. Unlike 5-hydroxytryptamine, which rapidly dissociates from the receptor, LSD dissociates quite slowly—up to one hour in some test systems (7). The kinetics of this dissociation may account for its prolonged action upon acute administration. On the other hand, serotonergic systems rapidly develop tolerance with repeated administration of 5-hydroxytryptamine. It is possible that the system develops tolerance even more quickly with persistent stimulation such as that produced by LSD.

Interactions with Dopaminergic Systems

Very recently several investigators have demonstrated that LSD has effects on dopaminergic systems as well (9). This work is not nearly as complete as that just described, but it shows promise. The data indicate that LSD acts as both agonist and antagonist on dopamine postsynaptic receptors, whereas the nonhallucinogenic analogue 2-bromo-LSD has no effect. *In vivo*, LSD alters motor behavior which is believed to involve dopaminergic pathways; *in vitro*, it affects dopamine-sensitive adenylate cyclase, which suggests a direct postsynaptic action on the dopamine receptor. While there are no data supporting a presynaptic

---

FIGURE 22-2. Correlations Between Clinical Potencies, Effects on Serotonergic Cells, and Molecular Steric Factors for Four Hallucinogens

I. Note that all four hallucinogens can form the indole nucleus. D-LSD, psilocin, and dimethyltryptamine also have the ethylamine sidechain. Thus, the first three hallucinogens contain the basic indoleamine structure (3,7).

II. Potencies are expressed in "mescaline units," based on the reciprocal of the dose required to produce effects which are comparable to those of mescaline (3).

III. Note that LSD is most potent and mescaline is least effective inhibitor of serotonergic cell firing. This correlates well with their clinical potency (6).

IV. The lower the E_H value, the better the electron donor. For example, LSD is a better donor than psilocin (3,8).

action of LSD at dopaminergic synapses, both the terminal fields in the caudate and the cell bodies in the limbic system appear to be sensitive to LSD (see Chapter 2). One of the problems with this work involves the fact that neither dopamine precursors nor receptor agonists can mimic LSD; however, dopamine receptor blockers do seem to be useful in inhibiting the effects of LSD. This work has yet to be integrated with that on 5-hydroxytryptamine to produce a comprehensive theory.

OTHER HALLUCINOGENS

PHENCYCLIDINE

Phencyclidine (PCP) was first used in 1957 as an anesthetic agent. Currently, it is approved only as an animal tranquilizer, because of its potent hallucinogenic properties. The molecule does not include the indole structure typical of many other hallucinogens (Fig. 22-3). Yet it is often contained in street hallucinogen preparations advertised as THC, mescaline, or LSD, and a large proportion of drug psychoses actually result from its use.

Little work is available on the mechanism of action of this agent. Both phencyclidine and a related compound, ketamine, are "dissociative" anesthetics. They reduce the effect of sensory input to the cortex but generate hallucinations, confusion, and disorientation (10). The specific neurochemical substrates for their effects are totally unknown. No clear antagonism of their central effects has been produced by any agent. To the contrary, the pressor effects of phencyclidine seem to potentiate the effects of sympathomimetic amines and anticholinergic agents alike (11).

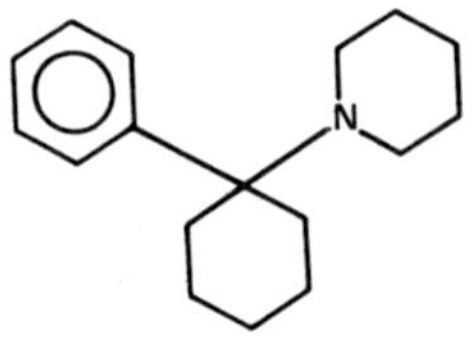

FIGURE 22-3. Phencyclidine

Phencyclidine is known to produce change in central catecholamine levels (12) and is reported to aggravate schizophrenia. Clinical reports of phencyclidine administration to schizophrenics emphasize that a large number of such patients become more psychotic, that most do not want to take the agent again, and that the effects on these patients far outlast those seen in normal individuals (13). It is tempting to speculate that alterations of brain catecholamines and the sensitivity of schizophrenics are related. Unquestionably, the actions of this potent and fascinating agent deserve further study.

CANNABIS

Cannabis sativa is a plant which provides a wide variety of cultures with a common drug of abuse. The active preparation is known by a variety of names—marihuana, hashish, charas, bhang, ganja to name a few. There are many good reviews of the pharmacology of cannabis (14,15). The symptoms produced by this agent range from a sense of well-being and euphoria, relaxation, and sleepiness at low doses to a psychotic reaction similar to that seen with LSD at high doses. The major active form is l-Δ^9-tetrahydrocannabinal (Δ^9-THC) (Fig. 22-4), although the l-Δ^8-tetrahydrocannabinol is also quite active. One current thesis is that the metabolite 11-hydroxy-Δ^9-tetrahydrocannabinol is also active (16). Although there are substantial behavioral similarities between LSD and high-dose cannabis, there is no evidence of cross-tolerance between them. Further differences between LSD and cannabis are reflected in the fact that LSD shows rapid tolerance, while tolerance to cannabis develops slowly, if at all.

The neurochemical basis of the mode of action of cannabis is poorly delineated. There is no major transmitter thesis which accounts for its

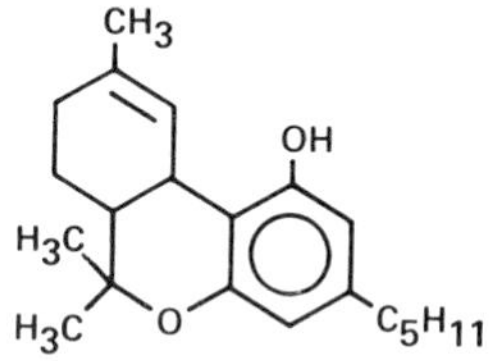

FIGURE 22-4. l-Δ^9-Tetrahydrocannabinol

action, but there are some hints that catechol- and indoleamines might be involved (17). For example, cannabis produces a small decrease in brain norepinephrine levels and turnover, while 5-hydroxytryptamine levels are increased with a decrease in turnover. The alterations in 5-hydroxytryptamine are very similar to those seen with LSD and may underlie a common mode of action. Although the evidence is inconsistent, cannabis may also interfere with cholinergic mechanisms in hippocampal and limbic structures, suggesting a mechanism for the influence of cannabis on memory and concentration (14). Yet a third line of investigation suggests that cannabis may have direct effects on nerve conduction. Thus, l-Δ^9-tetrahydrocannabinol produces a dose-related decrease in the action potential of nonmyelinated fibers of the rabbit (18). Clearly, no cohesive theory of the mode of action of cannabis has yet emerged. The lack of a firm hypothesis comes from the enormous complexity of the problem rather than from a lack of effort. It is unfortunate that we have so weak a neurochemical understanding of such a major drug of abuse.

ANTICHOLINERGICS

Drugs in this class have in common the ability to block muscarinic cholinergic receptors and are exemplified by agents such as atropine, scopolamine, and ditran (4) (Fig. 22-5). The main central symptoms produced by anticholinergics are confusion, amnesia, hallucinations, disrupted cognition, and poorly organized speech. Although they produce hallucinations, these agents differ from LSD in that the patient is severely confused and amnesic. Brawley and Duffield (3) refer to these agents not as hallucinogens but as *deliriants*, to indicate their ability to produce confusion and amnesia.

The peripheral symptoms of cholinergic blockade are related to the relative increase in sympathetic tone. They include rapid heart rate with palpitation, dryness of mouth, dilated pupils, blurring of vision, difficulty in swallowing, dry and hot skin, and difficulty with urination (Chapter 24).

It is interesting to note that although LSD-like agents have been associated with their effects on serotonergic receptors, the specific pharmacology of those receptors is not well understood. In contrast, the anticholinergic hallucinogens are known by the pharmacology of the

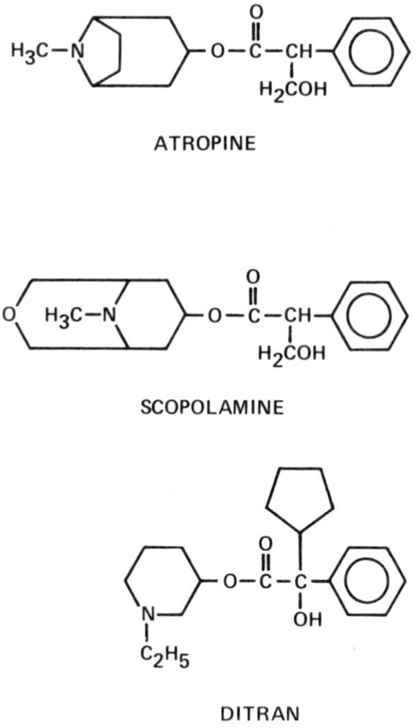

ATROPINE

SCOPOLAMINE

DITRAN

FIGURE 22-5. Common Anticholinergics

receptor they influence and are treated accordingly; but there is so little information about the anatomy of cholinergic systems in the brain that we have only a poor understanding of the connectivity and physiology of the systems involved (Chapter 3). However, we have gained some useful information from the use of these agents. It seems clear that the brain contains mainly muscarinic receptors, with relatively few nicotinic receptors. The behavioral effects from blockade of CNS muscarinic sites show that acetylcholine is intimately involved in coding and storage of memory: both anticholinergics and LSD produce hallucinations and confusion, but only the anticholinergics produce amnesia.

ORGANIC SOLVENTS AND GASES

In the last fifteen years there has been a tremendous expansion of abuse of various volatile organic solvents and propellant gases. These agents form a heterogeneous group ranging from gases like Freon, carbon dioxide, and nitrous oxide to liquids such as acetone, gasoline, ether, toluene, and carbon tetrachloride (Fig. 22-6). The problem of their abuse is exacerbated by the cheapness, general availability, and extraordinarily wide variety of preparations in which they can be found. Thus, glue, paint thinner, hair spray, paint, lighter fluid, nail polish remover, plastic cement, and gasoline have all been used for this purpose. The toxic syndromes produced by these agents are exemplified by a recent report on glue sniffers (19). Effects include "pleasant exhilaration, euphoria, excitement, ataxia, slurred speech, diplopia, and tinnitus." Chronic exposure to glue can also produce psychological dependence, habituation, and tolerance.

Unfortunately, there is no systematic pharmacological or biochemical information on the modes of action of these substances. However, the thread running through these gases and organic solvents is that they generally seem to be rapidly transported across biological membranes, e.g., in the lungs. It may be that lipid solubility is the key not only to their rapidity of action but also to their global effects on the brain. The

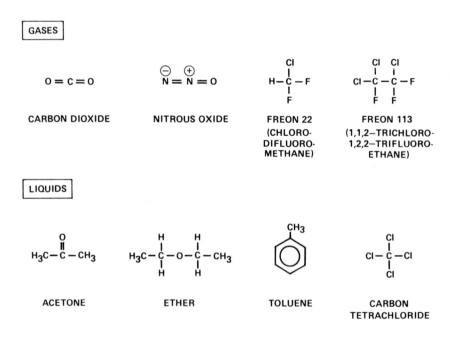

FIGURE 22-6. Commonly Abused Organic Solvents and gases

rising incidence of abuse should foster future studies on the mechanisms involving these substances.

CONCLUSION

While hallucinogenic agents represent a clinical problem to the physician (Chapter 24), they provide a useful and fascinating tool to the scientist and theoretician. As pharmacological agents, they have pointed to important differences between presynaptic and postsynaptic receptors in the serotonergic system. Furthermore, their dramatic effects on perception and emotion may provide a clue to the physiological basis for perceptual distortions in psychoses. Several theories of schizophrenia do, in fact, advance the concept that brains of psychotic individuals produce their own psychotomimetic agents (Chapter 8). Similarly, phencyclidine has been recently considered as a possible model for schizophrenia. Unlike the amphetamine-induced paranoid psychoses, "PCP" psychoses involve more complete disorganization and a wide variety of symptoms. Thus, hallucinogens continue to suggest interesting avenues for investigating the elusive interface between psychoses, physiology, pharmacology, and neurochemistry.

REFERENCES

1. Hofmann, A. The discovery of LSD and subsequent investigations on naturally occurring hallucinogens. *In: Discoveries in Biological Psychiatry.* F. J. Ayd and B. Blackwell, *eds.,* Philadelphia: Lippincott Co., 1970, pp. 93–106.
2. Gaddum, J. H. Antagonism between lysergic acid diethylamide and 5-hydroxytryptamine. *J. Physiol. 121:*15p, 1953.
3. Brawley, P. and Duffield, J. C. The pharmacology of hallucinogens. *Pharmacol. Rev. 24:*31–66, 1972.
4. Brimblecombe, R. W. Psychotomimetic drugs: biochemistry and pharmacology. *Adv. Drug Res. 7:*165–206, 1973.
5. Freedman, D. X. Effects of LSD-25 on brain serotonin. *J. Pharmacol. Exp. Ther. 134:*160–166 ,1961.
6. Aghajanian, G. K. and Haigler, H. J. Hallucinogenic indoleamines: preferential action upon presynaptic serotonin receptors. *Psychopharmacol. Comm. 1:*619–629, 1975.
7. Berridge, M. J. and Prince, W. T. The nature of the binding between LSD and a 5-HT receptor: a possible explanation for hallucinogenic activity. *Br. J. Pharmacol. 51:*269–278, 1974.
8. Snyder, S. H. and Richelson, E. Psychedelic drugs: steric factors predicting psychotropic activity. *Proc. Nat. Acad. Sci. U.S.A. 60:*206–213, 1968.
9. DaPrada, M., Saner, A., Burkard, W. P., Bartholine, G., and Pletscher, A. Lysergic acid diethylamide: evidence for stimulation of cerebral dopamine receptors. *Brain Res. 94:*67–73, 1975.
10. Burns, R. S., Lerner, S. E., and Corrado, R. Phencyclidine: states of acute intoxication and fatalities. *West. J. Med. 123:*345–349, 1975.
11. Eastman, J. W. and Cohen, S. N. Hypertensive crisis and death associated with phencyclidine poisoning. *J. Am. Med. Assoc. 231:*1270–1271, 1975.
12. Tonge, S. R. Catecholamine concentrations in discrete areas of the rat brain after the pre- and neonatal administration of phencyclidine and imipramine. *J. Pharm. Pharmacol. 25:*164–165, 1973.
13. Rainey, J. M. and Crowly, M. K. Prolonged psychosis attributed to phencyclidine: report of three cases. *Am. J. Psychiatry 132:*1076–1078, 1975.
14. Drew, W. G. and Miller, L. L. Cannabis: neural mechanisms and behavior–a theoretical review. *Pharmacology 11:*12–32, 1974.
15. Paton, W. D. M. Pharmacology of marijuana. *Ann. Rev. Pharmacol. 15:*191–220, 1975.
16. Hollister, L. E. Structure-activity relationships in man of cannabis constituents, and analogs and metabolites of Δ^9-tetrahydrocannabinol. *Pharmacology 11:*3–11, 1974.
17. Truitt, E. B. and Anderson, S. M. Biogenic amine alterations produced in the brain by tetrahydrocannabinols and their metabolites. *Ann. N.Y. Acad. Sci. 191:*68–72, 1971.
18. Byck, R. and Ritchie, J. M. Δ^9-Tetrahydrocannabinol: effects on mammalian nonmyelinated nerve fibers. *Science 180:*84–85, 1973.
19. Glaser, H. H. and Massengale, O. N. "Glue-sniffing" in children: deliberate inhalation of vaporized plastic cements. *J. Am. Med Assoc. 181:*300–303, 1962.

23 | Treatment of Abusers of Alcohol and other Addictive Drugs

PHILIP A. BERGER and

JARED R. TINKLENBERG

INTRODUCTION

The patient who abuses addicting drugs is a common and sometimes difficult problem in the emergency room. The drug involved can be an opiate, a barbiturate, one of the newer sedatives or minor tranquilizers, or alcohol. Often the patient is abusing more than one of these pharmacological agents. His symptoms may result from acute drug toxicity, from an abstinence syndrome, or from a variety of medical illnesses which are frequently associated with drug abuse. Thus, the care of the addicted drug abuser often entails both medical and psychiatric intervention. This chapter focuses primarily on the emergency management of patients who abuse addicting drugs, but also briefly summarizes current approaches to long-term treatment and rehabilitation.

Although there are a wide variety of addicting substances, they break down into three classes, based on clinical syndromes and pharmacological properties. These are opiates, sedative hypnotics, and alcohol (Table 23-1). Acute and long-term treatment of addicted patients is similar within each group. The patient who abuses drugs from more than one pharmacological group—the polydrug abuser—should probably be placed into a fourth category, since his acute treatment requires a somewhat different approach. The acute treatment of the polydrug abuser is described in Chapter 24.

OPIATES

Three major emergency-room problems caused by opiate abuse are: acute opiate toxicity, the opiate abstinence syndrome, and a variety of

TABLE 23-1.

REPRESENTATIVE POTENTIALLY ADDICTING DRUGS

GENERIC NAMES	REPRESENTATIVE BRAND NAMES
Opiates and Opioids	
Alphaprodine	Nisentil
Anileridine	Leritine
Dextropropoxyphene	Darvon
Dihydromorphinone	Dilaudid
Heroin	
Levorphanol	Levo-Dromoran
Meperidine	Demerol, Mepergan
Methadone	Dolophine
Morphine	
Oxycodone	Percodan
Sedative-Hypnotics	
Chloral hydrate	Noctec
Chlordiazepoxide	Librium
Diazepam	Valium
Ethchlorvynol	Placidyl
Ethinamate	Valmid
Flurazepam	Dalmane
Glutethimide	Doriden
Meprobamate	Equanil, Miltown
Methaqualone	Quaalude, Sopor
Methyprylon	Noludar
Oxazepam	Serax
Pentobarbital	Nembutal
Phenobarbital	Luminal
Secobarbital	Seconal
Ethyl Alcohol	
Numerous commercial preparations at varying concentrations.	

medical illnesses which are frequently associated with long-term opiate use. For a discussion of the pharmacology of opiates, see Chapter 18.

PATTERNS OF ABUSE

Opiate abuse has existed in the United States throughout its history. Intravenous administration of opiates dates back to the Civil War, when the hypodermic syringe was first commonly used. Before World War II, a significant percentage of opiate addicts were Caucasians from the southern states, and female users were common. Since then, an increasing proportion have been urban blacks, Puerto Ricans, and Mexican Americans. These groups probably account for half of all the addicts today. While most opiate addicts are young males, the number of female addicts is also increasing.

Addicts within the medical profession often use preparations manufactured by pharmaceutical companies, such as morphine, meperidine, and codeine, which they illegally obtain from hospital or office supplies. Others must seek "street" sources of illegally synthesized heroin. Typically, the heroin addict belongs to a drug subculture in a major urban area and obtains his daily supply from an illegal "pusher" or "connection." Many enter the heroin subculture with intermittent heroin use, called "chipping," which gradually escalates to daily injections or to chronic, intermittent use.

ACUTE OPIATE TOXICITY

Acute opiate toxicity results from an accidental or intentional overdose of opiates or from an allergic or hypersensitivity reaction to them or to adulterants. An addicted patient may develop acute toxicity if, after withdrawal, he returns immediately to his usual dose. Alternatively, family members—all too often children of patients on methadone maintenance—may inadvertently swallow an overdose of methadone, since it is frequently dissolved in a fruit juice or flavored syrup. In an adult, 60 mg of morphine, or an equivalent dose of another opiate, is dangerous; 240 mg of morphine may be fatal if the patient is not treated immediately. Patients with respiratory diseases or with hypothyroidism are more sensitive to opiate toxicity, as are children and the elderly (1).

Diagnosis
Acute opiate toxicity is similar for most natural and synthetic opiates. Common symptoms have been summarized in Table 23-2. If anoxia is severe, pupillary constriction may not be evident. Coma is often lighter than the degree of respiratory depression would suggest. Most opiates only occasionally induce convulsions when an overdose is taken. However, both meperidine and dextropropoxyphene have been reported to cause seizures (1,2). Although the diagnosis of opiate toxicity can

TABLE 23-2.
SYMPTOMS OF TOXICITY OR WITHDRAWAL IN THE ADDICTED PATIENT

	OPIATES AND OPIOIDS	SEDATIVE HYPNOTICS	ETHYL ALCOHOL
ACUTE TOXICITY	*General:* Respiratory distress, with apnea or slow, shallow breathing and cyanosis Unresponsiveness, areflexia, and pinpoint pupils Hypotension, tachycardia, and occasional pulmonary edema	*Mild to Moderate:* Confusion, talkativeness, emotional lability, and ataxia Lateral nystagmus, depressed tendon reflexes, and constricted pupils *Severe:* Respiratory depression and hypotension; can lead to deep coma and death	*Mild:* Talkativeness, exaggerated affect, and subjective sense of well-being *Moderate:* Sensory and motor impairment and emotional lability *Severe:* Slurred speech, ataxia, and severe sensory impairment Apathy and sleepiness Respiratory depression and hypotension; can lead to deep coma and death
ABSTINENCE SYNDROME	*Early (8–10 hours):* Restlessness, sleeplessness, increased respiration, yawning, tearing, nasal discharge, and sweating *Late (24–36 hours):* Agitation, chilling, and anorexia Fever, muscle and joint pain, vomiting, diarrhea, and abdominal cramps Tachycardia and hypertension	*Minor:* Insomnia, anxiety, sweating, anorexia, nausea, vomiting, muscular weakness, postural hypotension, and coarse tremors which worsen with anxiety or voluntary movement *Major:* Grand mal seizures, fever, and psychosis	*Alcoholic tremulousness (12–48 hours):* Insomnia, tinnitus, blurred vision, numbness, anorexia, nausea, vomiting, weakness, anxiety, hyper-vigilance, and coarse tremors which worsen with anxiety or voluntary movement *Alcoholic hallucinosis (12–48 hours):* Auditory or visual hallucinations *Alcoholic seizures (12–48 hours):* Grand mal seizures in groups of 2 to 6 *Delirium tremens (36–96 hours):* Tachycardia, hypo- or hypertension, sweating, fever Delusions, disorientation, hallucinations, and agitation

usually be made on the basis of its clinical syndrome, confirmation is often found in the form of a recent venipuncture site and scarred veins from multiple intravenous injections. Furthermore, the friends or family members who bring the patient to the emergency room can often help with the diagnosis and may be able to specify the time the overdose was taken.

Treatment

The first concern in treating a severe overdose is the same for all three classes of the addicting drugs, i.e., to stabilize cardiopulmonary function. As with the sedative hypnotics and alcohol, the opiates can produce profound respiratory depression and hypotension. Left untreated, the patient can slip into a coma and die. Thus, before resorting to specific measures for opiate toxicity, cardiopulmonary resuscitation may be necessary. The essential features of handling the initial emergency are summarized in Table 23-3. Since surface veins in addicts are often severely damaged, a venous cutdown may be necessary.

The second step in treating acute opiate toxicity involves the specific antagonism of the opiate effects. Until recently, intravenous injection of either N-allylnormorphine (Nalline) or levallorphan (Lorfan) were used for this purpose. However, since both of these medications can, themselves, induce respiratory depression, the treatment of choice is now naloxone (Narcan), a pure narcotic antagonist. Naloxone can even be used as a diagnostic test in a coma of unknown etiology. The

TABLE 23-3.
EMERGENCY TREATMENT FOR SEVERE TOXICITY FROM ADDICTING DRUGS

Stabilize cardiopulmonary status.
  Institute respiratory resuscitation measures, if necessary.
  Begin cardiac massage if no heartbeat is present.
  Intubate with a cuffed endotracheal tube if respiratory depression continues and
    begin mechanical ventilation.

Establish intravenous line.
  Draw blood gases.
  Inject 50 ml of 50% glucose, to counteract possible hypoglycemia.
  Keep line open for other drugs such as antihypotensive agents, if needed.

Monitor patient status frequently.
  Check pulse, blood pressure, electrocardiogram, and arterial blood gases and pH.

---

intravenous dose of naloxone is 0.4 mg—1 ml of the usual preparation—for adults and 0.01 mg/kg for children. If no arm vein can be found, the external jugular or the femoral vein can be used. If respiration fails to improve, this dose can be used twice more at three-minute intervals. Failure to respond after three doses suggests that the coma is due to factors other than, or in addition to, opiate toxicity. When naloxone is effective, the response is dramatic, and the patient sometimes wakes up disoriented and agitated. For this reason loose restraints should be placed on the patient as naloxone is administered (1,3–6).

After they respond to naloxone, patients must still be observed carefully. The drug has a short half-life, and respiratory depression may return in two to four hours. Thus, further doses of naloxone may be necessary, and patients should be continuously observed for twenty-four to forty-eight hours. This is particularly important for the child who has taken a toxic dose of methadone. Since it blocks opiate action, naloxone may also induce severe withdrawal symptoms, the medical management of which are described in the next section.

Patients with acute opiate toxicity may also have medical problems which result from attempts at resuscitation by well-meaning friends. One common technique is stimulation, such as slapping the face and either squeezing the nipples or testicles or applying ice to them. Another "street cure" calls for the injection of amphetamine, which may precipitate seizures in patients with hypoxia. In some areas, intravenous saline and milk are believed to "bind" heroin. The saline may disturb electrolyte balance, while the milk can probably cause lipoid pneumonia (1).

Opiate Abstinence Syndrome

Despite its popular reputation as a life-threatening condition, the opiate withdrawal syndrome is the least serious and most easily managed of the syndromes produced by drugs in the three major addictive classes. The morphine and heroin withdrawal syndrome has been studied carefully and can be described in detail.

Diagnosis

Common features of both the early and late components of the opiate abstinence syndrome are indicated in Table 23-2. For heroin and morphine, the syndrome severity usually peaks between forty-eight and seventy-two hours. However, milder symptoms such as weakness, anxiety, and sleep disturbances may persist for weeks or even months (1). Abstinence syndromes with other opiates differ primarily in their timecourse and intensity. For methadone, the syndrome is relatively mild, although it may last for about two weeks. The meperidine abstinence syndrome is characterized by earlier, milder symptoms and by a rapid recovery. Codeine withdrawal leads to delayed but mild symptoms which have a duration resembling that for heroin withdrawal (1,6).

As a general principle, the greater the daily dose, the more intense the abstinence syndrome. However, other factors also influence the adult patient's complaints and symptoms. It is possible that decreased tolerance for discomfort or a desire to obtain more opiates will lead an addicted patient to exaggerate his symptoms. Alternatively, an addicted patient who is in poor physical health may actually have a more complicated and severe withdrawal syndrome.

Opiate dependence has also been described in infants born to addicted mothers. The abstinence syndrome, which appears within forty-eight hours after delivery, can include extreme irritability; a shrill, high-pitched cry; vomiting; fever; coarse tremors; seizures; and respiratory disturbances, usually tachypnea (7,8).

Treatment

In treating the abstinence syndrome, one should first obtain a complete medical and drug-abuse history, a careful physical examination, a urinary screen for drugs of abuse, and a complete evaluation of routine laboratory chemistries. The best treatment is then to substitute oral methadone for the abused opiate, followed by gradual reduction of the methadone dose.

Several methods for pharmacological detoxification are available, most of which work fairly well. A commonly used technique begins with 20 mg of oral methadone. If the patient becomes intoxicated, the next dose is reduced to 10 mg and withheld until withdrawal symptoms begin. For most patients, a starting daily dose of 40 mg, given as 20 mg every twelve hours, is sufficient to prevent withdrawal symptoms. Some patients—for instance, those on methadone maintenance—will require larger doses. After a two- to three-day stabilization period, methadone can be reduced by 5 or 10 mg each day, as dictated by the severity of the symptoms. Usually, detoxification takes about two weeks; but patients ending a period of methadone maintenance often prefer a slower detoxification, lasting a month or more.

Psychological factors also play a role in the opiate abstinence syndrome, and anxiety reactions are common. The situation is complicated by the prevalence of malingering and persuasive complaining among opiate addicts. Some are experienced in such delinquent behaviors as forging prescriptions, stealing, and obtaining benefits or favors which were intended for other patients. For these reasons, opiate detoxification centers require adequate security and a vigilant staff which maintains a healthy skepticism. Probably, it is best to be sympathetic but firm. Complaints should be evaluated carefully, but it is rarely necessary to change the planned reduction of methadone. Predicting symptoms in advance can reduce anxiety in some patients, and antianxiety agents such as diazepam can also be helpful. Insomnia responds to flurazepam or chloral hydrate, and muscle and joint pains can be reduced with warm flow baths and massage (1).

Proper treatment of the infant of an addicted mother is somewhat more controversial. Infants with respiratory distress should be managed in a pediatric intensive care unit. Respiration should be supported as necessary, while a full diagnostic evaluation is obtained. Fluid and electrolyte balance must be monitored, and adequate caloric intake should be maintained when possible. Several pharmacological treatments have also been suggested. Paregoric (camphorated tincture of opium), 3–10 drops every four hours, or phenobarbital, 5–10 mg/kg/day in three or four doses, have been recommended for this purpose. No study has clearly demonstrated the superiority of either of these pharmacological treatments. In both cases, the dose should be adjusted to lessen hyperactivity, irritability, and other symptoms without causing significant sedation. This drug treatment can then be gradually decreased over a period of about five days (7,8).

ILLNESSES ASSOCIATED WITH OPIATE ADDICTION

As part of managing both the acute opiate toxicity and the opiate abstinence syndromes, it is important to diagnose and treat associated illnesses. Pulmonary edema occasionally presents as part of the overdose syndrome and can also occur at lower doses of opiates, particularly with "street" heroin. The cause of this pulmonary edema is not known but it may result from hypersensitivity (9). The patient should have a chest X-ray and arterial blood gas determinations. If hypoxia is evident, the patient should be hospitalized, kept in the sitting position, and given oxygen. If the pulmonary edema is severe, he may also require assisted ventilation, diuretics, and possibly rotating tourniquets.

Heroin addicts have an increased incidence of hepatitis and should have a laboratory evaluation of liver function. Pneumonia, tuberculosis, urinary tract infections, and venereal disease also occur more often in opiate addicts than in the general population (1). The frequent intravenous injections, often with contaminated syringes and unknown adulterants, add to the potential problems of the heroin addict, as indicated in Table 23-4. Finally, it is possible that a heroin addict may be unaware of an injury or an illness such as a tooth abscess or appendicitis, since the pain can be masked by the analgesic effects of the opiate (10). Clearly, opiate addicts require a careful and extensive medical evaluation, begun during the detoxification period and continued through long-term treatment and rehabilitation.

REHABILITATION

Although the actual prevalence of opiate addiction is unknown, there are probably between 300,000 and 600,000 addicts in the United States,

TABLE 23-4.
SOME MEDICAL COMPLICATIONS OF INTRAVENOUS DRUG ABUSE

Local infection:
  Skin abscess, thrombophlebitis, skin cellulitis, and folliculitis.

Distant infection:
  Septicemia; bacterial endocarditis; osteomyelitis; lung, bone and kidney abscess; malaria; serum hepatitis; and tetanus.

Foreign-body lung emboli:
  Cotton, talc, starch, and other substances.

Chronic destruction:
  Pulmonary fibrosis, acute and chronic polyneuropathy, glomerulonephritis, and nephrotic syndrome.

---

with 100,000 to 300,000 in New York City alone. Many addicts support their habit by selling drugs to others or with other illegal activities such as forgery, burglary, or robbery. Thus, the need for effective, long-term therapy of opiate addicts is clear. All treatments of overdose or withdrawal cases should include a vigorous effort to introduce the patient into a good rehabilitation program. For clarity, the pharmacological and drug-free approaches to treatment will be described separately. In practice, many centers use a combination of techniques or offer the addict a selection of them.

Pharmacological Treatments

Former addicts often experience a "narcotics hunger" or craving. Both of the pharmacological maintenance programs in current use try to relieve that "hunger." If the craving reflects a metabolic or biochemical defect, a cross-tolerant substitute such as methadone might fulfill that theoretical need (11). Alternatively, the craving might result from classical and operant conditioning. When a user returns to the setting of former drug use and withdrawal symptoms, he can develop some of the symptoms of withdrawal without being dependent, so-called conditioned withdrawal symptoms. Operant conditioning then takes place with the heroin injection as the response and the relief of either conditioned or physiological withdrawal symptoms as the reward (12). This response might be extinguished if the reinforcement were blocked by an opiate antagonist such as naltrexone. In practice, the biochemical and conditioning hypotheses are not clearly separated by methadone maintenance, since methadone both blocks heroin-induced euphoria and satisfies any theoretical metabolic need. Furthermore, the biochemical and behavioral components may work together. Whatever the mechanism, both methadone and narcotic antagonists help some addicts to abstain from heroin.

Oral methadone maintenance schedules vary among clinics. Typical programs begin with 40 mg/day, given in single or divided doses; then, over three to six weeks, this is increased to a single dose of 100 mg/day. There are recent suggestions that maintenance at 50 mg/day may be equally effective (13). Early side effects of sedation, mood swings, and anorexia gradually abate, although excessive sweating and constipation persist. To date, no serious sequelae to chronic methadone use have been found (1).

Methadone maintenance can be established on an outpatient basis. Two problems which arise are the need for daily administration and the growing use of illegal intravenous methadone injections. The first of these difficulties may be alleviated with the introduction of longer-acting methadone analogues, such as l-α-acetylmethadol. The second may be obviated by combinations of methadone and naloxone, which are effective orally but not intravenously (14).

The moral aspects of methadone maintenance are still being debated. Certainly, critics are correct in asserting that it merely replaces one form of addiction with another. However, there is a vast difference between the life-style of an addict who must continually seek funds for illegal, expensive, and probably impure heroin and a user who receives his oral methadone under clinical supervision. In addition, as used in treatment, methadone is not intended to produce euphoria. Furthermore, good programs are far more than drug dispensaries, since they also supply vocational and psychological counseling and support.

Maintenance with narcotic antagonists is a relatively recent approach to the long-term therapy of opiate addicts. We have already indicated that naloxone is the agent of choice in treating acute toxicity; however, its short half-life makes it impractical as a blocking agent. In contrast, naltrexone has a long duration of action. Early clinical trials with this compound are encouraging, since it can block the normal psychological effects of intravenous heroin (15). However, further research is required to establish what role, if any, this approach may have in the management of heroin addiction.

Drug-Free Treatments

A variety of good programs can provide a therapeutic environment for the opiate addict. Individual or group psychotherapy helps former addicts understand factors which may foster their drug abuse. Alternatively, some inpatient programs or communes provide short-term exposure to a drug-free environment of psychotherapy, peer group confrontation, recreation, and vocational guidance. A third approach offers a drug-free alternative to traditional society, with a permanent communal setting which makes extensive use of confrontation and therapy. Since each approach has particular advantages and disadvantages for specific individuals, it is important to help the addict find a program which is most closely aligned with his own needs.

SEDATIVE-HYPNOTICS

Identification of sedative-hypnotic abusers is often difficult, and users seldom seek treatment specifically for addiction. Since presenting symptoms may be erratic work performance, alcohol-like intoxication, depression, or other neurologic or psychiatric disorders, physicians should include sedative-hypnotic addiction in the differential diagnosis of such complaints. However, most patient-physician contacts initially occur in the emergency room as a result of acute toxicity or of the abstinence syndrome. Acute barbiturate toxicity causes about 1,500 deaths in the United States each year (1). Since 1952, a growing number of nonbarbiturate sedative drugs have been introduced as anti-anxiety agents and sleeping pills. Intoxication with these newer sedative-hypnotics is an increasing problem for physicians. Biological actions of the sedative-hypnotics are described in Chapter 19.

PATTERNS OF ABUSE

Sedative-hypnotic abuse occurs at all ages and in all classes but is slightly more common in women than in men. The use may be chronic, episodic, or acute. Chronic users are often Caucasians between thirty and fifty years old. Abuse crosses all socio-economic lines but is somewhat more common in the middle and upper classes. The conventional appearance and apparent social adjustment of the chronic user often masks the addiction and facilitates acquisition of multiple prescriptions and repeated refills. Chronic intoxication usually results from efforts to escape severe emotional stress.

Younger people, including teenagers, tend to use sedative-hypnotics episodically to obtain an alcohol-like intoxication. Many experience "disinhibition euphoria," a paradoxical excitation and exhilaration with increased activity and a sense of improved performance. Aberrant, sometimes violent behavior may occur, particularly among younger members of more violent social subcultures. Individuals who are deeply involved in the drug subculture may inject sedative hypnotics intravenously, primarily for a "rush"—an intensely pleasurable sensation of warmth and drowsiness. Intravenous abuse is probably the most dangerous form of sedative-hypnotic abuse, since the margin between intoxicating and fatal doses is dangerously narrow (16). Additional medical complications from intravenous injections are described in Table 23-4.

A third form of abuse is self-medication. Some individuals develop a stimulation-sedation cycle, using sedative hypnotics to counteract the effects of amphetamines, which are then used to overcome the sedatives. Others use sedative-hypnotics to combat the effects of alcohol or opiate withdrawal. In the drug subculture these drugs are used to treat such psychiatric symptoms as hallucinations and intense anxiety.

ACUTE SEDATIVE-HYPNOTIC TOXICITY

Suicide attempts account for most cases of acute toxicity, although accidental overdose and hypersensitivity reactions do occur. Severe depression is common among sedative-hypnotic users, and they are at high risk for both intentional and accidental overdoses. Overdoses are most common in individuals between thirty and fifty years of age and are more common in women than in men. Physicians, pharmacists, nurses, and other medical personnel are overrepresented in this group.

Diagnosis

The syndrome of mild to moderate barbiturate intoxication strongly resembles that of alcohol intoxication. Common symptoms are listed in Table 23-2. Severe barbiturate intoxication is a medical emergency, since the respiratory depression and hypotension can lead to deep coma and death. Mild to moderate intoxication with either the minor tranquilizers or sleeping pills produces a syndrome which is essentially identical to that for the barbiturates. Some, but not all, of these drugs also cause respiratory depression and death at higher doses. Thus, while both meprobamate and glutethimide have caused fatalities, oral doses of benzodiazepines such as chlordiazepoxide, diazepam, oxazepam, and flurazepam have not yet been implicated as the sole cause of a fatal overdose.

Treatment

Again, the first priority in treating the overdose victim is to stabilize cardiopulmonary function, using the procedures outlined in Table

23-3. Once the patient has been stabilized, efforts should be made to remove the intoxicating drug. In an alert, adult patient, syrup of ipecac, 15–40 ml orally, or apomorphine, 2.5–5.0 mg intravenously, can be used to induce vomiting (1,3,17). Intravenous naloxone, 0.4 mg, can stop this apomorphine-induced vomiting if it becomes prolonged. If the patient is comatose, gastric lavage should be attempted, after a cuffed endotracheal tube has been inserted to prevent aspiration of gastric materials. Stomach contents can be analyzed to help determine the cause of the intoxication. Activated charcoal, 30 g in 250 ml of water, can be administered after lavage and may absorb some of the remaining drug (17). If return from gastric lavage is poor, charcoal administration can be followed by a cathartic such as sodium sulfate; the catharsis may remove drug retained in the intestine. Finally, rapid, intravenous fluid loading, with or without diuretics, may hasten elimination of drugs which are excreted by the kidney. However, if fluid loading is used, serum and urinary electrolytes and urine volume must be carefully monitored (1,17).

Unfortunately, no specific antagonist exists for sedative-hypnotic toxicity. Following emergency treatment, patients who are comatose and require ventilatory assistance should be admitted to an intensive care unit and managed in consultation with an anesthesiologist, a neurologist, and other experienced specialists. If the intoxicating drug is dialyzable, hemodialysis may be necessary to hasten recovery. Clinical status should be monitored frequently. General and neurological examinations should be supplemented with data on vital signs, central venous pressure, electrocardiogram, blood gases and pH, serum electrolytes, fluid intake and urinary output. Once the patient's condition has been stabilized, it is important to take a detailed medical history. Every attempt should be made to determine the type, amount, and time of the overdose. Since the sedative hypnotics are metabolized by the liver or kidney, the functional status of these organs should be determined. Pre-existing cardiac or pulmonary disease may also complicate the treatment procedure, and allergies to antibiotics should be known in the event the patient develops an infection (3,17).

Glutethimide intoxication presents a particular problem during the recovery phase. Patients can improve, only to relapse later into a deep coma. The phenomenon has been ascribed to release from lipid stores; to delayed absorption; or to excretion in the bile, followed by reabsorption. Whatever its etiology, this potential for relapse demands increased vigilance by the treating medical staff (1,3,17).

Following recovery from overdoses of barbiturates or other sedative hypnotics, some patients will develop a toxic psychosis. Patients who are hospitalized for a sedative overdose are often depressed and have made suicide attempts. Thus, psychiatric evaluation should begin as soon as the patient is no longer confused and is able to communicate.

SEDATIVE-HYPNOTIC ABSTINENCE SYNDROME

The prototype abstinence syndrome for sedative hypnotics was described for pentobarbital (1). Chronic users of 400 mg per day had only mild withdrawal symptoms; those taking 600 mg per day often developed anxiety, tremors, and feelings of weakness. Abrupt discontinuation of 800 mg per day led to seizures and psychosis in the majority of patients. This withdrawal syndrome is a medical emergency and should be treated in the hospital.

Diagnosis

As indicated in Table 23-2, the abstinence syndrome with sedative-hypnotics has both minor and major components. For pentobarbital, patients frequently experience major symptoms of withdrawal after discontinuing a daily dosage of 800 mg for longer than six weeks. Of the major symptoms, grand mal seizures usually begin on the second or third day, while psychosis can appear any time from the third to the eighth day. This psychosis bears a strong resemblance to the delirium tremens of alcohol withdrawal. Hyperpyrexia occurs less frequently, but its appearance is an ominous sign. Table 23-5 lists the approximate, chronic daily doses which can produce abstinence syndromes with other sedative-hypnotics. Methaqualone abstinence is of particular note since a widespread myth that it is nonaddicting has recently led to a substantial increase in its abuse.

Treatment

Treatment of the sedative-hypnotic abstinence syndrome, which is essentially independent of the sedative involved, requires patient hospitalization and careful medical management. Care begins with a com-

TABLE 23-5.
ABSTINENCE SYNDROMES WITH SEDATIVE-HYPNOTICS

DRUG	DOSE THAT MAY PRODUCE ABSTINENCE SYNDROME (G/DAY) (for 2–6 months)	COMMENTS
Pentobarbital	0.4–0.8	Seizures appear on 2nd or 3rd day.
Meprobamate	3.2–6.4	Death in one patient receiving >10 g/day.
Glutethimide	2.5	Seizures appear as late as 6th day.
Ethinamate	13	
Ethchlorvynol	2.0	
Methyprylon	2.4	Death in one patient taking 7.5–12 g/day.
Methaqualone	1.8–2.0	
Chlordiazepoxide	0.3	Seizures may occur as late as 12th day.
Diazepam	0.12	Seizures may occur as late as 12th day.

Except for methaqualone (1) and diazepam (19), data were obtained from Essig (18).

plete medical and drug-abuse history, a careful physical examination, a urinary screen for drugs of abuse, and a routine battery of clinical laboratory tests.

Unfortunately, even fully cooperative patients may be able to provide only a poor estimate of the extent of their tolerance to sedative-hypnotics. Daily intake can vary markedly with time and is generally measured as the number of pills or capsules swallowed. The problem is futher complicated by the prevalent use of "street" drugs of unknown purity. Thus, it is often necessary to determine the degree of tolerance empirically. One simple test for this purpose utilizes a single, oral dose of 60 mg of phenobarbital. A nonintoxicated, supine patient is given the phenobarbital and observed one hour later. The following estimates of tolerance can then be made:

Minimal— Patient is asleep or grossly intoxicated with slurred speech, nystagmus, and ataxia. The abstinence syndrome should be mild.

Moderate— Patient is comfortable, has normal speech, exhibits no ataxia, and shows only a fine lateral nystagmus. Abstinence syndrome can be prevented with 200–300 mg of phenobarbital per day.

Strong— Patient shows no response to the test dose or shows signs of withdrawal. Prevention of the abstinence syndrome will require from 300–500 mg of phenobarbital per day.

Whatever the twenty-four-hour dose, it should be given in four equal doses at six-hour intervals. This test provides only an approximation of tolerance. Therefore, the first forty-eight hours of treatment should be used to make fine adjustments by looking for signs of abstinence just before or of severe intoxication one hour after each dose. It is probably best to keep the patient mildly intoxicated (1,20,21). Since the sedative hypnotics are all cross-tolerant, any of them could be used in place of phenobarbital, at the proper dosage. To date, there is no evidence to suggest either significant advantages or disadvantages to using the drug upon which the patient originally became dependent.

Once the patient has been stabilized for two to three days and after careful medical evaluation, the dose of phenobarbital can be reduced by 30 mg every other day. If abstinence symptoms appear, the reduction can proceed more slowly. Convulsions should not occur on this reduction schedule; but, if a seizure does occur, 100–150 mg of intramuscular phenobarbital can be given to reintoxicate the patient. There is some controversy as to whether phenytoin (Dilantin) is useful in preventing sedative-hypnotic withdrawal seizures. It should be used in a patient with a history of idiopathic epilepsy and possibly in patients with a history of previous withdrawal seizures.

If the patient initially presents with a fully developed psychosis, treatment is more difficult. Rapid intoxication with phenobarbital does not generally reverse the delirium but is valuable for decreasing agitation, insomnia, and fever. Phenobarbital can be given intramuscularly until the patient is sedated and vital signs are stable (1,20,21).

Naturally, the patient with sedative-hypnotic withdrawal has needs in addition to phenobarbital. A low bed with padded side rails can prevent injuries. Those who are unable to eat may require intravenous fluids, restoration of electrolyte balance, and vitamins. Like the heroin addict, the user of sedative hypnotics may have associated medical illnesses and will require a careful medical evaluation. Finally, and perhaps most important, the detoxified patient will require follow-up psychiatric treatment to prevent the all-too-common return to the dependent condition (1).

REHABILITATION

There may be as many as 1 million abusers of sedative hypnotics in the United States alone. Despite this, there are no systematic programs which are specifically tailored for long-term therapy of the sedative-hypnotic addict. In fact, many existing programs for opiate and alcohol addiction actually reject these addicts because they have a high relapse rate. Nevertheless, sedative-hypnotic abuse should be treated essentially as a chronic condition, with exacerbations and remissions. As such, the most realistic treatment goal appears to be reduction of the severity and frequency of those remissions. Regular follow-up should be an essential feature of any program. Thus, it is important for the physician to become familiar with voluntary and governmental resources within the community and, perhaps, to mobilize efforts to establish centers for long-term care of these patients.

Pharmacological Treatments

Occasionally life may become so painful for the abuser that drug treatment is necessary. Naturally, sedative hypnotics should be avoided; however, long-acting, nonaddicting antianxiety agents such as hydroxyzine may be of value in selected patients. Unfortunately, no specific antagonists of the sedative hypnotics are yet available.

Drug-Free Treatments

As suggested in the description of patterns of abuse, sedative-hypnotic addicts often have profound psychiatric disturbances. Appropriate treatment should be determined with a complete pharmacological, psychological, and social evaluation. As a group, these individuals appear to require a strongly supportive environment, and the confrontation techniques of many opiate addiction programs are not particularly effective (22). Approaches like those for alcoholism, combining attention to physical, vocational, and psychological needs, do appear to meet with some success (16).

ETHYL ALCOHOL

Alcohol is the most widely used drug of abuse. A significant proportion of mankind's energy is devoted to the production and consumption of alcohol and to the management of problems caused by the abuse of alcohol. Individuals who abuse alcohol are frequent visitors to hospital emergency rooms. They may present with alcohol intoxication, with the alcohol abstinence syndrome, or with a wide variety of medical and psychiatric illnesses that are associated with alcohol abuse. The biological effects of ethanol are described in Chapter 20.

PATTERNS OF ABUSE

Alcohol is the only addictive drug of abuse which can be used legally for recreational purposes. Nearly 100 million Americans drink alcoholic beverages; of these, from 6 to 10 million suffer from alcoholism. Although there are more detailed definitions, alcoholism can be briefly defined as a preoccupation with alcohol use which is sufficiently serious to become a significant impediment both to physical and mental health and to interpersonal relationships. Alcoholics are found at every socio-economic level and in most subcultures of American society, but the distribution is not even. Traditionally, the ratio of male to female alcoholics is about 5 : 1, but this may be decreasing. There is also an apparent tendency for alcoholism to cluster in families, and there are powerful cultural patterns in its social use. There seems to be a recent and disturbing increase in alcohol use among young people between the ages of twelve and eighteen.

Two of the most common of the multiple patterns of severe alcohol abuse are continuous or daily use and episodic but heavy "binge drinking." Although the "skid row" alcoholic who is unemployed and lives on the streets in well-defined areas of most cities is a popular stereotype of the alcoholic, he probably represents only 3 to 5 percent of the total number of alcoholics.

ACUTE ALCOHOL TOXICITY

Mild to moderate alcohol intoxication produces a syndrome that is familiar to most of us. It is one of the most easily studied syndromes in medicine, since classic cases of each stage of intoxication can be found at many social gatherings and nearly any bar or pub.

Diagnosis

Table 23-2 divides the common features of acute alcohol toxicity into mild, moderate, and severe symptoms, most of which are characterized by a loosening of inhibitions and a deterioration of sensory and motor skills. The degree of intoxication is related, at least roughly, to blood alcohol content (23). With moderate intoxication, wide mood swings through happiness, sadness, and irritability are common. "Pathological intoxication" refers to an excited, combative, and confused state which is seen in some individuals. Explosive or "epileptoid" personalities are thought to be particularly prone to this syndrome, even with the ingestion of only small amounts of alcohol; however, it probably occurs more commonly with more severe intoxication (23). As with other acute toxicity syndromes, the respiratory depression and hypotension resulting from severe alcohol intoxication can lead to coma and death and should be treated as a medical emergency.

Treatment

The mild to moderately intoxicated patient requires no specific treatment. If such a patient appears in the emergency room, the physician should perform a careful physical examination and laboratory evaluation and offer a referral to a long-term alcohol treatment program. It is often helpful to make the appointment for this treatment from the emergency room and to involve family members or members of the local chapter of Alcoholics Anonymous, since these measures increase the chances that the patient will accept the referral. "Pathological intoxication" can be a more difficult problem. The combative patient may require physical restraints. Parenteral administration of sedative hypnotics such as diazepam, 5–20 mg, may be necessary to prevent the patient from injuring himself on the physical restraints. However, the syndrome will pass as the alcohol is eliminated from the body.

In contrast to the earlier stages of alcoholic intoxication, the alcoholic coma is a medical emergency. As with severe toxicities from opiates or sedative hypnotics, specific aspects of the alcoholic intoxication should be treated only after the patient's clinical status has been stabilized, using the steps recommended in Table 23-3. Gastric lavage is important when other drugs may have contributed to the respiratory depression; but lavage is not usually helpful in removing alcohol, which is rapidly absorbed from the stomach.

Following emergency treatment, the patient should be admitted to the intensive care unit. Careful and frequent general physical and neurological evaluations are essential, as is attention to vital signs, central venous pressure, arterial blood gases and pH, serum electrolytes, and fluid intake and output. Despite the complicated literature on agents which reportedly hasten alcohol metabolism, there is little firm evidence that their use significantly reduces morbidity. Thus, although insulin, glucose, or fructose infusions appear to abbreviate alcohol intoxication, further studies of their use as adjuncts in treating alcoholic coma are required (24).

When a patient begins to recover from alcoholic coma, a psychiatric evaluation should be performed. Referral to a psychiatric or alcohol treatment program is usually indicated.

ALCOHOL ABSTINENCE SYNDROME

The alcohol abstinence syndrome is similar to that produced by the abrupt cessation of high doses of short-acting barbiturates. As with alcoholic intoxication, alcohol withdrawal is a familiar syndrome in many emergency treatment centers.

Diagnosis

To many medical personnel, laymen, and alcoholics, the "DT's" refer to any of the spectrum of symptoms produced by alcohol abstinence. Rigorously, however, delirium tremens is only the most severe of four stages of withdrawal, which are described in Table 23-3. The first stage, alcoholic tremulousness, usually appears within twelve hours. Although it generally subsides within three to four days, it may progress into the more severe forms of withdrawal. If they occur, alcoholic hallucinosis and convulsions normally appear by the second day. Alcoholic hallucinosis often progresses from a misinterpretation of auditory or visual sensations to frank hallucinations. Buzzing sounds, bells, and light and dark spots are common, while more severe cases may involve deprecatory voices or small creatures such as insects or mice scurrying about the room. Grand mal seizures are so typical of alcoholic convulsions that the presence of focal seizures suggests another source of pathology. As with tremulousness, both hallucinosis and convulsions may either subside spontaneously or develop into frank delirium tremens. This last stage appears from the second to the fourth day and is characterized by a massive autonomic discharge, agitation, and a profound confusion (24).

Treatment

Attempting to treat the alcohol abstinence syndrome on an outpatient basis is a common but dangerous practice, since the ultimate severity of the symptoms is difficult to predict in the early phases of withdrawal. Optimal treatment requires hospitalization, with the institution of complete medical management, including careful medical evaluations, psychological support, use of a drug which is cross-tolerant to alcohol, attention to fluids and nutrition, and prompt treatment of medical problems such as seizures or fever (23–25).

Alcoholics frequently present with a variety of associated illnesses, making essential a complete medical evaluation. Alcoholics have abnormally high incidences of several disorders (Table 23-6). Thus, the patient should receive complete physical and neurological examinations, skull and chest X-rays, routine hematological and blood chemistry screens, and a test for occult blood in the feces. Further clinical and laboratory procedures should be initiated as warranted. All serious problems should be treated in consultation with the appropriate specialists. In addition, the patient should be evaluated and treated for psychiatric disturbances, since alcohol is often used as self-medication for depression or mania.

Psychological support is important in the successful treatment of the alcohol abstinence syndrome. Many of the symptoms can produce severe anxiety, and the additional pain and discomfort of numerous tests is not comforting. Moderate amounts of light and noise are probably

TABLE 23-6.

SOME MEDICAL COMPLICATIONS OF ALCOHOL ABUSE

Trauma:
Falls, burns, subdural hematomas, and other injuries.

Liver disease:
Acute alcoholic hepatitis, cirrhosis, esophageal varices, and hepatic coma.

Gastrointestinal disease:
Gastritis, peptic ulcers, bleeding, pancreatitis.

Nutritional disease:
Malnutrition; anemia due to iron, B_{12}, or folate deficiency; subacute, combined neurological degeneration, from B_{12} deficiency; and Wernicke-Korsakoff syndrome, from thiamine deficiency.

Infections:
Tuberculosis and viral, pneumococcal, or klebsiella pneumonia.

Neurological disease:
Mononeuropathy, polyneuropathy, Marchiafava-Bignami disease, toxic amblyopia, cerebellar degeneration, and dementia.

---

best, since extremes in either direction can worsen perceptual distortions. Frequent reassurances and opportunities for reality testing are also helpful.

The alcoholic abstinence syndrome per se, is treated with a drug which is cross-tolerant with alcohol. Although many sedative hypnotics and tranquilizers have been used for this purpose, chlordiazepoxide and diazepam are probably best. Antipsychotics are not recommended: they lower the seizure thereshold and may produce hypotension. The dose should be individually titrated, and particular care should be given with cirrhotic patients. Patients should be mildly intoxicated but not oversedated. The amount of medication needed will depend on the severity of the withdrawal syndrome. For most patients with alcoholic tremulousness, 50 mg of chlordiazepoxide four to six times per day is sufficient. For patients with hallucinosis or alcoholic epilepsy, 100 mg of chlordiazepoxide four to six times per day may be necessary.

For the complete delirium tremens syndrome, even higher doses of cross-tolerant medications are needed. This required dose is often higher than the manufacturer's recommended therapeutic dose. One regimen begins with 50–100 mg of chlordiazepoxide, given orally or intramuscularly every one to two hours until the patient is sedated and then every four to six hours. A total of 800 mg or more may be necessary during the first twenty-four hours. Beginning on the second day, the original dose can be reduced by 10 percent each day, until the patient is detoxified ten days later. This reduction schedule can be increased to 20 percent each day if the patient is too sedated. Diazepam, in initial doses of 20–40 mg, can be used in a similar regimen. In both cases, absorption from intramuscular injections is somewhat unreliable, so oral medications should be instituted as soon as the patient can tolerate them. Successful development of a benzodiazepine which is absorbed from muscles more reliably should improve these treatment regimens.

Patients who are in alcoholic withdrawal often have serious fluid and electrolyte imbalances. Some alcoholics are dehydrated from vomiting, diarrhea, and anorexia; but many have an overall fluid excess. Cirrhosis can also disrupt electrolyte balance. As a result, fluid replacement must be individualized by monitoring fluid intake and urinary output, serum and urinary electrolytes, and urine specific gravity (25). Patients may have low total body potassium and magnesium levels, even if serum concentrations are normal. Magnesium sulfate, 2–4 ml of a 50 percent solution, should be given intramuscularly every six hours for a total of four to six doses (25,26). Patients who are eating probably do not need extra potassium; however, those on intravenous fluids should receive 60–80 mEq over the entire first twenty-four hours, with frequent assessment of serum potassium. Potassium is always given by continuous infusion—*never in a bolus*.

Alcoholics are also frequently malnourished and may have severe vitamin deficiencies. All patients should receive an initial intramuscular dose of 100 mg of thiamine, followed by oral doses of 50 mg, three times a day for four days. Multivitamins, including vitamin B_{12} and folic acid, should also be given daily. In addition, a prolonged prothrombin time should be treated with a single dose of vitamin K (24–26). Hypoglycemia can be another problem. Alcohol impairs gluconeogenesis and depletes liver glycogen stores. Patients who are eating should have no difficulties, but all intravenous fluids should contain dextrose. If a patient's level of consciousness drops suddenly, he should immediately receive an intravenous injection of 50 ml of 50 percent glucose.

A patient in delirium tremens may have several problems which require immediate treatment. In severe cases, peripheral circulatory collapse is a strong possibility and should be guarded against with frequent assessments of vital signs. If shock does develop, patients require the usual treatment for circulatory collapse (24). The grand mal seizures of alcohol withdrawal generally do not necessitate anticonvulsant medication, although a neurological examination and an evaluation of electrolytes, including calcium and magnesium, are probably indicated (24). As already mentioned, focal seizures are so uncommon in this syndrome that they require a more extensive neurological work-up. Frequent seizures should respond to slow intravenous infusion of 5–10 mg of diazepam or to an intramuscular injection of 100–150 mg of phenobarbital. Phenytoin may be of value as a preventative measure in patients with a history of withdrawal seizures. Seizure suppression probably requires two to three days of 100 mg of phenytoin, four times a day. It need not be continued for more than one week in alcoholics who have no history of idiopathic epilepsy (24,27).

Fever is also a common symptom during the alcohol abstinence syndrome. It can result from dehydration, hepatitis, or pancreatitis; but a complete search for infection should also be undertaken. Common sources include pneumonia, tuberculosis, urinary tract infections, and infections from intravenous or urinary catheters. If hyperthermia is severe, ice pack or cooling blankets should be used (24,26).

Finally, and perhaps most important, the alcoholic needs a referral to a long-term treatment program. Referrals are generally most successful if they are made as soon as the patient is coherent enough to understand what is being offered. Vigorous follow-up by the staff of that program is also extremely important in preventing the usual return to heavy alcohol use after hospital discharge.

REHABILITATION

Like the opiate addict, the alcoholic has available both pharmacological and drug-free treatment programs for long-term therapy. Although this addiction is not illegal, it is the source of untold anguish both for the addict and for his family and friends. In addition, alcoholism exacts an enormous toll upon society in the form of shattered families, lost wages, traffic accidents, and rehabilitative care, with economic costs estimated at $25 billion per year.

Pharmacological Treatments

The major pharmacological agent for combating alcoholism has been disulfiram (Antabuse). Disulfiram alone produces few clinical effects. However, by a mechanism which is discussed in Chapter 20, the combination of alcohol and disulfiram induces flushing, sweating, palpitations, dyspnea, hyperventilation, tachypnea, hypotension, nausea, vomiting, and drowsiness. Tolerance to these effects does not develop. The acute discomfort and relative safety of these symptoms forms the basis for disulfiram use in alcoholism. An early treatment paradigm attempted to establish an aversion to ethanol by repeatedly giving it to patients who had been pretreated with disulfiram. This has subsequently yielded to programs in which the patient is simply maintained on low doses of disulfiram as a means of discouraging alcohol use.

Patients who are starting on disulfiram maintenance should be fully advised of its action and of the consequences of alcohol ingestion. Treatment should never begin until twelve to twenty-four hours after the last intake of alcohol, so that the body is free of it. A typical schedule begins with no more than 500 mg/day, given as a single oral dose; after one to two weeks, this is reduced to a maintenance dose of about 250 mg/day. An initial drowsiness and loss of mental acuity usually disappear within one to two weeks; but other mild side effects such as fatigue, dizziness, skin eruptions, headache, impotence, gastrointestinal disturbances, and the presence of a peculiar taste and odor may require a dose reduction. The severe psychiatric disturbances that occasionally occur are discussed in Chapter 29. Disulfiram is clearly contraindicated by histories of heart disease and psychosis and should be used with caution in the presence of cirrhosis, nephritis, epilepsy, goiter, pregnancy, drug addiction, diabetes mellitus, asthma, and hematopoietic disorders. When disulfiram is used, paraldehyde is contraindicated, since it can interact with disulfiram. For best effect, disulfiram treatment should be only one aspect of an intensive effort on the part of the physician, the patient, friends, family, and formal groups to help the alcoholic with his problem (28,29).

As alcoholics recover from withdrawal, they may experience strong anxiety and complain of palpitations, epigastric discomfort, pain, and other symptoms. Antianxiety agents have been helpful in relieving such symptoms; however, as with sedative-hypnotic abusers, the alcoholic may be particularly susceptible to drug dependence, so great care must be taken (30).

Drug-Free Treatments

For alcoholics who seek treatment, a variety of inpatient and outpatient programs are available. Many are organized by professionals from various disciplines; others, such as Alcoholics Anonymous (AA), are run by nonprofessionals. Individual therapy is available, primarily in the form of behavioral conditioning and hypnosis. However, most treatments utilize group therapies, either alone or in conjunction with pharmacological and vocational support. The rich variety of available options has been reviewed elsewhere (31,32) and will not be described here.

Several common themes run through many of these programs. A supportive but firm attitude toward the addict is essential. The alcoholic must recognize that he has a severe problem for which there is no ready cure. Active involvement of close friends and family should be encouraged, since their understanding of and help with the recovery program can be a key factor to success. As with programs for opiate addicts, no single approach will work for all people. Even patients who repeatedly return to drinking should be encouraged to continue to seek ways of reducing the frequency and intensity of drinking episodes and of minimizing the effects their drinking might have on other phases of their private and public lives.

CONCLUSION

Abuse of addictive drugs causes profound problems for society and is a particular challenge to physicians. This chapter has focused primarily upon the emergency management of acute toxicity, abstinence syndromes, and associated medical illnesses. Careful medical management of these syndromes can produce dramatic recoveries. Unfortunately, long-term treatment and rehabilitation programs have been far less successful than have the acute treatment regimens. Thus, these recoveries are often only temporary, with the patient rapidly returning to drug abuse once he is released. Worse, neither physicians nor society as a whole have been able to prevent the introduction of drug abuse among young people. As clearly evidenced by the steadily increasing numbers of drug abusers, research efforts in both these areas deserve a high priority.

REFERENCES

1. Berger, P. A. Management of the addicted patient. *In: Psychiatric Treatment: Crisis, Clinic, and Consultation.* C. P. Rosenbaum and J. E. Beebe, *eds.,* New York: McGraw-Hill, 1975, pp. 161–171.
2. Rubin, Peter E. and Cluff, L. E. Differential diagnosis of emergency drug reactions. *In: A Treatment Manual for Acute Drug Abuse Emergencies.* P. G. Bourne, *ed.,* DHEW Publication No. (ADM) 75–230. U.S. Government Printing Office, 1974, pp. 8–10.
3. Greenblatt, D. J. and Shader, R. I. Drug abuse and the emergency room physician. *Am. J. Psychiatry 131:559–562,* 1974.
4. Green, M. H. and Dupont, R. L. The treatment of acute heroin toxicity. *In: A Treatment Manual for Acute Drug Abuse Emergencies.* P. G. Bourne, *ed.,* DHEW Publication No. (ADM) 75–230. U.S. Government Printing Office, 1974, pp. 11–16.
5. Kleber, H. D. The treatment of acute heroin toxicity. *In: A Treatment Manual for Acute Drug Abuse Emergencies.* P. G. Bourne, *ed.,* DHEW Publication No. (ADM) 75–230. U.S. Government Printing Office, 1974, pp. 17–21.
6. Green, A. I., Mayer, R. E., and Shader, R. I. Heroin and methadone abuse: acute and chronic management. *In: Manual of Psychiatric Therapeutics: Practical Psychiatry and Psychopharmacology.* R. I. Shader, *ed.,* Boston: Little, Brown and Co., 1975, pp. 203–210.
7. Reddy, A. M. The management of the narcotic withdrawal syndrome in the neonate. *In: A Treatment Manual for Acute Drug Abuse Emergencies.* P. G. Bourne, *ed.,* DHEW Publication No. (ADM) 75–230. U.S. Government Printing Office, 1974, pp. 27–28.
8. Kahn, E. J. The heroin withdrawal syndrome of newborn infants. *In: A Treatment Manual for Acute Drug Abuse Emergencies.* P. G. Bourne, *ed.,* DHEW Publication No. (ADM) 75–230. U.S. Government Printing Office, 1974, pp. 29–33.
9. Duberstein, J. L. and Kaufman, D. L. A clinical study of an epidemic of heroin intoxication and heroin induced pulmonary edema. *Am. J. Med. 51:*704–714, 1971.
10. Cherubin, C. E. Management of acute medical complications resulting from heroin addiction. *In: A Treatment Manual for Acute Drug Abuse Emergencies.* P. G. Bourne, *ed.,* DHEW Publication No. (ADM) 75–230. U.S. Government Printing Office, 1974, pp. 38–47.
11. Dole, V. P. and Nyswander, M. E. Methadone maintenance and its implication for theories of narcotic addiction. *Assoc. Res. Nerv. Ment. Dis. Proc. 46:*359–367, 1968.
12. Wikler, A. Conditioning factors in opiate addiction and relapse. *In: Narcotics.* D. M. Wilner and G. G. Kassebaum, *eds.,* New York: McGraw-Hill, 1965, pp. 85–100.
13. Garbutt, G. W. and Goldstein, A. Blind comparison of three methadone maintenance dosages in 180 patients. *Assoc. Res. Nerv. Ment. Dis. Proc. 46:*411–441, 1968.
14. Nutt, J. G. and Jasinski, D. R. Methadone-naloxone mixtures for use in methadone maintenance programs. I: Evaluation in man of phar-

macological feasibility. II: Demonstration of acute physical dependence. *Clin. Pharmacol. Ther. 15:*156–166, 1974.

15. Resnick, R. B., Volavka, ·J., and Freedman, A. M. Studies of EN–1639A (naltrexone): A new narcotic antagonist. *Am. J. Psychiatry 131:*646–650, 1974.

16. Wesson, D. R. and Smith, D. E. Barbiturate toxicity and the treatment of barbiturate dependence. *J. Psychedel. Drug 5:*159–165, 1972.

17. Hollister, L. E. Overdoses of psychotherapeutic drugs. *In: Psychiatric Treatment: Crisis, Clinic, and Consultation.* C. P. Rosenbaum and J. E. Beebe, *eds.,* New York: McGraw-Hill, 1975, pp. 145–154.

18. Essig, C. F. Newer sedative drugs that can cause states of intoxication and dependence of the barbiturate type. *J. Am. Med. Assoc. 196:*714–717, 1966.

19. Hollister, L. E. Diazepam in newly admitted schizophrenics. *Dis. Nerv. Syst. 24:*746–775, 1963.

20. Wikler, A. Diagnosis and treatment of drug dependence of the barbiturate type. *Am. J. Psychiatry 125:*758–765, 1968.

21. Smith, D. E. and Wesson, D. R. Phenobarbital technique for treatment of barbiturate dependence. *Arch. Gen. Psychiatry 24:*56–60, 1971.

22. Benvenuto, J. A., Lau, J., and Cohen, R. Patterns of non-opiate/polydrug abuse: findings of a national collaborative research project. Reported to the Committee on Problems of Drug Dependence, National Academy of Sciences, Washington, D.C., May 20, 1975.

23. Beebe, J. E. Evaluation and treatment of the drinking patient. *In: Psychiatric Treatment: Crisis, Clinic, and Consultation.* C. P. Rosenbaum and J. E. Beebe, *eds.,* New York: McGraw-Hill, 1975, pp. 115–144.

24. Victor, M. Treatment of alcohol intoxication and the withdrawal syndrome: a critical analysis of the use of drugs and other forms of therapy. *In: A Treatment Manual for Acute Drug Abuse Emergencies.* P. G. Bourne, *ed.,* DHEW Publication No. (ADM) 75–230. U.S. Government Printing Office, 1974, pp. 105–177.

25. Knott, D. H. and Beard, J. D. Diagnosis and treatment of acute withdrawal from alcohol. *In: A Treatment Manual for Acute Drug Abuse Emergencies.* P. G. Bourne, *ed.,* DHEW Publication No. (ADM) 75–230. U.S. Government Printing Office, 1974, pp. 118–123.

26. Greenblatt, D. J. and Shader, R. I. Treatment of the alcohol withdrawal syndrome. *In: Manual for Psychiatric Therapeutics: Practical Psychiatry and Psychopharmacology.* R. I. Shader, *ed.,* Boston: Little, Brown and Co., 1975, pp. 211–239.

27. Vincent, T. When to use Dilantin during withdrawal. *Res. Staff Phys. 22:*50–51, 1976.

28. Lundwall, L. and Baekeland, F. Disulfiram treatment of alcoholism. *J. Nerv. Ment. Dis. 153:*381–394, 1971.

29. Fox, R. Treatment of the problem drinker by the private practitioner. *In: Alcoholism: Progress in Research and Treatment.* P. G. Bourne and R. Fox, *eds.,* New York: Academic Press, 1973, pp. 227–243.

30. Hoff, E. C. Pharmacologic and metabolic adjuncts in alcoholism. *In: Alcoholism.* R. J. Catanzaro, *ed.,* Springfield: Thomas, 1968, pp. 175–185.

31. Catanzaro, R. J., ed., *Alcoholism.* Springfield: Thomas, 1968.
32. Emerick, C. A review of psychologically oriented treatment of alcoholism. II: The relative effectiveness of different treatment approaches and the effectiveness of treatment versus no treatment. *Quart. J. Stud. Alc.* 36:88–108, 1975.

24 | Treatment of Abusers of Nonaddictive Drugs

JARED R. TINKLENBERG and PHILIP A. BERGER

INTRODUCTION

Illegal, nonmedical use of psychoactive drugs is an increasing problem for clinicians. Frequently, physicians first encounter the drug abuser in the emergency room, as a result of adverse, sometimes life-threatening, reactions to the drug. The management problems of the acute toxicity and abstinence syndromes of addicting drugs are considered in Chapter 23. This chapter discusses the treatment of adverse reactions with nonaddictive psychoactive agents.

Nonaddictive drugs are defined functionally as substances for which abrupt cessation of chronic consumption does not produce severe physical withdrawal reactions. This diverse group of compounds can be clustered into five major pharmacological categories—hallucinogens, cannabis, central stimulants, anticholinergics, and volatile solvents. Since drugs within each of these categories produce similar clinical syndromes and adverse reactions, treatment regimens follow a similar pattern.

HALLUCINOGENS

The hallucinogens include a variety of substances, some derived from natural plants and others synthesized in the laboratory (Table 24-1). These substances have also been called psychotogens, dysleptics, phantasticas, psychotomimetics, and psychedelics. Drugs in this group satisfy the following criteria (1):

- Changes in thought, perception, and mood predominate.
- Stupor, narcosis, or psychomotor stimulation are not prominent.
- Autonomic nervous system side effects are not severe.
- Addictive craving is minimal.

TABLE 24-1.
REPRESENTATIVE NONADDICTIVE DRUGS

Hallucinogens–Lysergic acid diethylamide (LSD); peyote; mescaline; psilocybin; 2,5-dimethoxy-4-methylamphetamine (STP); dimethyltryptamine (DMT); tri-methoxyamphetamine (TMA); methylenedioxyamphetamine (MDA); phency-clidine (Sernyl, PCP).

Cannabis

Central Stimulants–Amphetamine (Dexedrine, Benzedrine); methamphetamine (Methedrine); methylphenidate (Ritalin); phenmetrazine (Preludin); diethyl-proprion (Tenuate, Apisate); cocaine.

Anticholinergic Agents–Scopolamine, atropine, hyoscyamine (datura, Jimson weed), ditran (JB329).

Inhalants–Acetone, toluene, gasoline and other petroleum products, ether, carbon tetrachloride, nitrous oxide, carbon dioxide.

Our current understanding of the modes by which these drugs exert their effects is summarized in Chapter 22.

ADVERSE EFFECTS

Many of the adverse reactions to the hallucinogens are in response to normal components of their somatic, sensory, and psychological effects, as exemplified by the LSD "trip." Somatic symptoms of LSD use include drowsiness, paresthesia, dizziness, weakness, tremor, and nausea. The drug also induces perceptual alterations of colors and shapes, increased auditory acuity, difficulty in focusing on objects, and synesthesia, in which stimulation of one sensory modality produces sensations in another. Thus, an LSD user may report that he can "see" a sound. Psychological effects of LSD include profound but labile shifts in mood, difficulty in expressing thoughts, distorted time sense, depersonalization, dreamlike feelings, and visual hallucinations. Reaction to these effects seems to be related to personal predisposition. For example, some individuals describe a sense of "universal insight" or a feeling of emotional ties with all other people and living things; others experience unpleasant, frightening images or disturbing thoughts.

Other adverse effects of hallucinogenic drug use involve transient aberrant behavior. Drug-induced feelings of omnipotence have led to fatal leaps from high places by users who felt they could fly. Loss of control of coordination, emotions, or intellect may lead to anger or panic. Severe panic can result in self-injury during a frenzied attempt to escape terrifying thoughts and sensations. While such events do occur, they are probably less common than popular press reports would lead one to believe. Hallucinogens have also been linked with persisting psychosis, prolonged depression, and clouded thinking and judgment with deficient social functioning. However these reactions may relate more to adulterants in "street" hallucinogens, such as anticholinergics, and to pre-existing psychological problems of the user (2).

The clinical syndromes produced by LSD, psilocybin, and mescaline are quite similar. The dimethyltryptamine syndrome is also similar, but it is of shorter duration and may involve more visual distortions. Phencyclidine produces a somewhat different clinical syndrome, which may include disorientation and exaggerated disturbances of motor skills, proprioception, and thought processes; acute adverse reactions may be more common among phencyclidine users (1).

TREATMENT

The acute adverse reaction to hallucinogens that leads to the emergency room is often called the "bad trip." Although lethal overdoses of hallucinogenic drugs are extremely rare, fatalities are more likely to occur when the hallucinogen has been mixed with adulterants, such as sedative hypnotics or anticholinergics. Management of the anticholinergic intoxication syndrome is described below, while treatment for sedative-hypnotic toxicity is detailed in Chapter 23.

General principles for treating "bad trips" with hallucinogenic drugs are also useful in treating adverse reactions to other types of nonaddicting, psychoactive drugs. The three overlapping treatment priorities are summarized in Table 24-2. Since reactions to these drugs are seldom life-threatening, emphasis is placed upon making the patient as comfortable as possible, while minimizing the risk of physical harm to either the patient or others. In addition, efforts must be made to determine which drug or drugs are involved, so that rational steps can be taken to decrease toxic effects and relieve behavioral disturbances.

The highest immediate priority for the clinician is to secure the

TABLE 24-2.
TREATMENT PRIORITIES FOR ADVERSE REACTIONS
TO NONADDICTIVE DRUGS

Secure the safety of the patient
  Arrange for someone to stay with the patient.
  Use gentle physical restraints to control combative or self-destructive behaviors.
Establish a working diagnosis
  Obtain history of drug use from patient and his friends.
  Look for characteristic physical signs.
Reduce toxic and behavioral effects

---

safety of the patient and those around him. The patient should not be left unattended while he is awaiting medical attention or during the diagnostic process. Combative, extremely agitated, or self-destructive patients may require gentle physical restraint. Vital signs should be taken immediately, so that prompt intervention can begin if the patient shows cardiovascular irregularities; they also provide baseline values for use in later decision-making.

Once the patient's safety is secured, priority should be given to establishing a tentative diagnosis. Information pertaining to the drug experience should be gathered from as many different sources as possible. People suffering from toxic reactions to psychoactive drugs are frequently brought in by friends who have pertinent information, especially regarding others who consumed the same drugs as the patient. By comparing the patient's reactions with those of other users, inferences about idiosyncratic reactions and approximate dosages can be made. It is particularly important to determine the approximate dosage; the mode of administration; the time the drug was taken; and, whether any other drugs were consumed by the patient, either during the initial episode or during attempts to treat the toxic reaction. Unfortunately, accompanying friends sometimes cannot provide valid information, either because they too are under drug influence or because they do not know exactly what happened. Sometimes, historical information can be supplemented with data about drugs which are currently being used in a specific geographic area. For example, some hospital emergency room staffs monitor the appearance of new drugs into the community and maintain descriptions of the alleged content, the actual content, and the appearance of the substance or pill. This information can be very helpful, but must constantly be updated, because illegal drug use is often faddish.

A definitive history is unusual in most cases involving toxic reactions to nonmedical drug use. Therefore, historical information should be integrated with a physical examination, which can often provide essential clues. Because of the problem of drug contamination, even a straightforward history that clearly identifies the drug should always be substantiated, if possible, by specific physical findings. For example, hallucinogens generally produce dilated pupils and hyperactive reflexes (Table 24-3).

After a tentative diagnosis has been established, the clinician can focus on reducing the toxic effects of the drug and managing any concomitant behavioral disturbances. Whenever possible, nonpharmacological forms of intervention should be used. The patient's surroundings should be arranged to avoid extremes of sensory input, which may

TABLE 24-3.
COMMON CLINICAL FINDINGS WITH DRUG ABUSERS

DRUG GROUP	EFFECTS	DRUG GROUP	EFFECTS
Hallucinogens	Dilated pupils Hyperactive reflexes Adequate mental orientation	Anticholinergics	Dilated, unreactive pupils, blurred vision, flushed face, warm and dry skin, dry mouth, foul breath, decreased or absent bowel signs, tachycardia, and fever
Cannabis	Tachycardia Dilated conjunctival blood vessels Normal pupil size		Disorientation, incoherence, bizarre delirium characterized by fluctuating levels of awareness, and memory impairment
Central Stimulants	Variable increases in blood pressure, sweating, and motor activity Paranoid behavior	Inhalants	Delirium characterized by impaired judgment, orientation, memory, and motor skills

worsen the syndrome. A quiet room with moderate light and sound is probably best. Talking should be subdued but understandable, and rapid or sudden movements should be avoided. The procedure known as the "talk down" is often effective when there is adequate time (3). The general principle is to maintain verbal contact with the patient in a soothing, almost parental, manner. The patient should be constantly reassured that he is experiencing an adverse reaction to a drug, that his problem is temporary, and that his distress will gradually subside. Repetition of orienting statements about person and place are useful, as is emphasis on the temporary nature of the experience. It may be helpful to have a patient verbalize his experiences, since this may give him a greater sense of control. In any event, the therapist should be flexible and pursue those topics of conversation which seem to reduce anxiety. As the effects of toxic reaction begin to diminish, the patient will often notice that symptom-severity is fluctuating. This should be explicitly anticipated by the therapist, who should also be duly cautious in deciding when the toxic reaction has subsided completely.

With most adverse reactions to hallucinogens, supportive treatment is all that is required. However, busy emergency room staff may not have time for the "talk down" procedure. If they do not, medication may be necessary to control the patient's anxiety and agitation. Antianxiety drugs such as the benzodiazepines, which have a wide margin of safety, are probably the drugs of choice. They should be given to reduce anxiety to manageable levels without undue sedation or depression of vital signs. For example, diazepam (Valium), 20–30 mg orally or 5–20 mg intramuscularly, may be given at three- to six-hour intervals as needed. For several reasons, phenothiazines or other antipsychotic agents are usually contraindicated. The narrow margin between effective behavioral sedation and serious depression of the cardiovascular system makes questionable the use of such potent drugs as sedatives for any clinical disorder in which the untreated course is usually benign. In this instance, the potential danger is increased because "street" hallucinogens frequently contain anticholinergic adulterants. Moreover, antipsychotic agents might mask an incipient schizophrenic psychosis, which could otherwise be detected and appropriately treated. Finally, the extrapyramidal side effects of these drugs are distressing for many patients and may increase agitation and anxiety.

Hospitalization for adverse hallucinogen reactions is rarely necessary, unless dictated by serious medical problems which can accompany drug abuse, such as hepatitis and bacterial endocarditis or other infections. Persistent impairment of cognitive functions or of perceptions for more than four to six hours, despite medication, is another adverse reaction which may require hospitalization. Otherwise, once brain functions and vital signs have returned to normal, the patient can be discharged to a responsible person. If a patient lives alone, it is probably best to help him find a place with friends or relatives for at least twenty-four hours. The patient and responsible person should be warned that lethargy, irritability, and depression are sometimes associated with recovery from an adverse drug reaction. A follow-up psychiatric consultation should also be offered.

Some users of hallucinogenic drugs report having "flashbacks" long after they last used the drug. Flashbacks are spontaneous reoccurrences of thoughts, feelings, and perceptions which were originally experienced during drug intoxication. The underlying mechanisms are not understood, but they seem to be psychological. Thus, flashbacks can occur months after all pharmacological effects should have dissipated and are usually triggered by fairly specific psychological factors such as certain emotions, thoughts, or environmental events. They are seldom a significant clinical problem. Treatment consists of advising the person to discontinue the use of all hallucinogens and any other psychoactive drugs which may be contributing to the difficulty; teaching the individual to avoid the events that trigger the phenomenon; and reassuring the person that under this regimen, the flashbacks will gradually diminish in intensity and frequency, until they eventually disappear altogether. In rare instances, low doses of antianxiety medications may be required.

CANNABIS

Cannabis is a generic term for psychoactive preparations of the plant *Cannabis sativa*. Marihuana is one common term used to describe a relatively weak preparation of cannabis. The strength of any given preparation depends upon its concentration of tetrahydrocannabinols, which possess most of the pharmacological activity. Little is known, as yet, about the biochemical mechanisms by which these substances exert their effects (Chapter 22).

ADVERSE EFFECTS

As with the hallucinogens, panic is an important adverse reaction to cannabis (4). The major characteristics of the panic reaction are anxiety, fear, and a sense of helplessness and loss of control. Certain susceptible individuals may manifest panic reactions at low doses; however, adverse reactions are usually associated with high doses or with naive individuals who are unprepared for the drug-induced alterations. Fleeting paranoid thoughts and hallucinations may also be present, particularly with high levels of intoxication. These more serious reactions occur less frequently and are usually of shorter duration than are those seen with LSD use.

Toxic psychoses from cannabis use are severe but transient reactions characterized by the sudden onset of confusion, delusions, visual hallucinations, emotional lability, excitement, disorientation, depersonalization, paranoia, and temporary amnesia (5). Some experienced clinicians consider impaired judgment to be a hallmark of the toxic psychosis (4). Individuals with a previous history of personality or psychiatric disorder may exhibit an intensification of underlying pathology after remission of acute drug effects. In addition, marihuana, even at low doses, may precipitate functional psychoses in vulnerable individuals (4). It has not been established whether the psychosis reflects individual premorbid pathology or a direct pharmacological effect of cannabis. Regardless of their origin, these conditions are treated with a standard regimen of psychotherapy, hospitalization, and antipsychotic, antidepressant, and antimanic drugs (see Chapters 9, 11, and 12).

An "amotivational syndrome" has also been described among cannabis users (6). This syndrome is characterized by passivity, an absence of conventional motivation, and a preoccupation with drug-taking and its subculture. The role of marihuana in this syndrome is unclear. There is no consistent evidence that marihuana induces organic brain changes which result in less assertive, less goal-directed personality characteristics (4,7). However, pre-existing personality traits, social factors, and other drugs might combine with regular cannabis use to contribute to some personality changes, particularly during the formative period of adolescence.

TREATMENT

The management of adverse reactions to cannabis generally follows the same principles described for the hallucinogens (Table 24-2). In securing the safety of the patient, one should remember that only an extremely high dose of cannabis will be lethal and that the untreated course of toxicity is usually benign (8,9). Unless other drugs are involved, death from inadvertent or intentional overdose is rare, in part because cannabis is nearly insoluble in aqueous media.

The history of the drug use should be supplemented with a physical examination. Although the acute physical manifestations of cannabis use are limited, two consistent physical findings are tachycardia and conjunctival suffusion (Table 24-3). Other physical effects of cannabis vary considerably among individuals. Therefore, the most important function of the physical exam may be to determine whether any drugs other than cannabis are involved. Unlike most psychoactive drugs, cannabis does not discernibly affect pupillary diameter; nor does it markedly alter respiratory rate, amount of sweating, or deep tendon reflexes.

Once it has been established that only cannabis was used, the main treatment is supportive and symptomatic. The use of emetics, gastric lavage, and central or respiratory stimulants is not indicated. High doses of marihuana may induce transient bradycardia and decrease blood pressure, but these symptoms are usually alleviated when the patient is placed in a supine position with legs elevated. In patients who have coronary artery insufficiency, angina pectoris can occur more readily during cannabis intoxication than normally; the standard regimen of oxygen, absolute rest, and reduced demands on cardiac output is indicated. The effective treatment of transient panic reactions and toxic psychoses usually require nothing more than verbal reassurance and the other forms of nonpharmacological intervention decribed for the treatment of hallucinogens. Although on rare occasions antianxiety agents may be needed, more potent medications are not justifiable.

CENTRAL STIMULANTS

The most common of the central nervous system stimulants are the amphetamines (Table 24-1). Other members of this class, such as cocaine and methylphenidate, are not amphetamines, but the characteristics of the adverse reactions and the principles of treatment are similar for all of these drugs. The basic biochemical effects of amphetamines are discussed in Chapter 21.

ADVERSE REACTIONS

The most severe adverse reaction to amphetamine generally occurs at high concentrations of the drugs. High concentrations often result from repetitive use of oral amphetamines, taken either to permit sustained efforts, such as truck driving, or to control weight or chronic depression. As tolerance develops with repetitive use, the dosage is increased. Alternatively, elevated blood levels may occur after repeated intravenous injections of large doses of amphetamines for several days or longer; again, as tolerance develops, the user increases the dose to regain the initial sensations of vigor and euphoria (10). Quite commonly, these high doses or a sudden increase in dose levels induce a paranoid psychosis which is characterized by suspiciousness, hostility, persecutory delusions, and visual and auditory misperceptions. This psychosis may also include hyperactivity, repetitive compulsive behavior, and tactile hallucinations of small insects crawling on or just under the skin. Clinically, amphetamine-induced paranoid states can be indistinguishable from nondrug paranoid reactions, except that spontaneous remission usually occurs when the amphetamine use stops (11,12). With abrupt cessation of drug use, irritability, profound fatigue, and marked depression usually ensue.

TREATMENT

As always, the first priority in treating adverse reactions to the central stimulants should be securing the safety of the patient and others (Table 24-2). The diagnosis of amphetamine psychosis can often be made by direct questioning of the patient and of other knowledgeable people such as spouse or friends about the use of any central nervous system stimulants. These drugs should be asked about not only by trade names but also by the colloquial terms, e.g., uppers, speed, bennies, whites, crystal, crank, and many others. The physical findings of a person suffering an adverse reaction to these drugs are variable. Since tolerance often develops to the sympathetic effects of stimulants, increases in blood pressure and sweating are not always present. Chronic amphetamine users may show weight loss and emaciation from the anorexic effects of the drug and may have cutaneous excoriations from constant picking at their skin. Urinary analysis is often useful, but not all central stimulants are detected in the standard tests.

Supportive treatment should include verbal reassurance, and the patient's surroundings should be arranged to reduce unnecessary or threatening stimulation. Paranoid tendencies call for careful clinical management. Personnel should not be unnecessarily close to or behind the patient, and confined spaces or other settings which might be overwhelming should be avoided. As with paranoid schizophrenia, amphetamine-induced paranoid behavior often includes assaultive tendencies.

Usually, individuals respond to these supportive nonpharmacological methods. In certain instances, more active intervention is required, particularly if paranoid behavior is extreme; if a large amount of amphetamine has been consumed, as can occur with deliberate overdose or accidental ingestion; or if the blood pressure, pulse rate, or temperature is rising. If these conditions exist, and if there is convincing evidence that amphetamines were the only drugs taken in clinically significant amounts, then the patient should be given a dopamine receptor blocker, e.g., chlorpromazine (Thorazine) or haloperidol (Haldol), to antagonize the toxic amphetamine effects (cf. Chapter 21). Initial doses of these drugs are determined by the size of the individual and not by the severity of toxic effects (13). In adults, the initial dose of chlorpromazine ranges from 50–150 mg orally or 25–50 mg intramuscularly; the haloperidol dose by either route is 2–5 mg. Subsequent doses are tailored to the patient's overall response, especially his vital signs, and depend upon timecourse of peak effects of the antipsychotics. If too much drug is administered, cardio-respiratory suppression and excessive sedation may appear. Changes in body temperatures may be useful in determining subsequent dosage schedules: rising temperatures may indicate that amphetamine toxicity is reaching life-threatening proportions and that larger doses of medication are necessary. Hyperpyrexia itself should be treated with standard techniques such as alcohol sponge baths, fans, and cold mattresses. Aspirin or acetaminophen (Tylenol) may also be necessary.

Hydration and the use of ammonium chloride, 500 mg every three to four hours, to acidify the urine will accelerate the excretion of amphetamines and hence shorten the duration of the amphetamine reaction. Urine pH should be kept below 5. Benzodiazepines are often useful when the adverse reaction to amphetamine is not life-threatening but the patient remains distressed despite calm reassurances.

In rare instances, the patient with an amphetamine reaction manifests markedly elevated blood pressure. This usually results from high doses of amphetamine, most often by intravenous injection. Immediate treatment is required if the systolic pressure exceeds 200 mm mercury or if there are indications of an impending cerebral vascular accident, such as visual disturbances or other transient neurological signs. Phentolamine (Regitine), 1–5 mg, should be given by intravenous drip over five to ten minutes, while the blood pressure is monitored. Care must be taken to reduce the systolic blood pressure to 160–170 mm mercury without precipitating hypotension. After the blood pressure is adequately titrated, a dopamine receptor blocking drug can be given cautiously.

Indications for hospitalization with adverse amphetamine reactions include: protracted paranoid behavior; elevated vital signs despite adequate levels of medication; severe suicidal tendencies, which sometimes follow discontinuation of amphetamine use; persistent impairment of perceptions or cognitive functions; and serious associated medical problems, such as hepatitis or bacterial endocarditis. If there are no indications for hospitalization and if brain function and vital signs are returning to normal, the patient may be discharged to a responsible person who can observe him closely for the next twenty-four hours. The patient and responsible person should be warned that lethargy, irritability, and depression are common features of amphetamine withdrawal. Since amphetamine use is associated with markedly increased morbidity and mortality (14), a follow-up visit should be arranged.

ANTICHOLINERGIC DRUGS

The anticholinergic intoxication syndrome can be produced by a variety of agents (Table 24-1). These substances are found in a wide assortment of nonprescription preparations for insomnia, colds, gastrointestinal problems, and asthma. Others, such as tricyclic antidepressants, antipsychotics, and antiparkinsonian drugs are used clinically (15). The intoxication syndrome may result from an accidental or intentional overdose or from use of an hallucinogen contaminated with anticholinergic agents, an anticholinergic hallucinogen, or a combination of a centrally acting anticholinergic compound and an antipsychotic agent. Biochemical effects of the anticholinergics are covered in Chapter 22.

Adverse Reactions

The clinical syndrome produced by the anticholinergics has pronounced physiological and psychological components (Table 24-3) (16). Many of the former result from blockade of the autonomic parasympathetic system. Several of the symptoms are captured in the following couplet:

> Mad as a hatter, dry as a bone,
> Red as a beet, and blind as a stone.

One of the most striking features of the anticholinergic syndrome is a profound impairment of memory. If a conscious patient is unable to recall the events of the immediately preceding one-half hour or is unable to remember his own name, the diagnosis of anticholinergic intoxication should be strongly considered.

Treatment

The treatment of the anticholinergic intoxication syndrome begins with a careful examination. The patient may be unable to give a history, but friends or relatives may be able to provide information on the source of the intoxication.

A patient who presents with the classical anticholinergic syndrome described above and who is hyperpyrexic, profoundly delirious, or acutely agitated should be treated with 2 mg of physostigmine salicylate, given either intramuscularly or intravenously; a second dose of 1–2 mg can be given fifteen minutes later (17,18). During this procedure, vital signs should be monitored carefully, and the patient should be connected to a cardiac monitor. A decline in pulse rate is evidence of the physostigmine effect on the cholinergic blockade. The relatively short duration of action of physostigmine may necessitate its readministration every two hours. This treatment regimen must be undertaken with considerable caution, since overtreatment will precipitate a cholinergic crisis. Medical contraindications to physostigmine include a history of heart disease, asthma, peptic ulcer, diabetes, mechanical obstruction of bowel or bladder, pregnancy, hyperthyroidism, and a previous allergic reaction to physostigmine. Not every patient will require physostigmine. Many can be treated with the nonpharmacological methods used to manage adverse reactions to other nonaddictive drugs. On recovery, the patient who has made a suicide attempt with anticholinergic agents should be evaluated psychiatrically, and psychiatric follow-up should be offered.

INHALANTS

Drug abusers sometimes inhale or "sniff" glues, lacquer, paints and paint thinner, kerosene, gasoline, industrial and household solvents, aerosols, nitrous oxide, and a wide variety of other compounds for their psychoactive effects (Table 24-1) (19). Users are often preadolescents from low socio-economic or otherwise disadvantaged backgrounds. Like most forms of nonmedical drug use, inhalant abuse is usually a peer-related activity and frequently takes place in a group setting. Inhalant use is faddish: within a given community, one specific inhalant will be used extensively by the youth for a specific time period; then, its use will subside only to be replaced in popularity by another substance.

ADVERSE EFFECTS

Although these substances have varying pharmacological modes of action, their behavioral effects are generally quite similar. In sufficient doses, they cause a diffuse impairment of brain function which is called delirium and which resembles the delirium of severe alcohol or barbiturate withdrawal. The individual demonstrates changing levels of awareness to surrounding events and impairments of judgment, orientation, memory, and motor functions.

TREATMENT

The treatment of the inhalant abuser is supportive and symptomatic. Physical restraints are sometimes required to curb agitated assaultiveness. Since some inhalants, such as the aerosols, induce alveolar-capillary blockade or otherwise impair pulmonary function, oxygen or enhanced ventilation may be necessary. Most of the inhalants are rapidly metabolized, so pharmacological sedation or other specific treatments are seldom required. Many inhalants are highly toxic, and sudden deaths do occur. Thus, those inhalant abusers who do reach medical attention should be evaluated thoroughly. Most clinicians find that inhalant abusers do not respond to psychotherapy, counseling, or other forms of direct intervention. Perhaps the best long-term treatment regimen is general education about inherent health risks attendant to the use of these substances.

THE POLYDRUG ABUSER

Poly- or multiple drug use, i.e., the simultaneous or sequential use of more than one psychoactive drug for nonmedical purposes, has been increasing in many parts of the world. Some polydrug users normally take just one of the psychoactive agents, using additional drugs only occasionally. Others cycle their drugs, using central nervous system stimulants in the morning, antianxiety agents during the day, and sedative hypnotics at night. Still others indiscriminately use whatever is available. Since specific combinations of drugs and patterns of use are virtually endless, this section will outline only general guidelines for the management of the polydrug user.

The highest priority in treatment is the immediate assessment of vital signs. Direct support of respiratory and cardiovascular functions may be necessary. Any cardiac arrhythmias should be monitored, and preparations should be made for defibrillation or other intervention. If opiates are involved, the intravenous injection of naloxone (Narcan), 0.4 mg, will reverse respiratory and central nervous system depression (Chapter 23). In fact, naloxone is so safe that it should be tried even when the combination of drugs is unclear, as long as opiate overdose is a possibility.

Once the patient's condition is stable, the physician should determine if addicting drugs were being used and whether the patient is susceptible to a withdrawal reaction. Treatments for individual abstinence syndromes are detailed in Chapter 23. The primary complication introduced by multiple drug abuse involves deciding which syndrome to treat first. If the patient combined only one addictive drug with any of the nonaddictive drugs, then withdrawal management can focus entirely upon the addicting agent. Since alcohol and the sedative-hypnotics are cross-tolerant, mixed dependencies to them can be managed as a unit. When alcohol or a sedative hypnotic has been used in combination with an opiate, initial attention should be given to managing the alcohol or sedative-hypnotic withdrawal. The patient is maintained on a stabilizing regimen of methadone (see Chapter 23), while he receives progressively smaller doses of sedative hypnotics. Once the sedative dose has reached a low level, methadone reduction can begin.

Guidelines for using anticonvulsant drugs in the treatment of polydrug abusers are still unclear. Evidence for their utility in situations where the drug abuser has no predispositions for seizure is equivocal. However, in most clinical situations, the medical history of the drug abuser is incomplete, so that an argument can be made for the prophylactic use of anticonvulsants. If long-acting anticonvulsants such as phenytoin (Dilantin) are used, an initial parenteral loading dose of 100 mg reduces the time needed to reach effective, steady-state levels. This can then be followed by oral doses of 100 mg, three to four times a day.

LONG-TERM TREATMENT AND REHABILITATION

In treating the drug abuser, the clinician should consider the possibility that the patient is taking the drug in an ineffective attempt to handle an underlying psychiatric disturbance which would respond to more specific treatment. For example, severely depressed individuals sometimes use stimulants to relieve their dysphoria, while hypomanic patients will futilely try to subdue their hyperactivity with sedative hypnotics or alcohol. In these patients, long-term treatment should obviously focus on the underlying disorder. Unfortunately, most nonmedical drug abusers do not have clearly treatable psychiatric problems. Instead, they show relatively enduring maladaptive patterns of behavior which are often diagnosed as personality or character disorders. The long-term management of these drug abusers is usually difficult and fraught with high rates of recidivism, regardless of the treatment regimen. At times, closely supervised hospitalization, or at least physical separation of the drug user from his usual milieu, is a necessary first step for treating the chronic amphetamine user. Tricyclic antidepressants such as imipramine (Tofranil) are sometimes useful to reduce the symptoms of depression which frequently accompany drug abuse, especially of the stimulants. These depressions usually subside spontaneously, but individuals may require up to a year of abstinence for return to predrug mood levels.

Almost invariably, there are marked deficiencies in the user's personal and social functioning; thus, during long-term management, treatment can appropriately be focused on these areas. A judicious blend of individual and group therapy can be helpful. Drug abusers often respond well to therapies that emphasize the development of coping skills for situations which are likely to arise in the user's immediate future. Systematic application of behavioral modification techniques is helpful with some patients, as are traditional insight-oriented approaches and confrontation or Gestalt-sensitivity techniques. All of these approaches have mixed results. Regardless of the approach, long-term follow-up is essential. An emphasis on day-to-day difficulties and on the development of social and vocational skills is often efficacious. Although the life history of the users of nonaddictive drugs is not well documented, most clinicians believe that life-long difficulties with drugs, particularly alcohol, are common.

REFERENCES

1. Hollister, L. E. *Chemical Psychoses*. Springfield: Thomas, 1968.
2. Smith, D. E. Personal Communication.
3. Taylor, R. L., Maurer, J. I., and Tinklenberg, J. R. Management of "bad trips" in an evolving drug scene. *In: Psychiatric Treatment: Crisis, Clinic, and Consultation.* C. P. Rosenbaum and J. E. Beebe, *eds.*, New York: McGraw-Hill, 1975.
4. Meyer, R. E. Psychiatric consequence of marijuana use: the state of evidence. *In: Marijuana and Health Hazards.* J. R. Tinklenberg, *ed.*, New York: Academic Press, 1975, pp. 133–152.
5. Chopra, G. S. and Smith, J. W. Psychotic reactions following cannabis use in East Indians. *Arch. Gen. Psychiatry 30:*24–27, 1974.
6. McGlothlin, W. H. and West, L. J. The marijuana problem: an overview. *Am. J. Psychiatry 125:*370–378, 1968.
7. Dornbush, R. L. Marijuana and the central nervous system. *In: Marijuana and Health Hazards.* J. R. Tinklenberg, *ed.*, New York: Academic Press, 1975, pp. 103–113.
8. Paton, W. D. M. Pharmacology of marijuana. *Ann. Rev. Pharmacol. 15:*191–220, 1975.
9. Nahas, G. G. *Marijuana: Deceptive Weed.* New York: Raven Press, 1973, pp. 105–108.
10. Kramer, J. C., Fischman, V. S., and Littlefield, D. C. Amphetamine abuse. *J. Am. Med. Assoc. 201:*305–309, 1967.
11. Connell, P. H. *Amphetamine Psychosis.* New York: Oxford University Press, 1958.
12. Snyder, S. H. Catecholamines in the brain as mediators of amphetamine psychosis. *Arch. Gen. Psychiatry 27:*169–179, 1972.
13. Espelin, D. E. and Done, A. K. Amphetamine poisoning: effectiveness of chlorpromazine. *N. Eng. J. Med. 278:*1361–1365, 1968.
14. Kalant, H. and Kalant, O. J. Death in amphetamine users: causes and rates. *Can. Med. Assoc. J. 112:*299–304, 1975.
15. Shader, R. I. and Greenblatt, D. J. Belladonna alkaloids and synthetic anticholinergics: users and toxicity. *In: Psychiatric Complications of Medical Drugs.* R. I. Shader, *ed.*, New York: Raven Press, 1972, pp. 103–147.
16. Ketchum, J. S., Sidell, F. R., Crowell, E. B., Aghajanian, G. K., and Hayes, A. H. Atropine, scopolamine, and Ditran: comparative pharmacology and antagonists in man. *Psychopharmacologia 28:*121–145, 1973.
17. Crowell, E. B. and Ketchum, J. S. The treatment of scopolamine-induced delirium with physostigmine. *Clin. Pharmacol. Ther. 8:*409–414, 1967.
18. Heiser, J. F. and Gillin, J. C. The reversal of anticholinergic drug-induced delirium and coma with physostigmine. *Am. J. Psychiatry 127:*1050–1052, 1971.
19. Kupperstein, L. R. and Sussman, R. M. A bibliography on the inhalation of glue fumes and other toxic vapors: a substance abuse practice among adolescents. *Int. J. Addict. 3:*177–198, 1968.

IV | Psychopharmacology for the Young and Old

The disorders of youth have long been neglected by psychopharmacologists. Anna Freud and others have provided brilliant insights into the psychological disorders of childhood that have been augmented by the development of a variety of treatment methods, including behavioral therapies. Indeed, the early recognition and treatment of childhood disorders may be one of the most successful areas of psychiatry. Nevertheless, for many aspects of childhood psychiatric disorders, present information is distressingly inadequate. Basic biological research on these disorders has developed only slowly and is complicated by severe ethical and legal dilemmas. The first three chapters in this part begin with an overview of the major psychiatric disorders of childhood, followed by more detailed descriptions of two major areas of interest—the hyperkinetic or minimal brain dysfunction syndrome and the childhood psychoses. Throughout these chapters, available pharmacological treatments are discussed, along with their limitations and problems.

The psychiatric problems of the aged have also been a neglected area in psychopharmacology. Only recently have we begun to recognize that some psychological changes in the aged are amenable to treatment. It is incumbent upon physicians to understand that many of the problems of the aged are neither inevitable nor irreversible. Often, effective treatment of these individuals requires special care in using familiar drugs such as the antipsychotics or antidepressants because of metabolic changes which accompany the aging process. Chapter 28 reviews these considerations in discussing the psychiatric problems of the aged and the pharmacological treatment of those problems.

25 | Psychopharmacology of Childhood Disorders

THOMAS F. ANDERS and

ROLAND D. CIARANELLO

CLASSIFICATION OF CHILDHOOD PSYCHOPATHOLOGY

The treatment of a disease assumes a nosology or capacity to define or diagnose that disease. In psychiatry, diagnoses have resulted largely from descriptions of behavior, rather than from etiological or structural explanations of disorder. Such a descriptive approach rests upon reliable observation and upon the ability to circumscribe the boundaries of normality. In an area as complex as human behavior, this has been almost impossible to achieve. Historical, cultural, socioeconomic, familial, interactional, and biological influences are only some of the many variables that influence definitions of normality.

In children, the boundaries of normality and pathology are particularly difficult to establish. On the one hand, the child's behavior is in a constant state of change, as development and maturation proceed and and as skills and capacities improve and decline. On the other hand, because of an enforced dependence on adult care-givers, the child is locked to an external environment far more than are adults. What may be normal for some children in their environment at a given age may be abnormal for others in a different one. As a result, perturbations in the environment are more likely to result in behavioral disturbances in children. Finally, the resilience of children seems to be greater than that of adults, so that what appears to be serious at one point in time may be transient, retrospectively. For all of these reasons, a uniform and generally accepted classification system of childhood psychopathology has been difficult to develop and is still needed.

Childhood behavioral disorders are most commonly classified according to the diagnostic and statistical manual of the American Psychiatric Association (DSM–II) (1). Since the manual was constructed for use with adults, it is largely unsatisfactory for classifying childhood disorders. The Group for the Advancement of Psychiatry proposed a classification scheme (GAP Report) which is more suited to the developing child (2). There are ten major categories of disorder, ranging from normal reaction to psychotic disorder. Both functional and biological disturbances are included. Although the GAP Report is more complete than DSM–II, it is already dated. At present, a special task force of the DSM–III Committee of the American Psychiatric Association has been formed to classify childhood disorders. The product of this group's effort is awaited eagerly by all those concerned with childhood psychopathology.

We emphasize the complexities and importance of classification in this section because, without a satisfactory scheme, promising directions in and legitimate progress of the therapeutic management of childhood disorders are confounded by controversy in diagnosis and by the lack of generalizability of results.

PROBLEMS OF PSYCHOPHARMACOLOGICAL RESEARCH IN CHILDREN

The development of a pharmacopoeia of drugs specific for childhood disorders has been delayed by a number of methodological and ethical problems. Although there are notable exceptions, research on the psychopharmacology of childhood disorders has lagged far behind that of research in adults. Drug studies in children are frequently limited by small sample sizes and by heterogeneous populations. As mentioned, uniform and reliable diagnoses are difficult to generate in child psychiatry, and the use of target symptomatology rather than diagnostic classifications does little to clarify the problem. Improvement is frequently measured on the basis of subjective rather than quantitative data.

Another problem in drug studies with children results from the different ages which are usually represented. Drug responses of adolescents may differ from those of preadolescents. Metabolic and clearance rates and processes of degradation depend upon the maturation of different enzyme systems, many of which vary according to age. Thus, particular drug effects reported in studies may be related to age rather than to disability.

Finally, few studies have been able to investigate responses in normal controls, to use placebos, and to measure rates of relapse following drug withdrawal. Ethical considerations limit these kinds of studies in human children. The issue of who can provide informed consent for children remains controversial.

GENERAL PRINCIPLES OF PSYCHOPHARMACOLOGY IN CHILDHOOD

In children, drugs should be used *sparingly* and for *specific purposes* only. Although this seems a truism, public furor over the alleged misuse of stimulant drugs to control classroom behavior has resulted only recently in tighter, centralized regulation of the use of psychopharmacological agents in children. Several reasons underlie a need for special caution with children. First, psychoactive agents generally have not been well studied in developing organisms. Thus, their side effects and adverse reactions are not as well known. A notable example is the short-term, growth-retarding effects of the psychoactive agents such as amphetamines in preadolescent children. Second, the psychological meaning of medication and of pills may be misunderstood by children, whose cognitive capacities are not fully developed. They may view medication as punishment, as a potion of magical strength, or as an added dimension of the self which is otherwise lacking. Guilt and anxiety are often associated with the taking of medication. Finally, as a corollary to psychological misunderstanding, the child may learn to associate pills with a life-style in which external methods are used to resolve life's conflicts.

With such admonitions for caution, there are, nevertheless, genuine indications for the use of psychoactive substances in childhood. When drugs are prescribed, both the parents and the child should be instructed about expected benefits and prepared for possible side effects and toxic reactions. Guilt and anxiety should be minimized, with careful exploration and clarification of unconscious fantasies. The medication should not become the focus of a power struggle between parent and child, nor should it provide false hope of a magical cure. Table 25-1 reviews the most frequently prescribed psychopharmacological agents

TABLE 25-1.
DRUGS COMMONLY USED IN THE TREATMENT OF CHILDHOOD DISTURBANCES

NAME		ORAL DOSAGE (MG/DAY)	NO. OF DIVIDED DOSES	INDICATIONS	SIDE EFFECTS AND TOXIC REACTIONS
GENERIC	REPRESENTATIVE BRAND				
Antipsychotics					
Phenothiazines				Psychosis, severe agitation, severe anxiety, emergencies, assaultiveness	Dystonic reactions, parkinsonian symptoms, blood dyscrasias convulsions
Chlorpromazine	Thorazine	9–200[1]	2–4		
Trifluptromazine	Vesprin	1–150	2–4		
Trifluorperazine[2]	Stelazine	1–20	1–2		
Thioridazine	Mellaril	10–200	2–4		
Butyrophenones and Thioxanthines					
Chlorprothixene[2]	Taractan	10–200	1–2		
Thiothixene[3]	Navane	1–30	1–2		
Haloperidol[3]	Haldol	2–16	1–2	Above, plus Gilles de la Tourette Syndrome	
Tricyclic Antidepressants					
Imipramine	Tofranil	6–200	1–2	Depressive states, enuresis, school phobia	Restlessness, ataxia, dry mouth, blurred vision,

		10–75	1–3		
...otriptyline	Aventyl				
Central Stimulants					
Dextroamphetamine sulfate	Dexedrine	5–40	2	Minimal brain dysfunction syndrome, narcolepsy	Anorexia, weight loss, irritability, stomach aches
Methylphenidate	Ritalin	10–80	2		
Pemoline	Cylert	25–100	1		
Antianxiety Agents					
Diphenhydramine	Benadryl	25–800[4]	1–4	Anxiety, insomnia, acute dystonic reactions, anxiety, sleepwalking, sleep talking, night terrors	Skin rash, dry mouth, drowsiness
Chlordiazepoxide[2]	Librium	25–100	1		
Diazepam	Valium	10–40	1		
Miscellaneous					
Chlorimipramine[5]		2–75	2–4	Cataplexy	Restlessness, ataxia, blurred vision
Lithium carbonate[3]	Lithium	450–1800	2–4	Hyperactivity, aggressivity	cardiovascular effects, blood dyscrasias
Triiodothyronine	Cytomel	10–75 μg/day	1	Autism, childhood schizophrenia	Hyperthyroidism
Chloral hydrate	Noctec	250–1000	1	Insomnia	

[1] Intramuscular dosage is a maximum of 40 mg/day for children under 5 and 75 mg/day for children under 12.
[2] FDA approval for children older than 6 years.
[3] FDA approval for children older than 12 years.
[4] Intramuscular dosage is 25–50 mg/day.
[5] Not approved for use in U.S.

in children, with accompanying dosage schedules, indications, and side effects (3).

The following sections of this chapter review some of the transient uses of drugs in emergency situations, some of the childhood disorders in which drugs may be useful as adjuncts to individual or family therapy, and some of the special symptom disorders in which specific medications seem to be therapeutic. The minimal brain dysfunction syndrome, the most prevalent childhood disorder requiring medication, is described in Chapter 26. The childhood psychotic disorders are discussed in Chapter 27.

PHARMACOTHERAPY OF THE EMERGENCIES OF CHILD PSYCHIATRY

Emergencies in child psychiatry are few. They are usually precipitated by a crisis, and crisis intervention techniques are often sufficient to resolve the acute symptomatology. When anxiety or aggression is so extreme as to be uncontrollable by environmental manipulation and intensive supportive psychotherapy, short-term medication is indicated. In children under six, diphenhydramine has been used with good results; in children over six, intramuscular phenothiazines have been effective. The behavioral disturbances generally assume one of the following forms: decompensation, with loss of reality testing; toxic states secondary to substance abuse; extreme agitation with hyperaggressive and homicidal outbursts; withdrawal and suicidal preoccupation or attempts; and severe anxiety or panic states.

Suicide attempts are uncommon in children younger than ten years of age; however, concern should be raised when young children are victims of frequent accidents or ingestions. For the very young, this may indicate a neglecting environment; for older, latency-aged children, this may represent an equivalent to suicidal behavior. Frequent misuse of alcohol and drugs may also indicate similar psychopathology. Suicide attempts increase in frequency during adolescence. All such attempts should be taken seriously and require sufficient evaluation to minimize the possibility of recurrence. A Lethality Index (Table 25-2), can be used to assess the nature of the crisis, the available support sys-

TABLE 25-2.
A LETHALITY INDEX FOR SUICIDAL TENDENCY

	SCORE "1"	SCORE "0"
Sex	M	F
Age	<12; >35	13–35
Successful suicide by family member or significant other	+	—
Previous attempt	+	—
Method	Gun Carbon monoxide Poisons	Razor blade Household pills
Preparation	Planned	Impulsive
Setting	Isolated	Safe
Premorbid personality	Depressed Borderline Schizophrenic	Neurotic Crisis
Suicide note	Short, to the point	Long, detailed
Support system	Absent	Available

tem, and the specifics of the suicide attempt. Scores below 3 suggest a low likelihood of immediate recurrence, whereas scores above 5 require caution. More formal research is required, however, before definitive conclusions can be drawn from this index. Currently, it serves as a useful guide for emergency room physicians and psychiatry trainees who are faced with the crisis of a suicide attempt and the need to make a disposition. Table 25-3 lists general rules and techniques to optimize the formation of a positive relationship in the emergency room setting, so that the evaluation is as complete as possible. These techniques derive from crisis intervention methodology.

Hyperaggressive and disorganized behavior secondary to substance abuse is becoming a more common emergency in child psychiatry. Tranquilizing and other depressant drugs are often contraindicated in states of obtunded consciousness. Seclusion, with reduction of extraneous stimulation, and sedation with chloral hydrate per rectum is often useful. Occasionally, acute dystonias and dyskinesias develop as side effects to phenothiazine usage, with symptoms such as wry neck (torticollis), dysphagia, aphonia, and occasionally respiratory difficul-

TABLE 25-3.

EVALUATION AND DISPOSITION OF SUICIDE ATTEMPTS

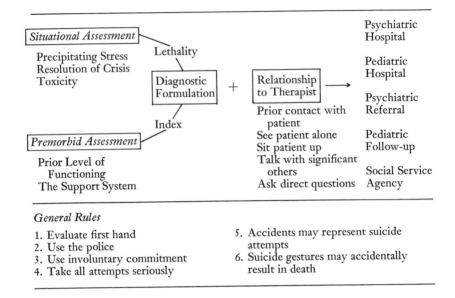

General Rules

1. Evaluate first hand
2. Use the police
3. Use involuntary commitment
4. Take all attempts seriously

5. Accidents may represent suicide attempts
6. Suicide gestures may accidentally result in death

ties. Intramuscular or intravenous diphenhydramine rapidly alleviates the acute symptomatology. Maintenance doses of antiparkinsonian agents minimize the chronic side effects of phenothiazines (Chapter 9).

PSYCHOPHARMACOLOGICAL AGENTS AS ADJUNCTS TO THERAPY

NEUROTIC DISORDERS OF CHILDHOOD

The neurotic disorders of childhood must be differentiated from the reactive disorders and from normal responses manifested by children during development. A neurotic disorder implies that the conflict is entirely intrapsychic and unconscious, rather than being related to observable environmental stresses. In contrast, a reactive disorder is symptomatic behavior associated with obvious stresses in the environment, even though the symptoms may appear to have a neurotic character. Likewise, some children utilize neurotic-like symptoms during normal development to master phase-specific tasks, as seen with compulsive rituals in some childhood games.

Psychoanalytic theorists ascribe the etiology of neurotic symptoms to unsuccessful resolution of an unconscious conflict. The painful anxiety, which signals the presence of the conflict, is reduced by the neurotic symptomatology. Behavior theorists relate symptoms to maladaptively reinforced responses. Whatever the theoretical frame of reference, the directly experienced anxiety or neurotic symptom may inhibit normal emotional development. Such children frequently are unable to succeed in school, have physical complaints, or experience difficulty in socializing with peers and family.

Individual, family, and group psychotherapy; behavior modification programs; and hypnosis are common treatment approaches to neurotic disorders. When necessary, pharmacotherapy should be used only transiently and as an adjunct to other forms of therapy. If symptom formation seriously impairs the child's capacity to interact effectively, the temporary use of medication may facilitate a return to more normal functioning. However, extreme caution must be employed in prescribing medication for children with neurotic symptomatology, since the unconscious fantasies and magical expectations described earlier are of particular concern.

Anxiety Neuroses

When anxiety attacks are the presenting complaint, the child is diagnosed as having an anxiety neurosis. Typically, the symptoms are those of autonomic arousal, characterized by increased breathing and heart rate, sweating, palpitations, and feelings of fear and dread. Somatic complaints are common. With extreme anxiety, hyperventilation may ensue. Severe temper tantrums, leading to breath-holding spells during the toddler period, may represent precursors of later full-scale anxiety attacks during latency. When neurotic symptoms are incapacitating, antianxiety agents such as diazepam or diphenhydramine are useful. For acute hyperventilation attacks, having the patient breathe into a paper bag and giving intramuscular diazepam are effective.

Hysterical Neuroses

Childhood hysterical neuroses are characterized most often by somatization, conversion reactions, and dissociative reactions. Acute states are best treated by uncovering the meaning or purpose of the symptom and resolving the crisis by environmental manipulation and by interpretation of the psychodynamic (behavioral) meaning of the symptom. An oral or intramuscular antianxiety agent like diazepam may be effective. Placebo effects are common (Chapter 31). Rarely, intravenous sodium amobarbital (Amytal) has been used for intractable hysterical symptomatology (cf. Chapter 16). Continued support should be provided to promote stability of the therapeutic relationship and to prevent recurrences of acute symptomatology.

Obsessive-Compulsive Neuroses

Obsessive-compulsive neuroses may become disabling when ritualistic behavior or obsessive ruminations prevent normal social interactions and lead to withdrawal. Antianxiety agents generally are not useful. Antipsychotics such as chlorpromazine or thioridazine may be necessary to alleviate the symptomatology sufficiently to permit development of a therapeutic relationship.

Summary

To repeat, psychopharmacological agents must be viewed as temporary and adjunctive therapy for neurotic symptoms, useful in returning the child to as normal a social situation as possible, as quickly as possible, while developing a therapeutic relationship.

SCHOOL PHOBIA

School phobia per se is not a single syndrome. Thus, although it may have neurotic components, it cannot be classified as a neurosis. School phobia has been called an "emergency" of child psychiatry. The emergency is not related to the life-threatening nature of the disorder but rather to the fact that the longer the child is out of the classroom, the more difficult the return will be. The disturbance is characterized by an unwillingness to attend school or a dread of it. It must be differentiated from school truancy. Typically, in school phobia, the child remains at home, whereas the truant child's whereabouts are unknown. Headaches, stomach aches, and other somatic complaints are common and disappear when the child is able to remain at home. Medical workups are negative for significant organic pathology. Symptomatology is typically worse following vacations and on Monday mornings and characteristically absent on weekends and during the vacation period. The precipitating events are diverse. Symptoms may follow a genuine traumatic incident in school, such as an encounter with a harsh teacher or with aggressive or sexually provocative peers. In such cases, school phobia resembles a traumatic neurosis. Alternatively, school phobia may follow a real illness, the death or loss of a parent, or the loss of a significant figure in the child's life, so that the behavioral disturbance more closely resembles a depressive reaction. Commonly, however, the precipitating stress is unknown, in which case, separation anxiety stemming from an overprotective, hostile-dependent, parent-child relationship is thought to be the source of the conflict.

The treatment of choice for school phobia is a speedy return of the child to school, by force if necessary. Sufficient parental support and preparation of school personnel are necessary if this treatment approach is to succeed. Mild antianxiety agents such as diphenhydramine have been recommended to alleviate the child's anxiety (4). Amphetamines and antidepressants have also been tried with some success. However, no psychopharmacological agents are sufficient without family and individual therapy. In the adolescent age group or when the child has been absent from school for long periods of time, the pathology is more resistant. In such cases, psychiatric hospitalization may be required to achieve adequate separation from home.

DEPRESSION

Depressive disorders in childhood have been difficult to define. Children generally do not become sad and withdrawn; rather, they frequently react by increased activity and inappropriate behavior, in order to escape the painful affects of hopelessness and helplessness. Neurotic depressions generally are associated with a significant loss, ranging from the loss of a parent through death, divorce, or emotional absence to the loss of self-esteem from poor grades or athletic performance or from rejection by peers. Symptomatology is wide ranging and includes recurrent physical complaints, sleep difficulties, fears, changes in behavior, and mood disturbances. When the symptoms become severe and disabling, neurotic depressions respond best to medication.

Tricyclic antidepressants (tricyclics) such as imipramine and amitriptyline frequently are used to treat severe neurotic depressions in children. The monoamine oxidase (MAO) inhibitors are used much less often, because of the many potential side effects. However, in one study, a combination of phenelzine and chlordiazepoxide was used in depressed children who were ill for up to five years (5). A significant number improved on this medical regimen.

Manic-depressive psychosis has been observed to occur only rarely before the age of twelve (6). The usefulness of lithium carbonate for treating children is still controversial. Similarly, retarded psychotic depressions are rare before young adulthood. Characterologic depressions, manifested by apathy, withdrawal, low energy level, and disinterest, are considered to result from severe deprivation in early childhood. Such deprivation may be either physical or emotional. Pharmacotherapy has been of little benefit.

ENURESIS

Enuresis, or bedwetting, is reported to affect approximately 7 percent of children. It is a symptom, rather than a single disease entity or syndrome. A careful history is required for proper etiologic diagnosis and therapeutic management. Most clinicians believe that an occasional episode of wetting is not pathological until after the age of seven, but frequent and regular wetting between ages three and seven should be investigated. The diagnosis of enuresis should be limited to those conditions in which a clear-cut organic diagnosis cannot be made. Thus, polyuria or incontinence associated with diabetes, urinary tract infections, urogenital pathology, and other endocrine or metabolic causes should not be classified as enuresis.

In obtaining a history of enuresis, the physician should determine whether the symptom occurs during the day, the night, or both and whether the symptom is primary, with the child never having had a period of dryness, or secondary, following at least six months of successful toilet training and night dryness. In addition, it is important to assess whether night wetting occurs during the first three to four hours of sleep or in the early morning, after six to seven hours of sleep.

Several types of enuretic patterns have been described (7). A useful classification scheme for enuresis is presented in Tables 25-4 and 25-5. Stage 4 non-rapid-eye-movement (non-REM) sleep-related enuresis (NREM dyssomnia enuresis) refers to wetting which occurs during

TABLE 25-4.

THE ORGANIC ENURESES

	TYPE*	AGE	TIME OF OCCURRENCE	TREATMENT
ANATOMIC/METABOLIC ENURESES	Primary or Secondary	Any age	Day and night	Surgery Specific medication
SLEEP-RELATED ENURESES				
NREM Dyssomnia Enuresis**	Primary	3–9	Night	Imipramine, 40–100 mg/day
Hypersomnia Enuresis	Secondary	>10	Night	Treatment of narcolepsy/sleep apnea syndrome
ENURESIS WITH MENTAL RETARDATION	Primary or Secondary	Any age	Day and night	Behavior modification, supportive psychotherapy

* In primary enuresis, the child has never had a period of dryness; secondary enuresis follows at least 6 months of successful toilet training and night dryness.
** Predominantly in males.

TABLE 25-5.

THE FUNCTIONAL ENURESES

	TYPE*	AGE	TIME OF OCCURRENCE	TREATMENT
SOCIOCULTURAL ENURESIS	Primary	3–12	Day and night	Education, support
SEPARATION-INDIVIDUATION ENURESIS**	Primary	3–7	Predominantly at night	Psychotherapy
REGRESSIVE ENURESIS	Secondary	3–10	Predominantly at night	Crisis intervention, behavior modification
ENURESIS WITH DEPRESSION	Secondary	3–12	Predominantly at night	Treatment of depression
ADOLESCENT ENURESIS	Secondary	12–20	Predominantly at night	Treatment of underlying disorder

* In primary enuresis, the child has never had a period of dryness; secondary enuresis follows at least 6 months of successful toilet training and night dryness.
** Predominantly in males.

the first hours of sleep, at the time of transition between Stage 4 non-REM sleep and the first REM period. NREM dyssomnia enuresis is familial, more common in males, and associated with autonomic arousal in the absence of elicitable mental activity. There is amnesia for the enuretic episode in the morning. Children with this disorder have a higher incidence of sleepwalking, sleep talking, and night terrors. Their bladder function is disturbed during the transition between Stage 4 non-REM sleep and REM sleep.

NREM dyssomnia enuresis responds well to a single daily dose of imipramine, administered prior to bedtime. The dosage should be increased gradually until the symptom disappears, then maintained for at least six months, followed by gradual tapering. Maximum doses of 150 mg are not uncommon. If the symptom does not improve significantly after two weeks of maximum dose levels, the case is considered to be a treatment failure. If the medication is terminated too soon or too abruptly and the symptoms return, a second course of medication is less likely to be successful. As bladder mechanisms gradually mature, the symptom subsides spontaneously. Medication should only be initiated when the enuretic symptom leads to behavioral problems which infringe upon the child's interpersonal relationships or school performance. When it is an isolated symptom in an otherwise well-functioning child, support and education for the parents usually suffice to reduce concern.

Enuresis which occurs later in the night or in the early-morning hours and which is associated with dream content is generally related to psychological stress. In cases of primary enuresis, a power struggle between the parent and child over toilet training often has not been resolved successfully. Secondary enuresis may appear if a child regresses to an earlier mode of functioning following a traumatic episode. Hospitalization, the loss of a parent, and the birth of a sib are examples of such stresses. These forms of enuresis generally do not appear to respond to the tricyclics. Instead, behavioral modification, crisis intervention, and individual psychotherapy are recommended.

SLEEP PROBLEMS

Adult sleep disorders are discussed in Chapter 14. Sleep problems in children include the hypersomnias, the insomnias, and the episodic disorders of sleep.

Episodic Sleep Disorders

The episodic sleep disorders include sleepwalking, sleep talking, and night terrors. Also called disorders of arousal and NREM dyssomnias, they are the most common of the sleep problems. Like NREM dyssomnia enuresis, they represent physiological dysfunction during Stage 4 non-REM sleep, at the point of transition to the first REM period. Table 25-6 portrays a common set of characteristics which seem to link these disorders. Detailed descriptions of these disorders have been published elsewhere (8).

If the episodic sleep disorder is persistent and intractable and leads to behavioral disturbances in other areas of functioning, diazepam is effective in controlling the dyssomniac pathology. Diazepam may act by reducing the amount of Stage 4 non-REM sleep. As with the treatment of NREM dyssomnia enuresis, dosages should be increased gradually until a therapeutic effect is noted. They should then be maintained for prolonged periods of time before gradual tapering. Maximum doses of 40 mg of diazepam, given as one dose several hours before bedtime, have been used.

Narcolepsy

Narcolepsy is a form of hypersomnia which occurs in children older than ten years of age (9). It is characterized by irresistible sleep attacks which impinge upon waking activity. Generally, the sleep attacks are brief; and upon awakening the individual feels refreshed. The pathology consists of episodes of REM sleep which spontaneously interrupt the waking state. Suppression of muscle tone alone results in cataplexy. Such cataplectic attacks are heightened by emotional outbursts such as laughter and rage.

The general syndrome of narcolepsy responds to the psychoactive agents such as methylphenidate and amphetamine. However, long-term maintenance with these agents has not been successful. For the isolated

TABLE 25-6.
CHARACTERISTICS OF EPISODIC SLEEP DISORDERS

Signs of neurological immaturity	Twin concordance	Automatic actions
Males > females	Paroxysmal	Nonresponsive to environment
Positive family history	Substitutive symptoms	Retrograde amnesia

symptom of cataplexy, chlorimipramine has been effective; but it is still classified as an investigational drug. MAO inhibitors almost completely suppress REM sleep and are being used experimentally in adults (Chapter 14). No significant deleterious effects on daytime personality functioning have been found after more than one year of REM deprivation by these agents, and narcoleptic pathology has been markedly reduced.

Sleep Apnea Syndrome

Another form of hypersomnia is the sleep apnea syndrome (9). In this condition, individuals arouse many times during the night, following spontaneous apneic episodes lasting up to thirty seconds. From two to three hundred of these spells may occur each night. With such sleep loss at night, drowsiness develops during the daytime. Long-term consequences of this syndrome include pulmonary hypertension and cor pulmonale. The syndrome has been seen in children as young as twelve. Since the serious apneic episodes appear to be associated with peritracheal obstruction, activated only during sleep, a definitive treatment is chronic tracheotomy. Following such a procedure, the symptoms disappear. During the day, the tracheotomies can be plugged and hidden behind a neckpiece (Chapter 14).

Insomnia

Insomnia is rare in children. Infants who delay sleeping through the night or manifest night-waking episodes have been described as insomniacs. Frequently, insomnia in children presents with problems related to going to bed or to having nightmares. Fear of the dark, delays in going to bed, and nighttime rituals are all common in children from age three to ten. Nightmares are common after the age of two. As isolated symptoms, nightmares relate more to daytime stressful or exciting experiences than to intrapsychic conflicts. Insomnia in childhood generally requires no medication. When disturbances of sleep behavior are crisis-related, such as following a serious illness or separation, children may benefit from short courses of chloral hydrate so that "bad sleep habits" will not develop.

GILLES DE LA TOURETTE SYNDROME

The Gilles de la Tourette syndrome is characterized by tics that begin as involuntary movements of the head and spread to the rest of the body. Vocal tics, including involuntary grunting, barks, or coprolalia, are present. The disorder begins in childhood, at age twelve to fourteen. Recent evidence has substantiated the effectiveness of haloperidol in alleviating the muscular and vocal tics (10). Supportive psychotherapy should also be provided. As yet, haloperidol is not approved by the Food and Drug Administration (FDA) for use in children under twelve. Experimentally, 5-hydroxytryptophan, a precursor of 5-hydroxytryptamine, has been tried. Preliminary results have been encouraging (11).

ORGANIC BRAIN SYNDROMES AND MENTAL RETARDATION

Some individuals with chronic organic brain syndromes or mental retardation have behavior which is characterized by agitation or hyperaggressivity. The cautious use of oral phenothiazines has been successful in alleviating these symptoms. Of course, reversible etiologies should be sought. The use of antipsychotics is symptomatic and does not affect the underlying pathology.

REFERENCES

1. American Psychiatric Association *Diagnostic and Statistical Manual: Mental Disorders II.* Washington: American Psychiatric Association, 1965.
2. Group for the Advancement of Psychiatry. *Psychopathological Disorders in Childhood: Theoretical Considerations and a Proposed Classification.* New York: Group for the Advancement of Psychiatry, 1966.
3. Campbell, M. and Shapiro, T. Therapy of psychiatric disorders of childhood. *In: Manual of Psychiatric Therapeutics.* R. Shader, ed., Boston: Little, Brown, 1975. pp. 137–162.
4. Gittleman-Klein, R. Pharmacotherapy and management of pathological separation anxiety. *In: Progress in Psychiatric Drug Treatment, Vol. 2.* D. Klein and R. Gittleman-Klein, eds., New York: Brunner/Mazel, 1976. pp. 454–467.
5. Frommer, E. Treatment of childhood depression with antidepressant drugs. *Br. Med. J. 1:*729–732, 1967.
6. Annell, A. Manic-depressive illness in children and effect of treatment with lithium carbonate. *Acta Paedopsychiatr. 36:*292–301, 1969.
7. Anders, T. and Freeman, E. Enuresis. *In: Comprehensive Textbook of Child Psychiatry.* J. Noshpitz, ed., in press.
8. Anders, T. and Guilleminault, C. The pathophysiology of sleep disorders in pediatrics. I. Sleep in infancy. *Adv. Ped. 22:*137–150, 1976.
9. Guilleminault, C. and Anders, T. The pathophysiology of sleep disorders in pediatrics. II. Sleep disorders in children. *Adv. Ped. 22:*151–174, 1976.
10. Shapiro, A., Shapiro, E., Wayne, H., Clarkin, J., and Bruun, R. Tourette's syndrome: summary of data on 34 patients. *Psychosom. Med. 35:*419–435, 1973.
11. Van Woert, M. H., Yip, L. C., and Balis, M. E. Purine phosphoribosyltransferase in Gilles de la Tourette syndrome. *N. Engl. J. Med. 296:*210–212, 1977.

26 | Pharmacological Treatment of the Minimal Brain Dysfunction Syndrome

THOMAS F. ANDERS and

ROLAND D. CIARANELLO

HISTORY

The minimal brain dysfunction (MBD) syndrome is known by many names. Diagnostic labels such as the "brain damage syndrome," the "hyperactive child syndrome," "minimal brain damage," "specific learning disability," and the "hyperkinetic syndrome" have all been used interchangeably and with confusion in the literature. The symptom picture is characterized by hyperactivity, impulsivity, distractibility, and excitability. Aggressive and antisocial behavior, specific learning problems, and emotional lability are also often considered to be part of the disorder.

Descriptions of variants of the above syndrome appeared in the medical literature at least as early as 40 B.C., when patterns of motor aphasia in children were first described (1). The neuropsychological studies of receptive and expressive aphasias, dyslexias, gross brain damage secondary to trauma and encephalitis, and cerebral palsy provided the foundations for our current state of knowledge. These studies of organic brain disorders have identified a wide range of behavioral, emotional, motor, perceptual, language, and other cognitive disorders in children who have suffered demonstrable insult to the central nervous system. A continuum of reproductive casualty, supported by extensive epidemiological evidence, additionally links abnormal maternal and fetal events with various disorders of language and behavior.

In a significant number of children, however, severe difficulty in acquiring spoken and written language cannot be accounted for by lack of intelligence; by primary sensory, motor, or emotional disorders; or by lack of environmental stimulation.

The hyperactive child syndrome was first described by the German physician Heinrich Hoffman in 1845 (2). Psychoactive medication for the control of symptoms was first attempted by Bradley, in 1934, when he used dextroamphetamine sulfate (Benzedrine) with good results (3). Amphetamines were again used for this purpose (4) in 1957; and in 1958 methylphenidate (Ritalin) was introduced into the treatment of hyperactivity (5).

INCIDENCE AND SYMPTOMATOLOGY

The prevalence of the minimal brain dysfunction syndrome varies according to the definition used, the type of examination provided, and the setting in which the examination occurs. The incidence is reduced when the diagnosis requires direct office observations, rather than a history of hyperactive behavior. Most symptomatology occurs in the classroom, so that office examinations frequently are not helpful. Nevertheless, epidemiologic studies generally agree that 4–10 percent of children demonstrate some of the critical symptoms of hyperactivity, impulsivity, distractibility, excitability, specific learning problems, and emotional lability. The male-female ratio is at least 4 : 1 (6).

Hyperactivity per se does not represent a syndrome; rather, it must be viewed as a symptom within a spectrum of diagnostic entities (Table 26-1). Children can manifest the symptom of hyperactivity under several conditions. First, excessive anxiety associated with emotional strain and conflict can lead to restless, "fidgety" behavior which may be labeled as hyperactive. Second, boredom due to understimulation may lead to "hyperactivity." For example, if children are brighter than their peers, they may not find sufficient stimulation in the normal

TABLE 26-1.
SOURCES OF HYPERACTIVITY AND LEARNING PROBLEMS

Excessive anxiety
Decreased environmental stimulation
Undernutrition
Mental retardation
Psychosis
Minimal brain dysfunction

---

classroom setting. Inadequate nutrition, hunger, mental retardation, and psychosis can also be associated with the symptom of hyperactivity. Finally, central nervous system deficits associated with minimal brain dysfunction may present with hyperactivity, "soft" neurological signs, or specific learning disabilities (Fig. 26-1) (7). The specific learning disabilities can be further subdivided into inability to read (dyslexia), inability to write (dysgraphia), inability to perform arithmetic manipulations (dyscalculia), and mixed deficits. Although this model is not complete, it leads to a rational approach to therapeutic management.

BIOCHEMICAL AND NEUROPHYSIOLOGICAL CORRELATES

Wender (8) has hypothesized biochemical abnormalities in the pleasure centers and in the reticular activating system of the brain in children with the minimal brain dysfunction syndrome. His formulations derive from clinical findings that these children appear to be hyper-aroused, with decreased attentiveness, inability to focus on relevant stimuli, and increased difficulty in figure-ground discrimination. They also have a diminished capacity for positive and negative affect—evidenced subjectively by a diminished ability to experience pleasure and pain and behaviorally by diminished sensitivity to positive and negative reinforcement. These children are difficult to discipline and react unfavorably to punishment.

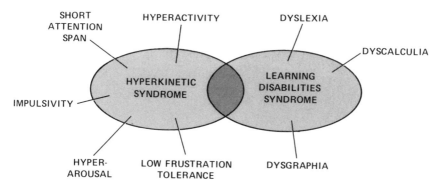

FIGURE 26-1. Minimal Brain Dysfunction Syndrome

To determine whether children with minimal brain dysfunction are hyperaroused requires operational criteria utilizing psychophysiological and electroencephalographic (EEG) techniques. Many studies have found an increased incidence of EEG abnormalities in hyperactive children. However, the prevalence of EEG abnormalities in the general population remains unknown; and in controlled studies the increased incidence of EEG abnormalities in hyperactive children remains controversial.

Satterfield and his group studied physiological arousal in hyperactive children (9). Criteria for arousal included skin conductance, amplitude and power of the EEG, and amplitudes and latencies of the auditory evoked response. Contrary to expectation, children with more severe problems of motor control, attention span, and impulsivity had lower levels of central nervous system arousal. Those hyperactive children with the greatest increase in central nervous system arousal level following stimulant medication demonstrated the best clinical improvement. To explain the high correlation between good drug responders and low central nervous system arousal, Satterfield has speculated that low arousal is associated with insufficient central inhibition. Insufficient inhibitory control of motor functions would then result in excessive and inappropriate motor activity. Similarly, lack of inhibitory control over sensory functions would result in easy distractibility and inattention to relevant stimuli.

Wender (8) suggests that 5-hydroxytryptamine decreases motoric activity and arousal, while dopamine and norepinephrine have the opposite effect. After synaptic release, catecholamines are inactivated by reuptake into presynaptic nerve terminals (Chapter 2). Amphetamines inhibit this reuptake, potentiating the action of the catecholamines (Chapter 21). This potentiation could, therefore, explain the ability of amphetamines to enhance central nervous system arousal in hyperactive children.

FAMILY AND GENETIC STUDIES

Sharp controversy exists about the relative contributions of inheritance and environment in the minimal brain dysfunction syndrome. Most studies agree that children with hyperactive symptoms live in families which have abnormally high incidences of psychopathology, including schizophrenia, affective disorders, and sociopathy. For example, a study of parents of children with hyperactive pathology and parents of controls showed an increased incidence of alcoholism, sociopathy, and hysteria in the parents of the former group (6). Fathers in this group tended to exhibit more psychiatric illness than did mothers, with 30 percent of the·fathers being labeled as alcoholic and 16 percent as sociopathic. Approximately 16 percent of the fathers of the hyperactive children were thought to have been hyperactive themselves as children. It is not clear from such studies, however, which came first. Was parental psychopathology enhanced as a result of dealing with a difficult child? Or did the chaotic environments of these children predispose to altered parenting and socialization?

Twin studies and adoption studies tend to suggest a genetic contribution to activity level, at least. Again, the definition of the symptomatology and the nature of the studies make rigorous conclusions difficult. A causal association between hyperactivity in childhood and adult sociopathy and alcoholism is particularly dangerous. Once a child is labeled as hyperactive, the significant members of his environment respond quite differently to him. A trend of expectation and response is established which, itself, may lead to later deviant behavior. To ascribe this path to genetic determination dooms the child unnecessarily, particularly since the data implicating a major role of genetic factors are incomplete.

CLINICAL EVALUATION

In evaluating the symptoms of minimal brain dysfunction, it is useful to keep the previously described model in mind. A careful interview with both parents about early development and current psychosocial functioning is critical. A complete physical and neurological examination and some special laboratory studies are also helpful. In addition, communication with the school is usually essential.

One important aspect of the history involves the point at which symptoms first appeared. Although behavioral problems may not become obvious until the child enters the classroom, precursors to hyperactivity frequently are present in the first year of life. Delays in sleeping through the night, fussy eating patterns, and irritable dispositions are common, i.e., the infant is not in "synchrony" with its environment. During the toddler period, the children also tend to "get into everything," to have difficulty adhering to limits, and to be unable to learn through positive reinforcement. Hyperaggressivity with sibs and peers also is described. A long-standing history of symptoms which suggest a diagnosis of the minimal brain dysfunction syndrome is clearly different from one in which there is an acute onset after a traumatic event such as divorce or illness. Other possible sources of conflict within the environment should be explored. It is important to attempt to differentiate the precipitating stresses leading to the onset of symptomatology from those leading to the referral.

A physical examination, a hearing test, and a speech and language evaluation should be obtained to rule out defects of vision or hearing, as well as abnormalities of speech. Minor physical anomalies such as large or low-set ears, widely spaced eyes, and curvatures of the fingers have been described in children with the minimal brain dysfunction syndrome. Growth rates for both height and weight should be plotted, especially in children who will receive psychoactive medications.

"Soft" neurological signs are difficult to confirm reliably. Furthermore, their incidence in the general population is unknown. Prechtl's sign of choreoathetoid movements in fingertips of hyperextended wrists has been reported to be positive in children with minimal brain dysfunction (10). Tests of fine motor coordination, of rhythm, and of laterality and spatial orientation may also be impaired. One carefully controlled study in which matched hyperactive, neurotic, and normal groups of children were tested with a standard neurological examination demonstrated an excess of minor neurological abnormalities in the hyperactive group, indicative of sensorimotor incoordination (11).

The mental status examination should pay particular attention to the child's baseline activity level, response to new situations, muscular tone, habitual mannerisms, attention span, persistence, distractibility, irritability, general mood level, speech and language, and response to frustration. Unfortunately, in a strange setting such as the doctor's office, the behavioral symptomatology may be suppressed. Several visits may be necessary before comfort and familiarity is achieved, so that the symptoms become demonstrable.

An abundance of standardized behavioral tests and rating scales have been designed to delineate and track the symptoms of the minimal brain dysfunction syndrome, as summarized elsewhere (12). Conners has developed three scales: a parent symptom questionnaire, a teacher questionnaire, and an abbreviated symptom questionnaire. Werry, Weiss, and Peters have developed an activity scale to measure motor activity and a continuous performance test to measure attention. Peterson and Quay have developed a symptom checklist to assess psychopathology. Specialized cognitive sensorimotor tests, such as the Lincoln-Oseretsky motor developmental scale, the Illinois Test of Psycholinguistic Aptitude (ITPA), the Frostig visual perception tests, the Porteus mazes, the Wepman test of auditory discrimination, the Benton right/left discrimination test, the Benton finger localization test, and a series of writing tests are all available for use in specific cases.

PSYCHOPHARMACOLOGICAL MANAGEMENT

Ideally, a drug used in the treatment of the minimal brain dysfunction syndrome should have several characteristics. Naturally, the drug should control hyperactivity; increase frustration tolerance and attention span; reduce impulsive and aggressive behavior; and improve deficits in visual and auditory perception, reading ability, and fine motor coordination. In addition, the drug should have few side effects or toxic manifestations. Though far from this ideal, central nervous system stimulants are currently the drugs of choice. Their side effects include insomnia and anorexia, and their toxic manifestations include psychotic-like thinking and behavior (Chapter 21).

As mentioned earlier, the amphetamines were used in the treatment of hyperkinesis more than thirty years ago, when Bradley (3) discovered their paradoxical calming effects in hyperactive patients. Since then, virtually every psychopharmacological agent has been tested in children with minimal brain dysfunction. Unfortunately, controlled studies are limited and reports conflict as to the type of child who is likely to respond favorably.

Currently, methylphenidate is considered to be the drug of choice for controlling hyperactive behavior, with dextroamphetamine sulfate being the second most successful drug. Both drugs have similar sites of action and behavioral effects, although methylphenidate has less tendency to produce anorexia. The dose of methylphenidate ranges from 5–100 mg daily. The maximum duration of treatment reported to date has been four years. Improvement in behavior occurs in an average of 83 percent of patients; worsening of hyperactivity may occur in approximately 5 percent. Doses of dextroamphetamine range from 5–40 mg daily, and the maximum duration of therapy reported for this drug has also been four years. Improvements in behavior occur in an average of 69 percent of patients, while deterioration is seen in 11 percent. The incidence of side effects for dextroamphetamine is slightly higher than that reported for methylphenidate. Dextroamphetamine is contraindicated in patients with hyperactivity associated with psychotic symptoms (Chapter 27).

A recommended treatment schedule for methylphenidate begins with an initial dosage of 0.25 mg/kg daily, divided into two doses given at breakfast and lunch. In children who are of average or below-average weight, the medication is given after eating, while in overweight children, it is given prior to mealtime. The dose is doubled during each successive week of treatment, up to an average optimal level of 2.0 mg/ kg daily. If side effects such as insomnia, anorexia, or severe depressive reactions develop, the dosage is reduced slightly or maintained constant until they disappear. The dosage is monitored on the basis of reports from parents and schoolteachers and by reexamination of the child after two to four weeks of treatment. Frequently, medication may be interrupted for weekends and during vacations, to help reduce side effects and toxic reactions. In children who show no response or who become tolerant to the effects of methylphenidate, amphetamine should be tried. When both drugs have proven to be without effect, tranquilizing agents may be tried.

Two other psychoactive agents which have been tested do not significantly improve upon the results of dextroamphetamine and methylphenidate. These are diethylaminoethanol (Deanol) (13), a drug which may be converted intraneuronally to acetylcholine, and pemoline (Cylert), a central stimulant which is structurally unrelated to amphetamine and methylphenidate (14). An advantage of this latter preparation is its long half-life, so that a single dose in the morning provides adequate blood levels.

When excessive anxiety seems to be the cause of the hyperactive symptomatology, antianxiety and antipsychotic agents should be tried. Chlordiazepoxide (Librium) relieves anxiety and tends to reduce aggressive tendencies. Thioridazine (Mellaril) is used chiefly in the treatment of mentally retarded children with hyperactivity. In one study, 57 percent of 308 patients were benefited, and only 2 percent experienced side effects of drowsiness. Extrapyramidal and sedative side effects are more frequent with chlorpromazine (Thorazine). Antidepressants and anticonvulsants also have been investigated in the treatment of hyperactive behavior. Generally, they are not effective, unless a depressive reaction or seizure disorder is associated with the hyperkinetic behavior. The barbiturates are always contraindicated, because they exacerbate hyperactive behavior.

Medication is usually not necessary after the age of twelve, since there is a tendency for the hyperactive disorder to improve with age. Thus, the need for drug treatment should be continually reevaluated over time.

The use of pharmacological agents in the management of minimal brain dysfunction has been associated with considerable controversy. The general principles of psychotic drug use in children, outlined in Chapter 25, apply with equal emphasis in this syndrome. The "antihyperkinesis" drugs are far from benign agents. Their abuse potential is considerable, and they have marked physiological effects. Whether or not they inhibit growth remains unresolved. Physicians, especially pediatricians, are often placed under intense pressure from parents or schools to use these medications. The casual use of these drugs in the absence of a thorough, careful diagnostic evaluation is to be avoided. The physician should feel confident that his use of these drugs is warranted and not simply a response to external exigencies. Frequent reevaluation of their continued need constitutes appropriate medical practice. However, when used appropriately, these agents can be extremely beneficial.

NONPHARMACOLOGICAL MANAGEMENT

Successful treatment of the minimal brain dysfunction syndrome requires a total approach. Educational evaluations are needed to permit design of remedial programs for each child. Learning consoles, special-education teachers, and small classes with highly structured curricula and individual attention are all useful in the school management of the learning-disabled child with a behavioral problem. Similarly, structure in the home setting, with well-defined tasks and limits, is useful. Parents and siblings require a great deal of support. Behavior modification programs are often useful in reducing disruptive and intrusive behavior. Finally, the child may require individual psychotherapy or play therapy, in order to understand and improve self-concepts and maladaptive behavior patterns. For successful treatment of children with minimal brain dysfunction syndrome, the teacher, the family physician, and the mental health professional need to work closely together around the specific needs of the child and the family.

REFERENCES

1. Strother, C. Minimal cerebral dysfunction: a historical overview. *N.Y. Acad. Sci. 205*:6–17, 1973.
2. Hoffmann, H. *Der Strumpelpeter: oder lustige Geschichtern und drollige Bilder.* Leipzig: Insel Verlag, 1845.
3. Bradley, C. The behavior of children receiving Benzadrine. *Am. J. Psychiatry 94*:577–585, 1973.
4. Laufer, M. and Denhoff, E. Hyperkinetic behavior syndrome in children. *J. Ped. 50*:463–474, 1957.
5. Knobel, M. Psychopharmacology for the hyperkinetic child–Dynamic considerations. *Arch. Gen. Psychiatry 6*:198–202, 1962.
6. Cantwell, D. Epidemiology, clinical picture, and classification of the hyperactive child syndrome. *In: The Hyperactive Child: Diagnosis, Management, Current Research.* D. Cantwell, *ed.*, New York: Spectrum Publications, 1975, pp. 3–15.
7. Kinsbourne, M. School problems: diagnosis and treatment. *Pediatrics 52*: 697–710, 1973.
8. Wender, P. *Minimal Brain Dysfunction in Children.* New York: Wiley-Interscience, 1971.
9. Satterfield, J. Neurophysiologic studies with hyperactive children. *In: The Hyperactive Child: Diagnosis, Management, Current Research.* D. Cantwell, *ed.*, New York: Spectrum Publications, 1975, pp. 67–82.
10. Prechtl, H. and Steinman, C. The choreiform syndrome in children. *Develop. Med. Child. Neurol. 4*:119–127, 1962.
11. Werry, J., Minde, K., Guzman, A., Weiss, G., Degen, K., and Hoy, E. Studies on the hyperactive child. VII. Neurological states compared with neurotic and normal children. *Am. J. Orthopsychiat. 127*:824–825, 1972.
12. *Psychopharmacology Bulletin: Pharmacotherapy of Children.* Washington, D.C.: U.S. Government Printing Office, 1970, pp. 24–29.
13. Conners, C. Deanol and behavior disorders in children: a critical review of the literature and recommended future studies for determining efficacy. *Psychopharmacology Bulletin: Pharmacotherapy of Children.* Washington, D.C.: U.S. Government Printing Office, 1970, pp. 188–195.
14. Millichap, J. Drugs in management of minimal brain dysfunction. *Ann. N.Y. Acad. Sci. 205*:321–334, 1973.

27 | Drug Treatment of Childhood Psychotic Disorders

ROLAND D. CIARANELLO and

THOMAS F. ANDERS

INTRODUCTION

Psychotic disturbances in children present a special diagnostic challenge to the psychiatrist. Because the child is developing and in a state of continuous transition, the age at which he or she first experiences psychotic symptoms is a major determinant in the clinical presentation. The signs displayed will be largely dependent upon the point in the maturational sequence at which psychosis interrupts or arrests development. The adult or adolescent whose cognitive growth is complete at the time schizophrenic symptoms appear will present with the typical signs of thought disorder, hallucinations, or a well-formed delusional system. In contrast, the psychotic child, whose illness may begin as early as age three, presents with an entirely different clinical picture. Therefore, diagnosis of childhood psychopathological syndromes necessitates an understanding of normal child development.

Child psychiatrists have disagreed about the diagnostic criteria which define the principal psychotic disturbances of childhood. Differing opinions have resulted from several factors. First, general psychiatrists often fail to understand that diagnostic criteria which are appropriate for adult disorders are largely inapplicable in children. Second, there is a paucity of rigorous scientific studies defining the major clinical syndromes in children. Finally, many psychiatrists are reluctant to burden children with serious diagnostic labels which may follow them through their lives, particularly when the outcome of the illness, as it is influenced by maturation, environment, and treatment, cannot be predicted precisely. Although this point is of concern, the use of appropriately derived diagnostic labels conveys in shorthand important information about etiology, clinical presentation, and prognosis. Diagnostic acumen is one of the most valuable skills physicians bring to the treatment team. Unless more rigorous diagnostic criteria are applied to childhood psychoses, we shall continue to be frustrated in our attempt to define, study, and treat them. Physicians should approach the diagnostic evaluation with the utmost gravity, and research in this area must make the elucidation of these disturbances its highest priority.

CLASSIFICATION OF PSYCHOTIC DISTURBANCES OF CHILDHOOD

The Diagnostic and Statistical Manual of the American Psychiatric Association (DSM-II) provides little help in classification of childhood psychotic disorders. The Group for the Advancement of Psychiatry (GAP) has attempted to meet the need for a classification scheme of childhood disorders, and has published a volume devoted exclusively to this area (1). This group defines psychosis in children as:

> characterized by marked, pervasive deviations from the behavior that is expected for the child's age. Psychotic disorder is revealed often by severe and continued impairment of emotional relationships with persons, associated with an aloofness and a tendency toward preoccupation with inanimate objects; loss of speech or failure in its development; disturbances in sensory perception; bizarre or stereotyped behavior and motility patterns; marked resistance to change in environment or routine; outbursts of intense and unpredictable panic; absence of a sense of personal identity; and blunted, uneven or fragmented intellectual development. In some cases, intellectual performance may be adequate or better, with the psychotic disorder confining itself to other areas of personality function.

This description recognizes the important interplay between symptoms and developmental sequence, and it stresses that the diagnosis of psychotic disorders differ at various developmental levels. According to the GAP classification scheme, psychoses are distinguished according to their occurrence in infancy and early childhood, in which ego disruptions occur in the development of those personality functions which concern individuation and relatedness to people; in later childhood, where failure of integration or personality disintegration with impaired reality testing may predominate; and in adolescence, where se-

TABLE 27-1.
CHILDHOOD PSYCHOTIC DISORDERS*

Psychoses of infancy and early childhood (birth–6 years).
  Early infantile autism
  Interactional psychotic disorders ("symbiotic psychosis")
  Other psychoses of early childhood
Psychoses of later childhood (6–12)
  Schizophreniform psychotic disorder
  Other psychoses of later childhood
Psychoses of adolescence (>12)
  Acute confusional state
  Schizophrenic disorder, adult type
  Other psychoses of adolescence

---

* As defined by the GAP Report (1).

vere impairment of social relationships or thought processes and of the individual's sense of identity may occur (Table 27-1).

This chapter will focus on the two major psychotic disorders of children: early infantile autism, in which symptoms appear before the age of two and a half years, and childhood schizophrenia, in which symptoms generally appear after the age of five to seven years.

EARLY INFANTILE AUTISM

FEATURES OF THE ILLNESS

The term "early infantile autism" was first proposed in 1943 by Leo Kanner, who differentiated autistic children from those with dementia or childhood schizophrenia and noted the preponderance of males to females (4 : 1) and the occurrence in the general population (4–5 per 10,000). According to Kanner's diagnostic criteria, early infantile autism is characterized by the development before the age of two and a half of the following: withdrawal, isolation, and aloofness; language delays; ritualistic activities; and an intense dislike of change. Withdrawal, isolation, and aloofness may be present at birth or become progressive thereafter. There is a failure to make affective contact and form social relationships. Such infants may not show appropriate "molding" behavior when held. They may lie soundless in their crib, gazing fixedly into space, or play with their fingers for hours at a time. Autistic infants appear to be disinterested in their environment, make infrequent eye-to-eye contact, and give little sign of attending to the people around them. Frequently, these infants are mistaken for deaf, since they often do not respond to sounds. Conversely, these children may spend hours crying or screaming uncontrollably in their crib. Language delays involve both expressive and receptive language and must be differentiated from aphasia and problems in motor speech. These delays represent a central deficit in the ability to process the sequential information encoded in language and, perhaps, in visual information. Autistic infants engage in various ritualistic activities, including flapping of hands and arms, twirling, rocking, and head-banging. They may form morbid attachments to inanimate objects. Finally, they exhibit an intense dislike of change and an obsessive need for sameness in the environment. New routes, trivial and minuscule disruptions of routine, or minute changes in the position of familiar objects may be met with screaming, tantrums, and manifestations of severe anxiety.

It is important to note that no symptom or set of symptoms is pathognomonic of infantile autism. Unevenness of the maturational course, with delays in some areas and advances in others, is typical. The diagnosis demands careful consideration of the entire behavioral presentation and exclusion of other organic brain diseases. The diagnosis is usually established around the age of three, when the language delay and communication defect become paramount. However, even with these deficits, one should be cautious about making the diagnosis unless some of the symptomatic panoply has been present prior to that age.

ETIOLOGY

The etiology of early infantile autism remains obscure. For many years the psychogenic view was that autism developed as the child's response to cold, aloof, unloving parents. In the face of parental detachment and lack of warmth, the child was thought to withdraw into an autistic shell, becoming preoccupied with his inner fantasies. However, many personality studies have failed to distinguish parents of autistic children from parents of language-handicapped or normal children. While some parents of autistic children do, indeed, demonstrate traits of aloofness and withdrawal from their affected child, they are warm and loving to their other offspring, so that their "defensiveness" may be associated more with the frustration of having to deal with an unresponsive, withdrawn infant.

In his original article on infantile autism, Kanner concluded that the illness represented a "pure-culture example of inborn autistic disturbances of affective contact" (2). Indeed, there is mounting evidence to suggest that the illness involves central nervous system dysfunction. Although no specific localizing signs have been found, current studies indicate that a major defect lies in the development of appropriate language skills. In addition, long-term follow-up of autistic children reveals a high incidence of epileptic seizures during adolescence. Moreover, a striking incidence of infantile autism is seen in the offspring of mothers contracting rubella in the first trimester of pregnancy.

The intellectual deficits in infantile autism appear to include an inability to comprehend and utilize concept-forming skills in information processing and a global defect in receptive, expressive, and conceptual language. The pattern of language abilities in autistic children differs from that of either mentally retarded or normal children. Autistic children are typically poor in information transfer from one sensory modality to another. Moreover, they make little use of concepts in memorization or problem-solving, although they may memorize well by rote. Recent evidence suggests that the defect in processing sequential or temporally encoded information may extend to visual input as well (3,4).

PHARMACOLOGICAL INTERVENTION

At present the use of medication in the treatment of infantile autism is designed to foster social and learning skills in a multidisciplinary treatment setting specialized in dealing with emotionally disturbed children. Drug therapy is used to control explosive behavior, minimize social withdrawal and apathy, and reduce hyperkinesis and excitability. It is especially important that this intervention not oversedate the child, if the primary goal of optimizing educational advancement is to be met. Pharmacological agents should be selected carefully and their dosage monitored closely. The drugs found to be most effective in the treatment of autistic symptoms are the antipsychotics and the tricyclic anti-depressants (tricyclics). Triiodothyronine (T_3) and lithium may also be useful, although these drugs are currently in the investigational stage (5).

Antipsychotics such as chlorpromazine (Thorazine) and thioridazene (Mellaril) are among the most commonly used drugs to control behaviors such as explosiveness and hyperactivity in autistic children. Unfortunately, many children appear to be especially sensitive to the sedating properties of these two drugs, while being relatively unresponsive to their intended properties. Thus, behavioral control is achieved by putting the child to sleep or by making him so drowsy that his function in an educational setting is impaired. The higher potency antipsychotics, such as trifluoperazine (Stelazine), thiothixene (Navane), haloperidol (Haldol), and fluphenazine (Prolixin) do not have the sedating properties of chlorpromazine and thioridazene (Chapter 9). In moderate doses, they are quite effective in controlling the explosivity or excitability of autistic children. They are, however, associated with a fairly high incidence of extrapyramidal side effects, and dosage must be carefully monitored.

Recent reports suggest that thiothixene is especially satisfactory in controlling autistic behaviors, since it has a number of desirable properties. It provides good symptom control without excessive sedation; in addition, it has a mild "energizing" property which it shares with haloperidol and fluphenazine and which makes it useful in treating apathetic withdrawal. Thiothixene also has a relatively low incidence of extrapyramidal side effects, compared to haloperidol and fluphenazine. Haloperidol is currently restricted to investigational use in children below twelve years of age.

There is no set optimal dose of antipsychotic which provides symptom control, since behavioral remediation is achieved over a wide dose range. Each child must be treated individually, because his response to the drug and the side effects he may display cannot be readily predicted. A useful guide is to start treatment with a single bedtime dose; if more drug is needed, a morning dose can be added. Additional drug increments can be attained by adding to the bedtime and morning regimen. Since all of the antipsychotics have relatively long half-lives, it is usually not necessary to administer the drug more often than twice ·daily.

Tricyclics have been effective in treating withdrawn autistic children. Both nortriptyline (Aventyl) and imipramine (Tofranil) have been shown to be effective in these cases. The dosage of nortriptyline ranges from 30–150 mg daily. In a few cases, nortriptyline has successfully controlled explosive and hyperkinetic behavior as well, without sedation.

In recent clinical trials, triiodothyronine (T_3) and lithium have been tried in autistic and schizophrenic children, with claims of partial success. Lithium may be effective in ameliorating aggressive behavior associated with explosiveness and excitability. In a study investigating the use of triiodothyronine, improvement in communication skills was observed. This drug is currently under active investigation.

Most other classes of drugs are either ineffectual or contraindicated in control of autistic behaviors. Benzodiazepines, anticonvulsants, and vitamins are all without evidence of therapeutic benefit. In fact, the benzodiazepines may exacerbate behavioral disintegration. Barbiturates, hallucinogens, and amphetamines promote behavioral disorganization and are contraindicated; the latter two drug classes also exacerbate psychotic symptoms.

At present, then, the antipsychotics are the most effective drugs available for control of most autistic behaviors. The high-potency antipsychotics achieve this control without sedation and are, therefore, superior to the low-potency medications. Thiothixene is probably the drug of choice in treating these behaviors, although trifluoperazine is also satisfactory. Haloperidol and fluphenazine are highly effective but are associated with a higher incidence of extrapyramidal reactions. Where sedation is desired, diphenhydramine (Benadryl) remains the drug of choice. If a sedating phenothiazene is indicated, mesoridazene (Serentil) is sometimes effective.

CHILDHOOD SCHIZOPHRENIA

FEATURES OF THE ILLNESS

There is considerable disagreement about whether early infantile autism and childhood schizophrenia are separate disorders or whether infantile autism is simply the earliest manifestation of childhood schizophrenia. The former viewpoint is advocated by Rutter (4) and by

Wing (6), while the latter is offered by Bender (7). Each viewpoint has its devoted adherents.

The idea that autism and childhood schizophrenia are distinct is derived from epidemiological and clinical data. Proponents of this view emphasize that the incidence of childhood psychosis is bimodally distributed, with one peak at age two to three years (infantile autism) and the other at ten to eleven years (childhood schizophrenia). Between these peaks, the occurrence of initial psychotic symptoms is relatively less frequent. Moreover, advocates of this philosophy believe that childhood schizophrenia more closely resembles the schizophrenic process in adults. Using adult diagnostic criteria, they find that disordered thought associations, thought blocking, and persecutory delusions each occur in about 60 percent of cases and that auditory hallucinations (80 percent) and affective blunting (70 percent) are also prominent features of the childhood schizophrenic process.

The incidence of schizophrenia in childhood is two and a half times greater in males; this sex difference diminishes through adolescence until it reaches the equal distribution which is characteristic of adult schizophrenia. Moreover, the incidence of schizophrenia in the families of schizophrenic children is around 10 percent, whereas the incidence of schizophrenia in families of autistic children does not differ from that seen in the general population.

The concept of a continuum of schizophrenic disorders has been advocated by Bender and others. They argue that early infantile autism is the earliest manifestation of schizophrenia in children and that autistic children develop symptoms of classical schizophrenia as they grow to adulthood. This hypothesis emphasizes that virtually all psychotic disturbances of childhood progress to adult schizophrenia and that children diagnosed as autistic in childhood develop schizophrenic thought disorder as adults (7). However, British investigators, led by Wing (6), have presented compelling evidence that the progression from infantile autism to adult schizophrenia is by no means guaranteed. In their case studies, autistic children grown to adulthood shared none of the features of classical chronic schizophrenia.

DIAGNOSIS

The diagnosis of childhood schizophrenia is more difficult to make than is a diagnosis of infantile autism, where Kanner's criteria are still

widely accepted. If one applies the accepted criteria for adult schizophrenia to children, it is plain that some psychotic children display
"classical" adult schizophrenic symptoms, even as early as seven years
of age. However, it is also clear that thought disorders in children present features which are unique to childhood, stressing the urgent need
for particular attention to developmental norms. Numerous attempts
have been made to establish criteria for the diagnosis of schizophrenia
in children. Most assume the inclusion of infantile autism as a component of the schizophrenic spectrum and do not provide assistance in the
resolution of the central issue as to whether these are separate disorders.

The earliest attempt to define diagnostic criteria of childhood schizophrenia was made by Potter in 1933 (8). The following criteria were
used:

- Generalized retraction of interests from the environment
- Dereistic thinking, feeling, and acting
- Disturbance of thought, manifested through blocking, symbol-
  ism, condensation, perseveration, incoherence, and diminution,
  at times attaining mutism
- Defect in emotional rapport
- Diminution, rigidity, and distortion of affect
- Alteration of behavior with either an increase or a decrease in
  motility, leading either to a relentless activity or total immobility, or bizarre behavior with a tendency to perseveration or
  stereotypy.

Bender (9) defined somewhat less restrictive criteria:

> The schizophrenic child reveals pathology at every level in every field
> of integration within the functioning of the central nervous system, be
> this vegetative, motor, perceptive, intellectual, emotional, or social.
> Furthermore, the pathology disturbs the pattern of every functional
> field in a characteristic way.

In 1961, the British Working Party (10) established nine criteria for
determination of what they termed the "schizophrenic syndrome":

- Gross and sustained impairment of emotional relationships with
  people
- Apparent unawareness of personal identity to an inappropriate
  degree

- Pathological preoccupation with particular objects or certain characteristics of them without regard to their accepted functions
- Sustained resistance to change in the environment and striving to maintain or restore sameness
- Abnormal perceptual experience in the absence of discernible organic subnormality, implied by excessive, diminished, or unpredictable responses to sensory stimuli
- Acute, excessive, and seemingly illogical anxiety
- Absence, loss, or developmental loss of speech skills
- Distortion in motility patterns
- A background of serious retardation in which islets of normal, near-normal, or exceptional function or skill may appear.

It is worth noting that many children who meet Kanner's criteria for infantile autism would be included in the British Working Party classification of "schizophrenic syndrome."

This diagnostic dilemma would be greatly relieved by the discovery of a biochemical or neurophysiological marker to classify childhood psychoses. So far, no clear-cut markers have been found. Recently, attention has been focused upon the metabolism of catechol- and indoleamines in the central nervous system and the use of blood platelets as a peripheral model for central neurons. Some nonspecific defects in platelet efflux of 5-hydroxytryptamine have been reported in psychotic children, but these do not provide distinction from genetic forms of mental retardation. The elucidation of psychotic disturbances in children might seem to present a hopeless muddle to clinicians who are inexpert in working with children. Fortunately, some operational clarification is obtained if infantile autism is conceptualized as a developmental retardation with profound perceptual deficits, particularly in language, while childhood schizophrenia is viewed as a disorder of affective and thought processes. A recent review by Ornitz and Ritvo expands these themes nicely (11).

ETIOLOGY

A familial basis for childhood schizophrenia has been proposed and is widely accepted. Bender (12) has followed children who were identified as schizophrenic in childhood throughout their lives. She reports a strikingly high incidence of "schizophrenic spectrum disorders" in the relatives of these children—evidence in line with findings in adult schizophrenics. Rutter (4) has suggested that childhood schizophrenia is the same illness as its adult counterpart and that schizophrenia is a separate entity from early infantile autism. Since most earlier studies did not make this distinction, it is frequently difficult to interpret outcome studies in childhood "schizophrenics." Nonetheless, Bender's data seem to substantiate a genetic contribution for childhood schizophrenia.

PHARMACOLOGICAL TREATMENT

As with infantile autism, primary treatment of childhood schizophrenia is aimed at remediation of the cognitive defects in specialized schools, using behavioral therapy techniques. Drug treatment is adjunctive and is intended to provide sufficient behavioral control to optimize the educational environment. However, in this instance, the use of antipsychotics is more specifically aimed at alleviating target symptoms. Psychotherapy also plays a somewhat more important role in the treatment of childhood schizophrenia than in the treatment of infantile autism.

The antipsychotic agents used for behavioral management of infantile autism are also the drugs of choice in the treatment of childhood schizophrenia. Indeed, most reviews of pediatric psychopharmacology discuss treatment of "childhood psychoses," rather than the more specific subcategories. The same considerations discussed earlier apply here in the selection of appropriate medications: use of the high-potency antipsychotics is attendant with better symptom control and a higher incidence of side effects. Here again, thiothixene appears to be a valuable therapeutic tool, particularly where withdrawal, apathy, and anergy are salient features. Haloperidol and fluphenazine are as effective as thiothixene, have a higher incidence of extrapyramidal reactions, and in general are similar to each other in therapeutic efficacy.

REFERENCES

1. Group for the Advancement of Psychiatry. *Psychopathological Disorders in Childhood: Theoretical Considerations and a Proposed Classification.* New York: Group for the Advancement of Psychiatry, 1966.
2. Kanner, L. Autistic disturbances of affective contact. *Nerv. Child 2:* 217–250, 1943.
3. Rutter, M. and Bartak, L. Causes of infantile autism: some considerations from recent research. *J. Autism Child Schizophrenia 1:*20–32, 1971.
4. Rutter, M. Childhood schizophrenia reconsidered. *J. Autism Child Schizophrenia 2:*315–337, 1972.
5. Campbell, M. Biological interventions in psychoses of childhood. *J. Autism Child Schizophrenia 3:*347–373, 1973.
6. Wing, J. K. Diagnosis, epidemiology, etiology. *In: Early Childhood Autism.* J. K. Wing, ed., New York: Pergamon Press, 1966.
7. Bender, L. Alpha and omega of childhood schizophrenia. *J. Autism Child Schizophrenia 1:*115–118, 1971.
8. Potter, H. W. Schizophrenia in children. *Am. J. Psychiatry 12:*1253–1270, 1933.
9. Bender, L. Childhood schizophrenia. *Nerv. Child 1:*138–140, 1942.
10. Creak, M. Schizophrenic syndrome in childhood. Progress report of a working party. *Cerebral Palsy Bull. 3:*501–504, 1961.
11. Ornitz, E. M. and Ritvo, E. R. The syndrome of autism: a critical review. *Am. J. Psychiatry 133:*609–626, 1976.
12. Bender, L. Schizophrenic spectrum disorders in the families of schizophrenic children. *In: Genetic Research in Psychiatry.* R. R. Fieve, D. Rosenthal, and H. Brill, *eds.,* Baltimore: Johns Hopkins University Press, 1975, pp. 125–134.

447

28 | Psychopharmacological Treatment of the Aged

GEORGE GULEVICH

INTRODUCTION

Current trends indicate that physicians in general and psychiatrists in particular will be increasingly involved in providing health care for the aging patient. America's elderly population has almost doubled in the last twenty-five years; by the early part of the next century, it will nearly double again. Presently, there are 22.4 million persons who are at least sixty-five years old, accounting for 10.5 percent of the population (1,2). Despite the fact that this group is the fastest-growing segment of the population, the aged often have been at the fringes of the health care system. However, the elderly should be of particular interest to psychiatrists, since the incidence of psychopathology rises with age. Depressions and paranoid states increase steadily with each decade, as do organic brain diseases after the age of sixty. Suicide also increases with age. Most clinicians are well aware that the rate of suicide is highest in elderly white men and that 25 percent of all known suicides involve people over sixty-five years of age (1,3). Thus, knowledge of the use psychopharmacological agents in treating the elderly should be of considerable importance.

This chapter briefly describes general principles of drug use in elderly patients. In addition, it discusses the five major classes of psychotropic drugs which are commonly used to treat geriatric patients. Since antipsychotics, antidepressants, lithium, and antianxiety agents and sleep medications are also commonly used to treat psychiatric disturbances in other age groups, more comprehensive discussions on the use of these agents are presented elsewhere in this volume. Another pharmacological class, which is used to treat the cognitive deficits of geriatric patients, is described in more detail.

GENERAL PRINCIPLES

With increasing age, humans undergo physiological changes which have important metabolic consequences upon the absorption, excretion, and activity of psychoactive drugs. In general, drugs tend to remain in the body longer and to have more prolonged biological activity, so that the clinical and toxic effects may be more pronounced. In older patients, one can anticipate a decrease in cardiac output and an increase in circulation time. In addition, renal blood flow, glomerular filtration rate, and tubular secretion are diminished. These factors tend to extend the biological activity of any given drug. In older people, the ratio of fat to parenchymal tissue is also increased. Thus, lipid-soluble compounds, including many of the psychoactive drugs, tend to accumulate in the fatty tissues. Many drugs are bound to protein in the plasma. Since plasma protein decreases with age, the amount of drug bound to the plasma protein fraction may be reduced proportionately (3). Furthermore, the ability of the liver to metabolize drugs decreases with advancing age. The decreased cerebral blood flow that often accompanies the aging process, along with changes in neurons in the brain and other biochemical changes which are only beginning to be studied, may produce increased sensitivity of the brain to the pharmacological actions of drugs. It is generally assumed that the homeostatic mechanisms of the component organs and of the system as a whole decrease with age. Consequently, the threshold for toxic side effects may be proportionately lowered (3,4).

As a result of the factors just described, psychotropic drugs should usually be prescribed at lower dosages for elderly patients. As a general rule, starting dosages for most drugs should be 33–50 percent of those for younger adult patients. Increases in dosages should be gradual. It is common practice with many psychotropic drugs to provide the entire dosage at bedtime. This generally provides maximum benefit from sedative effects and, for many patients, is more convenient. However, this practice should not be used routinely with aged patients, since they may be less able to tolerate the sudden absorption of a relatively large drug dose into their circulation. On the other hand, absorption of drugs from the gastrointestinal tract may be diminished in some aged persons. Poor absorption may result from reduced gastric acid output, reduced abdominal blood flow, and impairment of systems responsible for transport across gastrointestinal membranes. For this reason, if an elderly patient fails to respond to a tablet or capsule form of a psychotropic medication, liquid or parenteral forms should be tried. Because of the possibility of increased toxicity, these latter forms of medication should also be administered in decreased doses.

Prior to instituting active psychopharmacological therapy with the aged patient, the physician should conduct a thorough psychiatric evaluation and a complete medical examination. Assessment of blood pressure, both erect and supine, complete blood count, total protein evaluation, urinalysis, and electrocardiogram (ECG) will help the clinician to determine the possible presence of concomitant medical problems which may complicate treatment with psychotropic agents. It is also essential to determine current drug use. Multiple physical illnesses being treated with multiple drugs markedly increase the risk of toxic drug interactions. Side effects of these interactions in aging patients may be difficult to differentiate from organic brain syndromes, neurological disorders, and a variety of other conditions.

Most clinicians believe that it is wise to avoid polypharmacy. The simultaneous use of multiple drugs clouds clinical signs and obscures the therapeutic effect of a drug and its side effects. Aged patients often have several chronic conditions simultaneously and, therefore, over-medication is particularly common. Hospitalization may be necessary to discontinue unnecessary drugs, to evaluate the patient's physical and psychological baseline on a drug-free regimen, and to determine what medications are required.

In addition to evaluating current drug usage for possible concomitant medical problems, the clinician should be aware of the overall metabolic state of the aging patient. It is not unusual for even mild disturbances in electrolyte balance to act as a precipitant for psychiatric symptoms in the elderly. In addition, states of mild toxemia and fever, along with deficiencies in protein and carbohydrate metabolism, can act as precipitants of psychiatric symptoms. A thorough physical evaluation, along with a review of the patient's present and past medical history, followed by appropriate laboratory tests, will help to identify any of these possible situations as aggravating or precipitating factors in the development of psychiatric symptomatology.

When patients are maintained on psychotropic drugs, dosage and clinical progress should be reviewed regularly, as should the possible development of insidious and progressive side effects. Follow-up evaluation should include examination of pulse, blood pressure, complete blood counts, and neurological status. Family members are often helpful in assessing the progress that a patient may be making or in alerting the physician to the development of side effects. Thus, it is a good practice to inform both the patient and the relatives of drug dosage and potential side effects (3–5).

ANTIPSYCHOTIC DRUGS

Psychosis is a common problem in the aged. Psychotic behavior may result from schizophrenic, organic, or affective disorders. Most schizophrenic and psychotic processes begin during the patient's early adulthood and persist into old age. Psychoses may also result from arteriosclerotic disease or other organic disorders. In addition, elderly patients may develop "late paraphrenia," characterized by agitation, paranoid delusions, thought disorders, auditory hallucinations, grandiosity, and absence of organic dementia or sustained confusion (3,5,6). In general, the drug treatment of psychoses in elderly patients follows the same rules which apply to treatment of younger patients (Chapter 9). Antipsychotic drugs are effective in treating continuing schizophrenic psychoses, organic psychoses, and the paraphrenias of late life.

Low-potency antipsychotics, such as chlorpromazine (Thorazine) and thioridazine (Mellarill) have marked sedative and hypotensive effects. The sedative side effects may be useful for quieting an agitated patient and increasing nighttime sedation. However, this side effect can be undesirable if it keeps the patient asleep during the day and out of contact with therapeutic activities. Moreover, the hypotensive side effects of the drugs may predispose to acute cerebrovascular catastrophes in the aged patient. Here, as in children, diphenhydramine (Benadryl) may be a useful sedating agent (Chapter 27). High-potency antipsychotics, such as fluphenazine (Prolixin) and haloperidol (Haldol) produce less sedation than do the low-potency agents; however, they are more likely to produce extrapyramidal reactions, which are often poorly tolerated by the geriatric patient. Mesoridazine (Serentil) is sometimes a useful agent in the elderly because it has marked sedative action but is about twice as potent as chlorpromazine.

Selection of the appropriate antipsychotic from among the dozens available is often empirical. One should delineate those psychotic target symptoms to be treated and those side effects to be avoided. For example, haloperidol may be the drug of choice in treating psychotic symptoms of elderly patients in whom low blood pressures may be a significant problem. The dosage of antipsychotics for a geriatric patient should be 30–50 percent of the usual adult dose. Thus, if one were using chlorpromazine, the usual geriatric dosage would be 50–300 mg daily. If haloperidol were the drug of choice, the dosage would be approximately 1–8 mg daily. Current evidence suggests that most elderly psychotic patients do not benefit more from massive doses than they would from normal doses of antipsychotic medication.

The side effects of antipsychotic medications are detailed in Chapter 9. They are of particular importance in the elderly patient (3–5,7). This is especially true of certain cardiovascular and neurological side effects. Serious orthostatic hypotension may manifest itself as progressive confusion or as transient ischemic attacks. Postural hypotension may last for several weeks and may require bedrest to prevent stresses to the cardiovascular system. In the elderly, severe attacks of hypotension can expose the patient to cardiovascular or cerebral vascular insufficiency and may aggravate the symptoms of basilar artery insufficiency. However, one of the more serious consequences of hypotensive episodes may be fainting, leading to falls which can cause fractures of the extremities. Blood pressures, taken with the patient in supine and standing positions, often give the clinician an indication of the possible hypotensive effects that the patient may experience throughout the day. The patient should be warned about these possible effects, particularly about the increased danger of fainting. Epinephrine should not be used to counteract drug-induced hypotension, since it has been shown to create paradoxical lowerings of the blood pressure in some patients.

The antipsychotics can also cause tachycardia and arrhythmias (Chapter 9). Along with these side effects, ECG changes may occur, including prolongation of the QT interval, lowering and inversion of the T wave, and appearance of a biscupid T wave or a U wave. A pretreatment ECG, repeated measurements of the patient's heart rate and rhythm, and frequent ECG recordings and cardiac enzyme determinations may all be necessary in monitoring a patient who experiences these side effects and who requires a continued use of antipsychotic medication. Thioridazine is the antipsychotic most often associated with ECG abnormalities.

Geriatric patients appear to be more susceptible to some of the neurological side effects of psychotropic drugs than are younger adults (4). Extrapyramidal symptoms are the most common neurological side effects of antipsychotic medications (Chapter 9). The occurrence of dystonias, or muscle spasms, appears to diminish with increasing age; the occurrence of akathisia, or restlessness, is most frequent between the ages of forty and fifty; and the occurrence of the akinetic parkinsonian side effects increases with age. As described in Chapter 9, extrapyramidal side effects generally respond to antiparkinsonian drugs. However, these medications should not be used routinely. Not all patients develop extrapyramidal side effects during their course of treatment, and antiparkinsonian drugs have anticholinergic effects which may contribute to the risks of polypharmacy and drug toxicity. It is important to differentiate akathisia from anxiety states and agitated depressions, which occur frequently in the elderly, since the appropriate treatment for these latter states would be considerably different.

One of the most serious neurological side effects of antipsychotics is tardive dyskinesia. This syndrome is most commonly characterized by involuntary buccal, lingual, and masticatory movements (Chapter 9). Typically, tardive dyskinesia occurs in some patients who have received large amounts of medication for more than six months; and in general it is seen more frequently in elderly females than in males. At present, there is no specific treatment for this syndrome. The physician can reduce the possible development of tardive dyskinesia by minimizing the unnecessary use of antipsychotic medication (4,7).

In addition to their increased susceptibility to cardiac and some neurological side effects of antipsychotics, elderly patients also evidence increased incidence and severity of other central nervous system complications of these drugs, such as depression, paradoxical agitation, delirium, confusion, hallucinations, assaultiveness, and delusions. Many of these paradoxical effects may be due to the anticholinergic activity of these agents.

Many antipsychotics are also potent anticholinergics. Anticholinergic activity is manifested by symptoms such as dry mouth, loss of ocular accommodation, constipation, hypotension, vertigo, sweating, urinary retention, atonic bladder, and increased intraocular pressure. Since anticholinergic effects are additive, the concomitant use of antiparkinsonian agents with antipsychotics can be hazardous. It is not unusual for patients receiving antipsychotics and antiparkinsonian drugs to develop the so-called central anticholinergic syndrome. This syndrome is characterized by marked disturbance of short-term memory, impaired attention, disorientation, anxiety, visual and auditory hallucinations, and increased psychotic thinking (Chapter 24). In a patient who is already being treated for psychosis, the development of the central anticholinergic syndrome may not be recognized. Thus, the physician may increase the psychotropic medication and the psychotic symptoms. Clinicians may avoid this problem by remaining alert for signs of peripheral anticholinergic toxicity. The antiparkinsonian drugs are probably the most frequent cause of this central anticholinergic syndrome. The reduction of the dosage of the antipsychotic medication being used and the discontinuation of the antiparkinsonian drug will generally produce amelioration of this syndrome. For cases in which the diagnosis remains uncertain or the rapid alleviation of the anticholinergic symptoms is desirable, the use of physostigmine salicylate (Antilirium) has been advocated. The use of physostigmine in such patients is detailed in Chapter 24. In the geriatric patient, physostigmine should only be used for severe anticholinergic toxicity, because of possible cholinergic side effects such as bradycardia.

All allergic reactions to antipsychotics occur with greater frequency in the geriatric population than in young adults. It has been estimated that 70 percent of all cases of agranulocytosis from antipsychotics occur in patients between the ages of forty-eight and seventy and are largely attributable to the phenothiazines. Cholestatic jaundice has been reported in 4 percent of elderly patients who are receiving phenothiazine therapy. In addition, the incidence of sunlight-aggravated, drug-induced dermatitis and photosensitivity is especially high in the geriatric patient.

ANTIDEPRESSANT DRUGS

The most common psychiatric disorders of old age are affective disorders, especially depressions. Depression in the elderly may represent a recurrence of depressive patterns having occurred earlier in life. Alternatively, it may represent the initial depressive episode in the patient's life. It is not unusual to find classical depression in patients seventy to eighty years of age. In addition to using antidepressant medications, the experienced clinician must be skilled in helping the geriatric patient deal with a variety of psychosocial factors that are responsible for precipitating or aggravating depressive symptomatology (3,5,6). More than any other stage of life, old age is a period of repeated losses. As people grow older, they generally experience a decline in physical vigor and stamina, a gradual decline in mental agility, job retirement with a decrement in personal income, increasing social isolation as friends and loved ones die, and the almost absolute necessity to deal with one's mortality. While this picture may seem gloomy and foreboding, aged people suffering from depression can be markedly responsive to appropriate care and treatment.

The presence of any severe depression in the aged may be an indication for use of antidepressant drug therapy. The symptoms of severe depression in the elderly include withdrawal and isolation, early-morning insomnia, severe anorexia and weight loss, fatigue, constipation, psychomotor retardation or agitation, somatic delusions, and suicidal ideation or behavior. As mentioned previously, the depressed elderly white male is an especially high suicidal risk. Depressed elderly patients occasionally present a clinical picture of pseudodementia or pseudosenility, masking the underlying depression (3,6). Such patients are often severely perplexed, disoriented, confused, and hostile. Patients with pseudosenile depression frequently display a recent and abrupt onset of defects of memory, defects in judgment, and depressive symptomatology. In such patients, negativism is common. In contrast, confabulation is more typical of the true organic brain syndrome.

The most important group of drugs for the treatment of depression in both the elderly and the young adult patient are the tricyclic antidepressants (tricyclics). The use of these drugs is detailed in Chapter 11. It is important to remember that, like the phenothiazines, the tricyclics have anticholinergic activity.

For elderly patients, tricyclics are initiated at lower doses than are used for younger adults; and the increments in dosage are smaller and made at a slower rate. For example, with a geriatric depressed patient, imipramine (Tofranil) treatment would begin with approximately 50 mg per day in divided doses. This dose could be increased by 25–50 mg per week with an outpatient, possibly faster if the patient were hospitalized and under close supervision. The eventual therapeutic dose range in the geriatric patient is 75–150 mg per day. Like all general guidelines, there are exceptions that are encountered in clinical practice. Some elderly patients may require and tolerate doses of 250 mg. But, patients given these high doses should be hospitalized. The dosage level for outpatient maintenance is about 50–65 percent of that used in the hospital setting. Many clinicians use the sedative effects of amitriptyline (Elavil) for patients in whom agitation, restlessness, and anxiety are prominent. Conversely, less sedating tricyclics, like protriptyline (Vivactil) and nortriptyline (Aventyl), may be useful in treating the apathetic, depressed individual. The single dose of tricyclic medication at bedtime, which is often used for younger patients, should be avoided in the elderly because of excessive morning sedation.

If there is no amelioration of target symptoms by the end of three weeks with appropriate levels of tricyclics, other treatment should be considered, including the possibility of monoamine oxidase (MAO) inhibitors (Chapter 11) or electroconvulsive therapy (ECT) (Chapter 33). MAO inhibitors should be used with great caution in the elderly because of increased potential for side effects.

When a patient responds, drug therapy is generally continued on a maintenance basis for at least several months. It may then be gradually reduced, as the patient's mental status is carefully monitored. During treatment, the patient is followed closely to provide continuous assessment of therapeutic results of the presence of severe side effects, and of the need for appropriate psychotherapy. In the follow-up, the danger of suicide should always be kept in mind, particularly when the patient seems suddenly to get better. An abrupt decrease in depressive symptomatology may indicate that the patient has decided to commit suicide. Overdosage of tricyclics is a serious clinical situation, often producing coma, clonic movements or seizures, respiratory depression, hyperpyrexia, and disturbances of cardiac rhythm (Chapter 11).

The important side effects of tricyclics have been reviewed in Chapter 11. Several of them are particularly important in the elderly (3,4, 7–9). Tricyclics cause more side effects at lower doses in older patients than in younger ones. The development of mild hypomanic excitement can occur in patients being treated with tricyclics, even in the absence of a previous history of hypomania or schizophrenia. In addition, tricyclics can exacerbate schizophrenic symptomatology and mania. The use of modest doses of antipsychotics and a reduction in the dosage of the tricyclic will usually ameliorate these conditions.

Since tricyclics have anticholinergic activity, they can cause side effects similar to those already described for the antipsychotics. Cardiovascular side effects that are of concern include the development of ECG and myocardial changes and both increases and decreases in blood pressure. A pretreatment ECG will assist in assessing the degree of severity of any cardiovascular side effects. Hypotensive episodes can be treated with reduction in medication, bedrest, and general supportive measures. The seriousness of hypotensive episodes in the elderly patient has been emphasized in the previous section on antipsychotics. Paradoxically, tricyclics can also induce increased blood pressure, particularly in the hypertensive patient. Since many elderly patients suffer from high blood pressure, it is important to keep this consideration in mind. It is also important to note that the tricyclics can block the antihypertensive effects of guanethidine (Ismelin). Doxepin (Sinequan) may produce less blockade than do other tricyclics. When cardiovascular side effects become apparent, tricyclic dosage should be reduced or these medications should be discontinued.

Stimulant drugs, such as the amphetamines or methylphenidate (Ritalin) probably have no role in the treatment of depression in the elderly (3,4,7). Antipsychotics can be used to treat severely agitated depressed patients. Antianxiety drugs have been used to reduce mild or moderate depression associated with anxiety, as well as in combination with tricyclics to attenuate the anxiety component of some more severe depressions in the elderly. These drug combinations should be used with caution and only when clearly indicated, to avoid the dangers of polypharmacy.

ANTIMANIC DRUGS

Even though the depressive psychoses predominate among the affective disorders in late life, manic psychoses do occur in old age (3,5,6). Elderly patients can present either with recurrent manic episodes or with recurrent manic-depressive episodes. While the onset of this disorder generally occurs in younger patients, rare instances have been reported of individuals having their first manic episode after the age of sixty. The symptomatology of manic conditions, including grandiosity, hyperactivity, lack of judgment, and inappropriate behavior, can cause serious disruption for the patient and his family. Until the introduction of lithium carbonate for the treatment of mania, the prognosis for mania in old age was generally quite poor. Often, continued institutionalization was necessary. The two main classes of drugs that are available for the treatment of the acute manic episode are the antipsychotics and lithium carbonate (Chapter 12).

Doses required to achieve a given blood level of lithium may be lowered in elderly patients. Elderly patients can also develop side effects with lower blood concentrations. The half-life of lithium in the middle-aged adult is approximately twenty-four hours. In the aged, the half-life of lithium is thirty-six to forty-eight hours. Thus, in treating the elderly manic patient, physicians should start with lower doses of lithium and should carefully monitor blood lithium concentrations. For example, lithium may be started at 300 mg daily, and serum lithium levels can be obtained three times a week. Increases in lithium dosage should be very gradual. In an elderly patient, one might only need 600–900 mg of lithium per day to achieve an effective blood level of 0.8–1.5 mEg per liter (4,7).

Aged patients are more susceptible to all of the side effects that are produced by lithium, including the gastrointestinal side effects, central nervous system side effects, and neuromuscular toxicity (7). The mild side effects of lithium in the elderly are the same as in the younger adults and include anorexia, nausea, vomiting, diarrhea, and fine tremors. The serious side effects of lithium toxicity include polydipsia and polyuria, ataxia, speech disturbance (dysarthria), hyperreflexia, confusion, and coma. Unsupervised use of lithium, along with improper dietary habits and lack of proper salt and potassium intake, can result in severe electrolyte imbalance. Patients with cardiac or renal disease should be monitored especially closely during lithium therapy, since malfunctions in these organ systems can dramatically increase lithium blood levels, leading to severe toxic states. The major sign of lithium toxicity is increasing confusion. Thus, lithium toxicity is another possible cause of pseudosenility. Family members or community facilities caring for patients on lithium therapy may attribute the increasing confusion to the senile state and delay treatment for the patient. For this reason, if confusion develops in an elderly patient on lithium, the patient should be evaluated for lithium toxicity.

ANTIANXIETY AGENTS AND SLEEP MEDICATIONS

Anxiety is common in the elderly (3,5,8). It is often associated with many of the real threats and losses which they experience. The development of hypochondriasis, also a common symptom of the aged, increases the sense of threat and anxiety. Chronic anxiety also commonly contributes to depression, insomnia, and other behavioral reactions. While the use of antianxiety drugs will play a role in the treatment of anxiety in the elderly, it is often not the primary treatment modality. Psychotherapy, family counseling, appropriate medical consultation, and environmental manipulation are all important in the management of the anxious elderly patient. Whenever possible, anxiety should be treated promptly. Persistent anxiety can have a marked alienating effect on others in the old person's environment. Chronic anxiety, with its concomitant irritability, tends to evoke negative or rejecting reactions from those persons around the aged individual, often increasing his sense of isolation and estrangement. Neurotic disturbances, including anxiety, depression, and obsessive-compulsive behavior, typically arise at a younger age, although they can occur as new symptoms for the geriatric patient.

Benzodiazepines, propanediols, diphenylmethanes, and barbiturates are used to treat anxiety and tension in the aged (3,4,8,10,11). The benzodiazepines have proven to be effective and safe in treating anxiety in the elderly. For this reason, they have largely replaced other drugs which were used earlier, such as meprobamate (Miltown) and phenobarbital. Many of the physical symptoms associated with anxiety, such as headaches, gastrointestinal distress, and fatigue, respond well to the benzodiazepines. Chlordiazepoxide (Librium), diazepam (Valium), and oxazepam (Serax) are similar in their sedative and muscle relaxant properties. They differ somewhat with regard to dosage and duration of action. Oxazepam is the shortest acting of these drugs. The usual initial geriatric dose of chlordiazepoxide is 5–10 mg three times per day; a high dose would be 20 mg four times per day.

The propanediols include meprobamate (Miltown) and tybamate (Solacen). Generally, these drugs are somewhat less effective than the benzodiazepines. In the elderly, the dosage of meprobamate ranges from 200 mg three times per day to a maximum of 800 mg four times per day. Tybamate is used in an initial dose of about 250 mg three times per day; the maximum dose is about 350 mg four times per day. One advantage to using meprobamate in older people is that it does not cause muscular instability which may occur with the benzodiazepines.

The diphenylmethane antianxiety agents include diphenhydramine (Benadryl) and hydroxyzine (Vistaril). Diphenhydramine is a widely used antihistaminic drug which has sedative qualities. It is frequently used in the elderly patient to induce sleep, because it has minimal side effects and no addiction potential. However, its value for treating anxiety is quite limited. Diphenhydramine can often be successfully used to treat the extrapyramidal symptom of akathisia produced by antipsychotic medication without increasing the overall anticholinergic effect that the patient will experience. Hyroxyzine may also be classi- fied with the antihistaminics and has primarily sedative qualities. The usual starting dose is 25 mg three times per day, ranging up to about 100 mg four times per day. It is relatively safe, with a low incidence of side effects.

For decades the use of low doses of barbiturates, primarily pheno- barbital, for the treatment of anxiety has been rather commonplace. However, with the introduction of the newer antianxiety agents, bar- biturates have been used much less frequently for this purpose. There is evidence that the barbiturates should not be used with elderly pa- tients, since they often produce delirium in this group (3,7,10).

Some phenothiazines, especially thioridiazine, have been used in small doses for anxiety and tension. Prescribed this way, they often effectively control anxiety and tension; but they have the disadvantage of lowering blood pressure to a much greater degree than do the benzodiazepines. Their sedative effects are usually more prominent than are those of the benzodiazepines. In addition, the danger of tardive dyskinesia should be kept in mind.

Of the antianxiety agents mentioned, the benzodiazepines appear to be the safest (Chapter 13). They are less commonly implicated in fatal overdoses than are the barbiturates and meprobamate. Confusional states and paradoxical agitation following barbiturate use are well known in the elderly; they are much less common with the benzodiaze- pines. Meprobamate, barbiturates, and benzodiazepines all produce ad- diction and habituation, especially when they are taken in large doses for a long period of time (Chapter 23). Meprobamate and the barbiturates have a high addiction potential, and withdrawal seizures are not unusual, following abrupt termination of these drugs. The benzodiazepines can also produce withdrawal reactions. However, the risk of addiction and withdrawal seizures is less with the benzodiazepines than with meprobamate or barbiturates.

The usual side effects of antianxiety drugs include drowsiness and unsteadiness of gait at the lower dose levels of these drugs, with ataxia, nystagmus, and incoordination at larger, chronic doses. Very high doses of these drugs can produce severe unsteadiness of gait, drowsiness, orthostatic hypotension, and coma. The possibility of falls, with resultant fractures, must be considered in any patient who is receiving the larger doses of antianxiety agents which might produce ataxia and incoordination. These side effects are generally not as severe or as common as are those for the antipsychotics and tricyclics (3,4,10).

Many people taking antianxiety agents also use other drugs which have sedative effects. A particularly dangerous combination is alcohol and antianxiety agents such as the barbiturates and the benzodiazepines. Acutely, alcohol can potentiate the effect of antianxiety agents. However, the chronic alcoholic may require higher doses of these drugs, because of cross tolerance.

One of the most frequent complaints of the elderly is that of insomnia (3–5). Insomnia may be attributed to daytime napping, anxiety about the future, or physical distress. The elderly generally have less total sleep time than do normal young adults. The percentage of rapid-eye-movement (REM) sleep is slightly less in the elderly, but Stage IV sleep tends to be considerably less and is sometimes absent (cf. Chapter 14). Older people have a longer sleep latency and, once asleep, tend to awaken more readily. In the clinical conditions of anxiety, depression, and psychosis, sleep disturbances are often the first to appear and the last to disappear. In addition to their high frequency, sleep disorders present complex problems in management (Chapter 14). Chronic usage of drugs to treat insomnia may complicate the problem by producing drug-dependent insomnia. In the treatment of the elderly patient with a sleeping disorder, hypnotics should be used judiciously, as should all psychoactive drugs. The most appropriate indication for medication is for the short-term treatment of situational insomnia which is not associated with depression, psychosis, or pain from physical distress. If these latter conditions are producing insomnia, they should be treated specifically.

Many agents have been used for the treatment of insomnia and other sleep disorders (3,4,10,11). The barbiturates, long a traditional favorite for the treatment of insomnia, have the undesired side effect of occasionally producing delirium in the aged patient. Because of this untoward effect and because of the possibility of respiratory depression, the barbiturates are inappropriate for the treatment of insomnia in the elderly. Recently, the benzodiazepines, particularly flurazepam (Dalmane), have been widely used for the treatment of insomnia. Of the more commonly used sleep medications, flurazepam is suggested to produce the least suppression of REM sleep. A drug with a long tradition of use as a hypnotic is chloral hydrate. It is generally conceded to be relatively safe, does not significantly suppress REM sleep, leaves little hangover or ataxia, and has less risk of habituation than the barbiturates. Other sedative-hypnotic drugs commonly used in the treatment of insomnia include methyprylon (Noludar), glutethimide (Doriden), ethchlorvynol (Placidyl), and methaqualone (Quaalude). None of these drugs has any significant features to make it more desirable than the benzodiazepines.

One of the most usual undesired consequences of nighttime sedation occurs when old people awaken at night in a state of fearfulness or in order to use the bathroom. Confusion and unsteadiness of gait can be produced by any of the sedative hypnotics. Falls resulting from this can further complicate the medical picture of the elderly patient. The use of side rails for the bed, subdued lighting to help the patient become oriented to his surroundings, and minimal drug dosages for nighttime sedation will reduce the possibility of confusion, unsteadiness, and subsequent falls as a hazard for the elderly patient.

DRUGS AFFECTING COGNITIVE FUNCTION IN THE ELDERLY

Deteriorating intellectual function, brought about by degenerative neuronal disease, cerebral atherosclerosis, or systemic illness occurs with increased frequency in the geriatric population. The patient with senile organic brain syndrome is a common visitor to psychiatric emergency rooms. These patients typically present with signs of memory loss, intellectual deterioration, confusion, disorientation, and, less frequently, agitation. Often, they are brought in as "emergencies" because they are management problems at the custodial facilities in which they reside or because their families can no longer provide an appropriate level of care. The acute pharmacological management of such patients has been covered earlier in this chapter. In this section, the use of the "cognitive-acting" drugs will be described. Such agents have become increasingly popular in recent years; their use has been the result of an active search for agents which will reverse or retard the intellectual deterioration and behavioral regression seen in elderly patients with organic brain syndromes (12).

STIMULANT DRUGS

There is some evidence that stimulant drugs such as amphetamines, methylphenidate (Ritalin), and pemoline (Cylert) are useful in counteracting lethargy and withdrawal in elderly patients. These drugs have also been reported to increase activity level, enhance alertness, and promote memory recall. While promising, such findings have not yet been verified in carefully controlled clinical trials.

Analeptic agents, such as pentylenetetrazol (Metrazol) are sometimes used in elderly patients, although reports of their effectiveness have not been well documented. In certain patients, a clear and dramatic improvement is seen, suggesting that the use of pentylenetetrazol should be considered in selected cases. Like other drugs of this class, its use is contraindicated in patients with seizure disorders.

VASODILATORS AND ANTICOAGULANTS

Both vasodilators and anticoagulants have been investigated as a means of making more oxygen available to the brain, by direct action on blood vessels to increase blood flow and reduction of hemostagnation and thrombus formation, respectively. No clear-cut evidence of efficacy exists with either class of agents. Nor has it been proven that a substantial increase in the oxygenation of the blood, brought about by hyperbaric oxygenation, is associated with a reversal of cognitive deterioration. Of the vasodilators, papaverine (Pavabid) has been shown to improve cerebral blood flow without an attendant improvement in cognitive function. Cyclandelate (Cyclospasmol), another such drug, has been suggested to increase long-term memory and cognitive function in mildly impaired patients. There appears to be no clearly demonstrable benefit from the use of anticoagulants, such as bishydroxycoumarin (Dicumarol) in geriatric patients without a clear medical indication for anticoagulation. The potential hazards of using anticoagulants in this age group probably outweigh their alleged benefits in patients with cognitive deficits.

Ergot Alkaloids

A mixture of ergot alkaloids (Hydergine) has been used to increase cerebral blood flow by direct ganglionic action. In some studies, administration of this combination has been associated with improvements in social abilities and general activity, but it has not produced any improvement in cognitive function. The most beneficial outcomes of the use of this ergot alkaloid combination has been observed in patients who have marked motor retardation, apathy, withdrawal, insomnia, and dysphoric affect. Since these symptoms can be associated with depression, it is possible that the treatment may be acting as an antidepressant in these patients. The ergot alkaloids inhibit norepinephrine reuptake *in vitro*—an action compatible with an antidepressant effect (Chapter 8).

Other Drugs

A variety of drugs have been tested in elderly patients. With few exceptions, none has been shown conclusively to be effective. Of the more promising leads under current investigation, propranolol (Inderal), procaine amide, and a combination of B-complex and C vitamins hold some interest. The long-term beneficial effects of these agents remain to be established, as do the mechanisms by which they are acting (12).

REFERENCES

1. Pfeiffer, E.   Interacting with older patients. *In: Mental Illness in Later Life.* E. W. Busse and E. Pfeiffer, *eds.,* Washington, D.C.: American Psychiatric Association, 1973, pp. 5–17.
2. Butler, R. N.   Psychiatry and the elderly: an overview. *Am. J. Psychiatry 132:*893–900, 1975.
3. Verwoerdt, A.   *Clinical Geropsychiatry.* Baltimore: Williams & Wilkins, 1976.
4. Saltzman, C., vander Kolk, B., and Shader, R. I.   Psychopharmacology and the geriatric patient. *In: Manual of Psychiatric Therapeutics.* R. I. Shader, *ed.,* Boston: Little, Brown, 1975, pp. 171–185.
5. Weinberg, J.   Geriatric psychiatry. *In: Comprehensive Textbook of Psychiatry II.* A. M. Freedman, H. I. Kaplan, and B. J. Saddock, *eds.,* Baltimore: Williams & Wilkins, 1975, pp. 2405–2421.
6. Pfeiffer, E. and Busse, E. W.   Mental disorders in later life—affective disorders; paranoid, neurotic, and situational reactions. *In: Mental Illness in Later Life.* E. W. Busse and E. Pfeiffer, *eds.,* Washington, D.C.: American Psychiatric Association, 1973, pp. 107–144.
7. Davis, J. M., Fann, W. E., El-Yousef, M. K., and Janowsky, D. S.   Clinical problems in treating the aged with psychotropic drugs. *Adv. Behav. Biol. 6:*111–125, 1973.
8. Klein, D. F. and Davis, J. M.   *Diagnosis and Drug Treatment of Psychiatric Disorders.* Baltimore: Williams & Wilkins, 1969.
9. Prange, A. J.   Use of antidepressant drugs in the elderly patient. *Adv. Behav. Biol. 6:*225–237, 1973.
10. Gershon, S.   Antianxiety agents. *Adv. Behav. Biol. 6:*183–187, 1973.
11. Lifshitz, K. and Kline, N. S.   Psychopharmacology in geriatrics. *In: Principles of Psychopharmacology.* W. G. Clark and J. del Guidice, *eds.,* New York: Academic Press, 1970, pp. 695–705.
12. Raskind, M. and Eisdorfer, C.   Psychopharmacology of the aged. *In: Drug Treatment of Mental Disorders.* L. L. Simpson, *ed.,* New York: Raven Press, 1976, pp. 237–266.

V | Special Topics in Psychopharmacology

Psychopharmacology interacts both with other areas of psychiatry and with medicine. Part V examines some of the broader issues arising from this interaction. Chapter 29, for example, reviews a variety of drugs which are given for nonpsychiatric purposes but which have powerful effects on the psychological well-being of the patient. Not infrequently, these effects go unrecognized, so that they pose problems for physicians in all areas of medicine. Such psychiatric side effects are also of theoretical interest, since by uncovering the underlying mechanisms we may expand our understanding of the actions of drugs on the brain.

Drug administration per se has psychological effects which are essentially independent of their pharmacological actions and which have a strong impact on the relationship between the psychiatrist and the patient. Chapters 30 and 31 examine these issues. Since psychopharmacological agents are only one aspect of the practice of psychiatry, it is essential to consider ways in which their use affects other elements of clinical practice. One key feature of this broad issue is the placebo effect. Both chapters emphasize that medicines represent far more than many physicians believe, and they attempt to bridge what is too often a wide gap between psychotherapeutic and psychopharmacological considerations.

Two other chapters in this part are unusual for a psychopharmacology text. Chapter 32 deals with statistical methods in the field, concentrating upon approaches to the evaluation of clinical reports and research studies rather than upon specific statistical tests. Chapter 33 discusses convulsive and coma therapies. These treatments frequently involve the use of psychopharmacological agents; and some, such as electroconvulsive therapy (ECT), are still used as adjuncts to psychopharmacological treatments. With improved psychopharmacological and psychological therapies, convulsive and coma treatments now have a smaller role in psychiatry. For a limited number of patients, however, these therapeutic modalities continue to be not only helpful but even essential.

29 | Psychological Effects of Nonpsychiatric Drugs

KENNETH L. DAVIS

INTRODUCTION

A review of the literature on the psychological effects of nonpsychiatric drugs often reveals little more than a series of case reports in seldom-read journals. In attempting to determine the substance of such articles, one must consider the following problems. First, potentially any drug can have psychological side effects. The problem is to distinguish between idiosyncratic reactions and relatively common side effects. Second, most reports are uncontrolled, so that correlation need not imply causality. For example, side effects such as fatigue, drowsiness, and insomnia are often spontaneous occurrences, with no specific relationship to the drug. Third, psychological side effects may result as much from the illness of the patient as from an interaction with medication. Finally, diagnostic criteria are rarely explicit. Therefore, what one clinician defines as "delirium" may be "psychosis" to another investigator.

Despite these difficulties, information is available about important effects of nonpsychiatric drugs on brain function. This chapter considers only major drugs for which frequent reports of psychological complications are available. Wherever possible, the information is drawn from studies using matched control populations. Where appropriate, the possible relevance of underlying diseases is clearly noted. Finally, the same diagnostic criteria are used throughout the chapter (Table 29-1).

ANTICHOLINERGICS

Anticholinergic agents are present in a huge number of medications. They are major components of a variety of nonprescription remedies

Table 29-1.

Definitions Used to Evaluate Psychological Effects of Nonpsychiatric Drugs

---

Depression
   dysphoric mood for one month plus five of the following symptoms: poor appetite or a weight loss, sleep difficulty, loss of energy, agitation or retardation, decreased libido, guilt or self-reproach, poor concentration, suicidal thought.

Schizophrenia
   formal thought disorder and delusions or hallucinations

Delirium
   disorientation, memory impairment, disordered intellectual function, slowing of electroencephalogram (EEG), impaired judgment, labile and shallow affect, reversibility, nocturnal exacerbation, visual hallucinations.

---

for colds, insomnia, motion sickness, and other problems. They are also used in treating Parkinson's disease, asthma, and some gastrointestinal disturbances. As a result, patients can receive anticholinergic medications from a number of sources without realizing it. Prompt recognition of anticholinergic toxicity is of particular benefit in emergency room consultations. Prominent symptoms include blurred vision, warm and dry skin, foul breath and dry mouth, fever, and tachycardia. The diagnosis and treatment of this syndrome are described in Chapter 24.

ANTIHYPERTENSIVES

A comprehensive prospective study of patients with hypertension compared the incidence of psychiatric complications with methyldopa (Aldomet) and guanethidine (Ismelin) (1). Of patients receiving methyldopa, 75 percent complained of tiredness, 10 percent experienced mild depression, and 7 percent had severe depression. Complaints of tiredness were virtually absent among patients receiving guanethidine; and, while 20 percent of these patients reported mild depression, none noted severe depression. Thus, both tiredness and severe depression appear to be generally more troublesome with methyldopa than with guanethidine. This difference may reflect the ability of methyldopa to cross the blood brain barrier, which guanethidine cannot.

In early trials of reserpine (Serpasil) as an antihypertensive agent, a large number of patients were reported to develop depressive symptoms. Additional symptoms included delirium with visual hallucinations, organic brain syndrome, anxiety, and phobia. Today, there are far fewer reports of reserpine depression. This may represent a decreased enthusiasm about reporting a well-known complication; however, it may also reflect increased caution in giving the drug to patients who have a past history of depression and careful adherence to a usual maximum daily dose of 0.5 mg.

Most severe depressions which are associated with reserpine occur at doses over 0.5 mg per day and after two to eight months of drug treatment. The best predictor of depressive symptoms is a past history of depression. In a summary of several studies, dysphoria was found to occur in 20 percent of patients, while 7 percent had a severe depressive syndrome; however, 9 percent of the patient population had past histories of endogenous depression (2). Thus, in 75 percent of all cases of reserpine-induced depression, the major symptoms appear to be overtranquilization, with psychomotor retardation; at most, only 25 percent of such depressions are identical to severe depression (Table 29-1). In addition, reports comparing hypertensive patients taking reserpine to hypertensive patients not taking the drug suggest that the incidence of severe depression is virtually identical for the two groups. These reports indicate that a small group of hypertensives, probably between 3 and 10 percent, can develop a significant "endogenous" depression on reserpine. Generally, these patients will have had a past history of depression.

Guidelines for treatment of reserpine-induced depressions are complicated by the frequent absence of a clear distinction between severe depression and dysphoric mood. The number of patients who have a few depressive symptoms without endogenous depression is unknown. However, a logical first step in any treatment plan would seem to be simple discontinuation of reserpine. Pharmacological treatment of depression is described in Chapter 11.

ANTITUBERCULAR AGENTS

Isoniazid (INH), iproniazid (Ipronid), cycloserine (Seromycin), and ethambutol (Myambutol) are the antitubercular drugs most often associated with psychiatric symptoms. Numerous case histories attest to the frequency of isoniazid psychosis. Symptoms include auditory and visual hallucinations, disorientation, agitation, delirium, delusions, and paranoid ideation. Another set of psychiatric symptoms seen following isoniazid treatment consists of formal thought disorder, depression, and acute organic brain syndrome, sometimes with peripheral signs of vitamin deficiency. Treatment includes the discontinuation of isoniazid and prescription of nicotinamide and pyridoxine, both contained in a vitamin B complex. Isoniazid is structurally similar to nicotinamide, so that isoniazid administration produces a deficiency in essential nitocinamide containing cofactors. Pyridoxine is often given with isoniazid to avoid such a deficiency state (3).

Like isoniazid, iproniazid has strong psychotropic properties (Chapter 10). It produces euphoria in many patients and more fulminant hypomanic symptoms in others. Acute brain syndromes have also been reported, often including paranoid delusions. All of these side effects may be related to the drug's ability to inhibit monoamine oxidase (MAO). Cycloserine produces a large number of psychiatric symptoms and is known to be one of the most toxic antitubercular agents. As many as 30 percent of patients receiving cycloserine may have mild side effects, while an additional 20 percent experience severe toxicity (4). All of the following symptoms have been reported: irritability, sleep disturbance, anxiety, confusion, disorientation, paranoia, hallucinations, and convulsions. However, confusion is the symptom mentioned most frequently. These symptoms have been variously labeled as schizophrenia, hypomania, depression, and delirium. Ethambutol may also cause psychiatric side effects—most commonly depression. Unfortunately, all reported cases of ethambutol-induced depression have been complicated by the simultaneous administration of other antitubercular agents.

CORTICOSTEROIDS

The administration of corticosteroids is an increasingly common medical practice. In addition, hyperadrenalcorticism can result from Cushing's disease. In both cases, psychological complications have been observed. Incidence of such side effects among patients on long-term corticosteroids may be as high as 40 percent. Depression is more common in hyperadrenalcorticism, while euphoria is more frequently associated with exogenously administered corticosteroids. Other symptoms include delirium, poor concentration, visual and auditory hallucinations, somatic delusions, and impaired cognition. In one study of hospitalized patients receiving prednisone, 3 percent described psychological symptoms (5). None of the affected patients had a prior history of emotional instability, yet about one-third displayed inappropriate euphoria and the remainder had psychosis, with hallucinations, delusions, and violent behavior. These effects were markedly dose-dependent: 75 percent of the side effects occurred with patients receiving more than 40 mg/day of prednisone. Incidence of psychological effects among patients on less than 40 mg/day was 1 percent; for those receiving more than 80 mg/day, it was 18 percent.

Psychiatric consultation is often requested in cases of hyperadrenalcorticism. Major concerns should be the patient's suicide potential and the necessity for corticosteroid treatment. Small doses of phenothiazines, benzodiazepines, or antidepressants may be useful in individual cases, but gradual reduction of the corticosteroid dose is probably the most effective treatment. In cases of depression, reduction of the corticosteroid therapy produces a more rapid response than would institution of an antidepressant (6). Some investigators have suggested that patients with a previous history of depression or psychosis may be more likely to develop psychiatric symptoms than are those without such histories. However, the absence of prior psychiatric illness in no way assures a trouble-free course of corticosteroid treatment.

DIGITALIS

When Wethering first described the properties of digitalis in 1785, he pointed out that "the foxglove, when given in very large and quickly repeated doses, occasions sickness, vomiting, purging, giddiness, confused vision, [and] objects appearing green or yellow." This has been referred to as "foxglove frenzy delirium." Unfortunately, any interpretation of the effects of digitalis is complicated by the cardiac disease for which it is given. Digitalis intoxication may produce visual or auditory hallucinations, delirium, depression, apathy, various visual disturbances, and nausea, vomiting, or diarrhea. These symptoms often precede dangerous cardiac arrhythmias (7). Approximately 10–20 percent of patients receiving digitalis manifest some symptoms of toxicity, with an incidence of psychiatric symptoms of 3–8 percent (8).

The following psychiatric symptoms have now been ascribed to digitalis: fatigue, apathy, depressions, memory loss, confusion, irritability, labile mood, delusions, hallucinations, violence, excitement, mania, insomnia, and belligerence. The patient experiencing delirium is typically conscious and responsive; but both cognitive processes and perception are impaired. The patient may be either excited or lethargic, with a fluctuating level of arousal. Nocturnal exacerbations are most typical. The syndrome is reversible. Underlying cardiac disease contributes to this syndrome but to an unknown extent. Older patients with more advanced atherosclerotic heart disease appear to be most vulnerable to digitalis delirium. Other conditions which lower the threshold of toxicity include acute ischemia or infarction, hypothyroidism, and potassium depletion. Impaired renal function is also a contributing cause, since compromised clearance causes excessive accumulation and higher blood levels of digitalis.

Regular determination of serum levels can be of great benefit in avoiding toxic reactions. Serum levels of digoxin greater than 2 ng/ml are likely to be toxic. If delirium does appear, the drug should be stopped immediately.

DISULFIRAM

Disulfiram (Antabuse) was introduced as an aid in the treatment of alcoholism in 1948. It produces a violent but reasonably safe reaction to alcohol (Chapter 23). The drug is thought to act by blocking aldehyde dehydrogenase, thus causing an accumulation of acetaldehyde following alcohol ingestion (Chapter 20). Disulfiram also blocks a number of other enzymes, including dopamine-β-hydroxylase, the enzyme which converts dopamine to norepinephrine (Chapter 2). The major psychological side effect of disulfiram is the disulfiram "psychosis." In the early days of disulfiram use, when patients commonly received large doses of the drug, the incidence of disulfiram psychosis was estimated to be as high as 20 percent. With the lower doses now in use, the incidence is much lower.

Disulfiram psychoses have been divided into three types (9). Group I patients present with only symptoms of delirium (Table 29-1). Group II patients have some symptoms of delirium and also exhibit signs of depression, delusion, mania, or paranoia. Group III patients are acutely manic, depressed, or schizophrenic and have no signs of delirium. Using this classification, one study reported the following distribution of disulfiram psychoses: Group I, 39 percent; Group II, 37 percent; and Group III, 24 percent (9). Of the patients in Group III, most had predominantly depressive or manic symptomatology. Without comparison to a matched group of abstinent alcoholics, it is difficult to attribute any of these Group III psychoses to disulfiram, because the expected occurrence of psychoses in this population is unknown. This is not to minimize the significance of these conditions, since 17 percent of the patients in this study attempted suicide with over half of the attempts being successful.

Treatment for these patients consists primarily of sedation with antianxiety agents and discontinuation of disulfiram. In the study just cited, patients in Group I generally obtained complete recovery less than one week after disulfiram was discontinued, while Group II and III patients required one to three weeks. A similar recovery period was necessary for the patients with pure psychosis. Antipsychotic medications are contraindicated, since they seem to worsen the delirium and do little for the psychotic elements (10). Reinstitution of disulfiram therapy produced psychiatric side effects in less than one-third of the Group I and II patients. Similar data for Group III patients are not available.

L-DOPA

L-DOPA is the immediate precursor of dopamine (Chapter 2). Its major medicinal use is in the treatment of Parkinson's disease. Analysis of patients receiving L-DOPA reveals an average incidence of psychiatric side effects of 20 percent (11). About 4 percent of patients experience delirium, depression, overactivity, restlessness or agitation, and delusions or paranoia; 1.5 percent report hypomania; and 1 percent, hypersexuality. Other side effects include lethargy, insomnia, vivid dreams, and anxiety. L-DOPA-induced "delirium" most closely resembles a senile dementia, with confusion, poor memory, and even disorientation. Occasionally it is a true delirium (Table 29-1). Clearly, the true incidence of side effects from L-DOPA is complicated by the increased frequency of organic brain syndrome in the parkinsonian age group.

The occurrence of depression is an interesting and significant side effect of L-DOPA, particularly in light of the catecholamine hypothesis of affective disorders (Chapter 10). L-DOPA is commonly associated with an improvement in mood, but whether this is a direct result of increased catecholamines or a secondary effect of improvement in the disease is unresolved. Many studies find no evidence of depression, while others report that it is one of the two most common side effects. This variability is hard to explain, but predrug psychiatric state may contribute to the postdrug psychiatric response.

Psychomotor activation is a desired clinical effect of L-DOPA. However, some patients are troubled by overactivity, restlessness, and agitation. It is not clear if these symptoms are dose dependent. A closely related side effect is hypomania, which differs from overactivity in being accompanied by nonmotor behavior such as euphoria, anger, pressured speech, grandiosity, or flight of ideas.

When given to patients with a diagnosis of schizophrenia, L-DOPA exacerbates their psychotic symptoms (Chapter 8). In patients with Parkinson's disease, psychotic side effects usually take the form of paranoid delusions, with visual hallucinations. Again, predrug psychiatric state probably influences the occurrence of delusions and hallucinations with L-DOPA.

Certain generalizations can be made about psychiatric complications following L-DOPA treatment (12). Side effects do not occur when therapy is initiated; rather, several months of treatment precede their appearance. Patients with pre-existing psychiatric illness or organic brain syndrome are at high risk for exacerbation of their condition with L-DOPA treatment. When these complications occur, they can usually be treated by decreasing or discontinuing L-DOPA treatment.

Increasingly, psychiatrists are called upon to consult on abnormal involuntary movements, due mainly to greater awareness of tardive dyskinesia. Thus, any discussion of the side effects of L-DOPA should include L-DOPA-induced dyskinesia, which is more common than any of the other psychiatric complications of this drug. Typically, the dyskinesia is a buccolingual masticatory movement much like tardive dyskinesia (Chapter 9). Decreasing the dose of L-DOPA is the most effective treatment, although, theoretically, drugs which increase central cholinergic activity should be helpful.

ORAL CONTRACEPTIVES

Numerous psychiatric symptoms have been attributed to oral contraceptives. Most frequently encountered is depression. Estimates of the incidence of this side effect range from 0 to 34 percent, with the actual incidence probably being about 7 percent (13). Depressive episodes occur more frequently in women with a past history of depression. Some studies have concluded that the majority of side effects noted with oral contraceptives are related more to psychological implications of birth control than to pharmacological effects of the drug. A study involving several thousand women found no definite evidence that oral contraceptives either cause depression or aggravate the condition in women with depressive histories (14). The women were divided into three categories: never users, current users, and past users. Never users and current users reported similar scores on depression scales. History of past depressions was an important predictor of current depression for all groups.

Some investigators have attempted to determine whether estrogen or progesterone is involved in the depressant side effects of oral contraceptives. One study concluded that oral contraceptives which contain mainly progesterone are more likely to precipitate depression (15). However, a double-blind placebo study involving pills of varying estrogen-progesterone combinations concluded that women who received mainly estrogen showed slightly greater adverse mental changes and more psychiatric symptoms than did women who also received progesterone (16). The progesterone group exhibited mainly dysphoric symptoms, while the estrogen group also reported depression, anxiety, and tension.

Psychosis has also been reported to accompany either administration or withdrawal of oral contraceptives in some patients. This appears to occur most frequently in women who have a prior history of psychosis. As already mentioned, for many women the use of oral contraceptives involves strong psychodynamic factors which may contribute to the occurrence of any particular psychiatric symptom. In addition, any medication used as widely as oral contraceptives may be blamed inaccurately for a large number of problems. Thus, items such as change in sexual interest, fatigue, irritability, and increased well-being are difficult to evaluate. Pharmacological effects, psychological effects, and effects of other medications can only be differentiated in appropriately controlled studies.

PROPRANOLOL

Propranolol (Inderal) is a β-adrenergic blocking agent (Chapter 2). It has been an exceptionally useful agent to cardiologists. Unfortunately, the drug is also psychoactive, usually producing unpleasant side effects. Propranolol has been implicated in psychiatric symptoms, including nonspecific complaints of weakness and lassitude, vegetative signs of depression, hallucinations, and organic brain syndromes. Estimates of the incidence of psychiatric disturbances range from the manufacturer's statement of virtually none to one report of 50 percent after three months of therapy (17).

In one survey, less than 1 percent of patients taking propranolol had significant neurological disturbances (18). Symptoms included drowsiness, fatigue, lightheadedness, dizziness, headache, nausea, and blurring of vision. It should be emphasized that reduced cardiac output could be responsible for these nonspecific symptoms. Depression is the most common psychiatric complication of propranolol treatment. In one study of hypertensives receiving propranolol, 30 percent had depressive symptomatology; two of these patients attempted suicide and another three required antidepressants (17). Both duration of propranolol therapy and dose were positively associated with the incidence of depression. Treatment of this side effect has not been studied. Most clinicians simply discontinue propranolol, if possible.

CONCLUSION

Psychological side effects of nonpsychiatric medications can be a major source of concern both to the patient and to his physician. In addition to the obvious discomfort they produce, these symptoms can also become life-threatening, either through direct toxicity or through secondary effects such as suicide. Prompt intervention with appropriate measures almost always reverses the side effects, making it imperative that physicians be familiar with the diagnosis and treatment of these toxicity syndromes.

REFERENCES

1. Prichard, N. C., Johnston, A. N., Hill, I. D., and Rosenheim, M. L. Bethanidine, guanethidine and methyldopa in treatment of hypertension: a within-patient comparison. *Br. Med. J. 1*:135–144, 1968.
2. Goodwin, F. K., Ebert, M. H., and Bunney, W. E., Jr. Mental effects of reserpine in man: a review. *In: Psychiatric Complications of Medical Drugs.* R. I. Shader, ed., New York: Raven Press, 1972, pp. 73–101.
3. Jackson, S. L. O. Psychosis due to isoniazid. *Br. Med. J. 1*:743–746, 1967.
4. Lewis, W. C., Calden, G., Thurston, J. R., and Gilson, W. E. Psychiatric and neurological reactions to cycloserine in the treatment of tuberculosis. *Dis. Chest 32*:172–182, 1957.
5. The Boston Collaborative Drug Surveillance Program: Acute adverse reactions to prednisone in relation to dosage. *Clin. Pharmacol. Ther. 13*: 694–698, 1972.
6. Carpenter, W. T., Jr., Strauss, J. S., and Bunney, W. E., Jr. The psychobiology of cortisol metabolism: clinical and theoretical implications. *In: Psychiatric Complications of Medical Drugs.* R. I. Shader, ed., New York: Raven Press, 1972, pp. 49–72.
7. Ellis, J. G. and Dimond, E. G. L. Newer concepts of digitalis. *Am. J. Cardiol. 17*:759–767, 1966.
8. Greenblatt, D. J. and Shader, R. I. Digitalis toxicity. *In: Psychiatric Complications of Medical Drugs.* R. I. Shader, ed., New York: Raven Press, 1972, pp. 25–47.
9. Liddon, S. C. and Satran, R. Disulfiram (Antabuse) psychosis. *Am. J. Psychiatry 123*:1284–1289, 1967.
10. Knee, S. T. and Razani, J. Acute organic brain syndrome: a complication of disulfiram therapy. *Am. J. Psychiatry 131*:1281–1282, 1974.
11. Goodwin, F. K. Behavioral effects of L-DOPA in man. *In: Psychiatric Complications of Medical Drugs.* R. I. Shader, ed., New York: Raven Press, 1972, p. 149.
12. Barbeau, A. L-DOPA therapy in Parkinson's disease: a critical review of nine years experience. *Can. Med. Assoc. J. 101*:791–800, 1969.
13. Herzberg, B. and Coppen, A. Change in psychological symptoms in women taking oral contraceptives. *Br. J. Psychiatry 116*:161–164, 1970.
14. Kutner, S. J. and Brown, W. L. Types of oral contraceptives, depression, and premenstrual symptoms. *J. Nerv. Ment. Dis. 155*:153–163, 1972.
15. Grant, E. and Pryse-Davis, J. Effects of oral contraceptives on depressive mood changes and on endometrial monoamine oxidase and phosphatases. *Br. Med. J. 3*:777–780, 1968.
16. Cullberg, J. Mood changes and menstrual symptoms with different gestagen/estrogen combinations. *Acta Psychiatr. Scand., Suppl. 236*: 1–86, 1972.
17. Waal, H. J. Propranolol-induced depression. *Br. Med. J. 2*:50, 1967.
18. Greenblatt, D. J. and Koch-Weser, J. Adverse reactions to propranolol in hospitalized medical patients: a report from the Boston Collaborative Drug Surveillance Program. *Am. Heart J. 86*:478–484, 1973.

30 | Psychotherapy and Psychopharmacology

ADOLF PFEFFERBAUM

INTRODUCTION

The advent of modern psychopharmacology may have begun with Sigmund Freud's introduction of the drug cocaine. His initial optimism that cocaine would relieve psychic distress was based on his personal use of this drug during his own depressions. In 1884 he wrote, "in my last severe depression, I took coca again and a small dose lifted me to the heights in a wonderful fashion" (1). He went on to promote its use for depression, neurasthenia, and morphine addiction.

However, Freud's initial enthusiasm was soon tempered by the recognition that cocaine could be addicting and could cause a toxic psychosis. Furthermore, it failed to afford lasting psychological relief from depression. Thus, what had begun as a panacea soon became regarded as poison. Ultimately, Freud's enthusiasm for cocaine brought him considerable personal distress and professional ridicule. This unfortunate experience with cocaine may have contributed to the early psychoanalytic bias against psychotropic medications.

The continuing development of new pharmacotherapies set the stage for further polarization of ideologies. During World War II, the use of barbiturates in narcotherapy was demonstrated to be effective in the abreactive treatment of traumatic war neuroses, while amphetamines were used in the symptomatic treatment of depression. With the introduction of meprobamate (Miltown) and chlorpromazine (Thorazine) by the mid-1950's, pharmacological treatment for anxiety, depression, and schizophrenia became readily available. However, as the potential for effective psychopharmacology was beginning to be realized, resistance to it began to appear.

CONFLICT BETWEEN PSYCHOTHERAPY
AND PSYCHOPHARMACOLOGY

Joost Meerloo published a paper in 1955 entitled "Medication Into Submission: the Danger of Therapeutic Coercion" (2). The title of this paper conveys some of the prevailing concerns about the use and potential misuse of psychopharmacology. Although some of Meerloo's concerns may have been overstated, several continue to be germane. One of them is the observation that "magical thinking" about drugs frequently influences the behavior of both patient and therapist. The unconscious search for a quick and effortless solution to psychological problems whose origins are likely to be insidious and complex is seen as a real deterrent to therapeutic progress. Only recently have physicians begun to accept the fact that the hope for pharmacological agents which will solve all emotional problems cannot be realized. Nonetheless, the widespread abuse of meprobamate in the 1950's and 1960's and the current extensive use of diazepam (Valium) suggest that resistance to this desire dies hard.

In the same article, Meerloo also described the social dangers of psychotropic medication, the most pressing of which included exploitation of the patient's desire for rapid relief from psychic distress. This creates an urgency which can be exploited by the unscrupulous for pecuniary or political gain. Drawing analogies to Nazi Germany and to communist bloc "brainwashing," Meerloo warned of the potentials of "menticide." Although his examples may now seem extreme, the drug cults of the 1960's and the persistent escalation of drug abuse today give Meerloo's warning more cogency.

In 1957, Szasz (3) made one of the first references to the use of "chemical strait jackets." When a patient's behavior is disturbing and unacceptable to those around him—particularly to therapists in psychiatric hospitals—steps are taken to control him. Prior to the introduction of potent tranquilizers, this was accomplished by the use of physical restraint such as hydrotherapy, cold packs, and straitjackets. The advent of tranquilizing antipsychotics facilitated the chemical control of unacceptable behavior. As Szasz points out, however, such "treatment" may be aimed more at benefiting the therapist than at helping the patient.

Early criticism of psychotropic drug use also came from those concerned about the effects of the medication-taking process on the psychotherapeutic interaction. The concern was frequently raised that drugs interfered with transference formation and reduced the anxiety which was a necessary accompaniment of psychological work. This was felt to apply especially to neurotic patients in analytically oriented psychotherapy. Hoch (4) countered these criticisms with the observation that psychotropic drugs can facilitate psychotherapy rather than hinder it, particularly when severe anxiety impedes therapeutic progress. In addition, it is unclear exactly how uncomfortable and anxiety-provoking psychotherapy must be in order to be effective. Hoch also questioned whether the resistance to the use of psychotropic medication came from psychiatrists who had either forgotten or had never learned how to use them.

Zetzel (5) claimed that the use of antipsychotics was an important adjunct to psychotherapy in treating schizophrenics. She maintained that pharmacological intervention reduced the formation of projections and delusions and thus facilitated psychotherapy. She also thought that, under certain circumstances, antipsychotic medications might actually improve the patient's ability to form a therapeutic alliance.

Today, there are still many psychiatrists who view all psychopathology as primarily psychogenic in origin, although they may concede a hereditary organic predisposition. This group maintains that drugs merely remove symptoms. While acknowledging the adjunctive efficacy of drugs, they advocate psychotherapy as the primary treatment, even for schizophrenia (6). By the late 1960's, however, the general attitudes toward psychotropic drug use and its relationship to psychotherapy had changed somewhat. The recognition was growing that psychotropic medications might also be useful adjuncts and facilitators of psychotherapy in the psychotic disorders and in some of the more severe neurotic disorders.

COMBINED USE OF PSYCHOTHERAPY AND PSYCHOPHARMACOLOGY

Much of the initial resistance to psychopharmacological agents was based on the assumption that they would interfere with the psychotherapeutic process. This concern lessened as the effectiveness of these drugs became increasingly apparent. However, while acceptance of pharmacotherapy as an adjunct to psychotherapy was growing, the assumption that psychotherapy was the principal treatment factor continued unchallenged, even though the basis for this assumption went unproven. It was only a matter of time before voices were raised in challenge and proponents of the opposing view began to question whether psychotherapy alone, or in conjunction with drug usage, offered any significant benefit over drug use alone.

Some controlled clinical studies addressing this question in the treatment of neurotic disorders have been carried out. For example, a study comparing psychotherapy to a combination of psychotherapy and pharmacotherapy in treating a group of predominantly psychoneurotic outpatients failed to show differences between the treatment groups (7). A follow-up to this study, comparing chlordiazepoxide and placebo, with or without psychotherapy, revealed only one significant interaction: chlordiazepoxide was more effective than placebo in relieving symptomatic discomfort (8). However, after six months of psychotherapy, patients who were treated with psychotherapy alone, with psychotherapy plus placebo or chlordiazepoxide, or with chlordiazepoxide did equally well (9). Each of these groups did better than patients who received no treatment of any sort or only placebo. From these studies there appeared no clear indication that the combination of psychotherapy and pharmacotherapy was superior to either treatment singly. A recent review of a large number of controlled psychotherapy and pharmacotherapy outcome studies concludes that combined psychotherapy and pharmacotherapy is often better than pharmacotherapy alone (10). This conclusion is derived primarily from studies with schizophrenic and depressed patients, however, and has not been supported by studies on neurotic or anxious patients.

The evidence for the efficacy of psychotropic drugs in the treatment of schizophrenia is impressive (Chapter 9). While there are some questions about the effectiveness of antipsychotic agents on the long-term outcome of schizophrenics, the immediate effects of these drugs are truly remarkable. Psychotherapeutic approaches with schizophrenic patients have had less dramatic success. For example, in a comparison of patients receiving psychotropic drugs, psychotropic drugs with psychotherapy, electroconvulsive therapy (ECT), placebo, or no treatment, drug treatment and drug treatment with psychotherapy were equally effective, and both were superior to treatments without drugs (11). The data did not show any significant statistical interaction between drugs and psychotherapy.

The above study has been criticized because the psychotherapy was provided by relatively inexperienced therapists. In fact, when any study maintains that "psychotherapy" was provided it is often difficult to know what the psychological treatment actually was. In comparison, pharmacotherapy can be specified much more precisely. In partial answer to this criticism, another study compared the effects of psychotherapy alone with those of psychotherapy and phenothiazines in a group of chronic schizophrenic patients (12). This study is unique in that patients were treated for two years by experienced, psychoanalytically oriented psychiatrists who initially saw each patient at least twice weekly. These investigators concluded, "Psychotherapy alone (even with experienced therapists) does little or nothing for chronic schizophrenic patients in two years' time." It may be that some uniquely talented psychotherapists can have profound psychological impact on some patients with schizophrenia; however, it has not been possible to demonstrate convincingly the efficacy of insight-oriented psychotherapy as an adjunct to psychotropic medication in the treatment of schizophrenia.

More recently there has been a shift in the emphasis of psychotherapy with schizophrenic patients away from insight-oriented approaches and toward "social functioning." There are significant psychological and psychosocial issues that can be dealt with in psychotherapy, and these may improve the outcome of the combined drug and psychotherapeutic treatment of schizophrenia. These issues include the problems of day-to-day living faced by the schizophrenic patient, and the impact of the patient's illness on himself and on his family. One approach in helping the patient handle these problems is called "major role therapy," referring to the kind of active social intervention generally thought of as psychiatric social work, such as job advice, assistance in filling out forms and managing finances, and intervention in family crises (13,14). With this therapy, the outcome variable of "social functioning" is defined as the "interpersonal relationship out of the home" and "overall functioning." In studies of this aspect of the long-term sequelae of schizophrenia, major role therapy was shown to be an effective adjunct to drug therapy and to provide a better adjustment for many patients. The beneficial effects of this social intervention did not become apparent, however, until eighteen to twenty-four months of treatment. These investigators concluded that drugs and social therapy are an important and effective combination in the treatment of schizophrenia, with medications controlling symptoms and preventing relapse and social therapy increasing the patient's social functioning.

Perhaps a more promising role for the combined use of pharmacotherapy and psychotherapy is seen in the treatment of depression. Amitriptyline (Elavil) has been compared to placebo or no drug treatment, both with and without psychotherapy, in a group of depressed women, all of whom initially responded to the antidepressant effects of amitriptyline (Elavil) (15,16). A retrospective classification of this group of patients revealed that about 70 percent of them would be classified as having "anxious depression." Psychotherapy showed a significant effect on "social adjustment," but only after six to eight months of treatment. The "social adjustment" was defined as involving six areas in the patient's life: work performance, anxious ruminations, interpersonal friction, inhibition of communication, submissive dependence, and family attachment. Although effective in treating the depression, amitriptyline alone did not improve the patient's social adjustment; and there was no evidence of an interaction between drugs and psychotherapy. The conclusions of this study are similar to those described with major role therapy for schizophrenics. That is, a patient whose depression responds to tricyclic antidepressant drug therapy can benefit from the combined use of pharmacotherapy and psychotherapy. Although these two treatment modalities do not appear to be interacting, the pharmacotherapy alleviates presenting symptoms and prevents relapse, while psychotherapy increases interpersonal and social adjustment.

Modern psychiatry began with the psychodynamic discoveries of Freud, and these have been refined and expanded upon in the years that followed. The development of effective pharmacotherapy has led some to regard dynamic psychiatry as superfluous and even irrelevant. There are others who still regard psychodynamic principles as the mainstay of treatment. This has resulted in two major competing theories of the cause of psychiatric disturbances. One view is strictly biological, stating that psychiatric disturbances result from a disorder in a metabolic, endocrine, or biochemical system. The other is strictly psychodynamic, arguing that psychiatric disturbances reflect a defect in psychosexual or interpersonal psychological development. These two polar views are frequently seen as competitive and mutually exclusive. Those supporting one view advocate the exclusive use of psychoactive medication; adherents of the other restrict themselves to psychological and behavioral intervention.

In practice, most psychiatrists do not limit themselves to either of the views as described. Instead, they choose psychoactive drugs, psychotherapy or a combination of the two, on pragmatic, rather than ideological, bases. The Group for the Advancement of Psychiatry (17) has suggested that "prototheories" are developed to aid in resolving theoretical positions with clinical practice and reality. These prototheories are partial theories which allow the proponent of one polar view to utilize the therapeutic tools derived from other theoretical frameworks. For example, the psychotherapist who understands a patient's distress in terms of an intrapsychic conflict may still prescribe psychotropic medications. He can describe the medication's function as symptom reduction, rather than in psychodynamic terms, so that he will not find it necessary to have a psychodynamic explanation of their efficacy. Use of the prototheories allows for the most pragmatic treatment of a wide variety of psychiatric disorders. Perhaps the psychodynamic and biological theoretical extremes will eventually converge and foster combined therapies which are based on a unified theory.

INTERACTIONS BETWEEN PSYCHOTHERAPY AND PSYCHOPHARMACOLOGY

The pragmatic practice of psychiatry often results in the combined use of psychotherapy and pharmacotherapy. Four theoretical possibilities for interactions exist: positive or negative effects of pharmacotherapy on psychotherapy and positive or negative effects of psychotherapy on pharmacotherapy.

EFFECTS OF PHARMACOTHERAPY ON PSYCHOTHERAPY

The positive effects of pharmacotherapy on psychotherapy include the reduction of severe anxiety and affective discomfort, thus enabling the patient to engage in and benefit from the psychotherapy. In addition, drugs may enhance primary autonomous ego functions such as verbal skills, memory, attention span, and concentration. Furthermore, the symbolic importance of the medication-taking process itself should not be minimized. In addition to providing a positive "placebo effect" (Chapter 31), medications may also meet the need of some patients to define themselves as "medically ill," so that they can accept psychiatric treatment.

The process of taking medications may also have negative consequences. For some patients, prescriptions may enhance dependency on the physician and contribute to the fantasy that the physician is a magically endowed and potent figure. When this occurs, the process of drug taking may bring about a deterioration of some aspects of the patient's psychological functioning. In spite of the drug's positive effects, the patient may become more dependent and less able to function autonomously. This phenomenon is sometimes referred to as the "negative placebo effect." The rapid relief of psychological discomfort and anxiety may also reduce the motivation to work for psychological insight and change. Finally, patients who come from a sociocultural group that values insight highly may view drugs as a "crutch" and may interpret the prescription for medication as evidence that the physician believes they have inadequate psychological resources.

EFFECTS OF PSYCHOTHERAPY ON PHARMACOTHERAPY

Some pharmacotherapists would maintain that, at best, psychotherapy satisfies Hippocrates' admonition, i.e., it does no harm. Others would argue that, indeed, it can do harm. They suggest that conflicts should not be "stirred up," especially with psychotic patients. Instead of encouraging psychological exploration, they believe that the emphasis should be placed on the "medical-model" treatment of a biological disorder. However, the relationship between physician and patient clearly contributes to the positive or negative placebo effects which accompany the pharmacological actions of all medicines (Chapter 31). Nonetheless, for many psychotic patients, a "psychotherapy goal" is the patient's recognition that he needs medication. While this may seem to be a minor point, the maintenance of psychotic patients on pharmacologic agents is frequently a difficult task, requiring considerable therapeutic skill (Chapter 9).

Psychological characteristics of both the patient and the physician, along with their interpersonal interaction, also have an influence on the process of pharmacotherapy. The giving and taking of the medication can be quite symbolic and it can serve as a means of either direct or distorted communication. Some patients see the prescription as a sign that the physician is concerned about them and is caring for them. Issues about medications frequently become a vehicle for the expression of transference feelings. While they are often positively directed, negative or hostile attitudes can also be generated. Reporting of unpleasant drug side effects can be the result of unconscious anger directed at the physician. An extreme form of this anger may appear as suicide attempts using the medications given to the patient by the physician. Fortunately these conflicts are usually acted out at less lethal levels. Should the physician be reluctant to prescribe a drug, the patient can ensnare him in a psychological battle. If the physician relents and prescribes the medication, the patient may feel that he has defeated the physician. Thus, both taking and refusing medication can be a significant part of the relationship between the physician and his patient and can reflect a wide range of transference phenomena.

The physician's personality, biases, and distortions also affect his prescribing habits. He, too, can endow medication with special meaning. This may be called the "countertransference" aspect of drug use. The unrealistically optimistic and positive attitude that many physicians exhibit adds to the positive placebo effects of medication (Chapter 31). This positive attitude can be carried to an extreme, however, leading to the belief that pharmacotherapy can solve all the psychological problems one might encounter. This may limit the physician's ability to accurately assess the efficacy of his pharmacotherapy regimens. The primary reliance on medication can also be used by both the physician and patient to avoid a meaningful psychological encounter, especially if the issues of psychotherapy are unpleasant to either of them. The patient may focus the psychotherapy sessions on medication, in order to avoid the discomforts of self-scrutiny. Likewise, the physician can participate in this defense by overemphasizing medication, thus allowing himself to avoid psychological issues. An extreme example of such behavior is seen with physicians who use medication to dismiss troublesome patients.

The many psychological components involved in drug-taking behavior and drug-prescribing behavior provide the opportunity for abuse, misuse, and overuse of psychotropic medications. Blackwell (18) has addressed this issue and notes that there were 144 million prescriptions written in 1972 for daytime psychotropic drugs; 70 percent of these were for antianxiety agents, and over 30 percent of the total was for diazepam. The use of diazepam has been steadily increasing at the rate of 7 million prescriptions per year. There has been no such increase in the use of antipsychotics or antidepressants. Does this rapid increase in the use of antianxiety agents reflect overuse and misuse of these drugs or the spiraling stress of our urban technological society? The majority of diazepam prescriptions written in 1971–1972 were written by non-psychiatrists, and only 30 percent were written for "mental disorders" (17). It is speculated that a large percentage of patients seen in general practice are actually suffering from psychological disturbances and anxiety, manifested as psychosomatic disorders. Perhaps the general practitioner has discovered this fact and now has an effective antianxiety agent at his disposal. Patients requesting these agents are frequently described by nonpsychiatrists as having "nothing really wrong with them." Perhaps these patients are requesting the medications to treat anxiety states which are not apparent to the clinician but do indeed exist.

Some patients do become psychologically habituated or even physiologically addicted to antianxiety agents (Chapter 24). In some cases, use of these drugs represents an attempt to cope with unpleasant life stresses for which psychological and interpersonal solutions would be more appropriate. Whatever the reasons for misuse, when it occurs, the resultant doctor-patient interaction can be quite unpleasant. The blame is passed back and forth between the patient and the doctor. The doctor sees the patient as dependent, inadequate, demanding, manipulative, and even immoral. The patient views the doctor as cold, withholding, and uncaring. These disparate views often lead to a struggle over whether or not the physician will prescribe the medication. If he does, he often feels that he has transgressed, particularly now that antianxiety agents have been reclassified as controlled substances.

At the other extreme the physician may enter into a collusion with the patient. He will readily overprescribe these agents at the patient's request in order to avoid conflict, and he will then employ many rationalizations for his prescribing habits. This may reduce friction with the patient, giving the physician the illusion that he is rendering aid.

Usually, however, the drug only temporarily reduces the patient's psychic distress, and further conflict and frustration follow when the physician finally is forced to question the continued overuse of medication. The immediate withdrawal of medications from the patient suspected of abuse can become a punitive countertransference phenomenon generated by the physician's anger with himself or with the patient, rather than by a desire to help the patient. Dealing with this problem requires considerable time and effort on the physician's part, as well as insight into the psychological significance of medications to both himself and the patient.

CONCLUSION

Our knowledge of psychological responses to the pharmacological process comes from astute observations by clinicians. These phenomena are not universal and take varied forms depending on the psychopathology and personality structure of each individual. Perhaps this variety makes the task of "proving" an interaction between psychotherapy and pharmacotherapy so difficult. To date, it has not been possible to demonstrate this interaction, especially with insight therapies; but clinical experience and observations leave many convinced that it exists. It is also intellectually appealing to recognize that there must be an interaction between the mind and the brain. There must be neurophysiological and neurochemical counterparts to thoughts and emotions. By the same logic, the actions of psychopharmacological agents on biological substrates should influence the effects of psychotherapy on psychological substrates. Perhaps some psychiatric disorders begin with changes in the psychological substrate, thus altering biological mechanisms, while in others the process is reversed. Unraveling this interaction is one of the great challenges of psychiatry, as Sigmund Freud recognized when he wrote: "In view of the intimate connection between the things that we distinguish as physical and mental, we may look forward to a day when paths of knowledge and, let us hope, of influence will be opened up, leading from organic biology and chemistry to the field of neurotic phenomena" (19).

REFERENCES

1. Jones, E. *The Life and Works of Sigmund Freud.* New York: Basic Books, 1953, p. 84.
2. Meerloo, J. Medication into submission: the danger of therapeutic coercion. *J. Nerv. Ment. Dis. 122:*353–360, 1955.
3. Szasz, T. Some observations on the use of tranquilizing drugs. *Arch. Neurol. Psychiatry 77:*86–92, 1957.
4. Hoch, P. H. Drugs and psychotherapy. *Am. J. Psychiatry 116:*305–308, 1960.
5. Zetzel, E. Discussion. *In: Psychiatric Drugs.* P. Solomon, *ed.,* New York: Grune and Stratton, 1966, pp. 75–85.
6. Arieti, S. An overview of schizophrenia from a predominantly psychological approach. *Am. J. Psychiatry 131:*241–249, 1974.
7. Lorr, M., McNair, D., and Weinstein, G. Early effects of chlordiazepoxide (Librium) used with psychotherapy. *J. Psychiatr. Res. 1:*257–270, 1962.
8. Lorr, M., McNair, D., Weinstein, G., Michaux, W., and Raskin, A. Meprobamate and chlorpromazine in psychotherapy. *Arch. Gen. Psychiatry 4:*381–389, 1961.
9. Roth, I., Rhudick, P., Shaskan, D., Slobin, M., Wilkinson, A., and Young, H. Long-term effects on psychotherapy of initial treatment conditions. *J. Psychiatr. Res. 2:*283–297, 1974.
10. Luborsky, L., Singer, B., and Luborsky, L. Comparative studies of psychotherapies. *Arch. Gen. Psychiatry 32:*995–1008, 1975.
11. May, P. and Tuma, H. Treatment of schizophrenia: an experimental study of five treatment methods. *Brit. J. Psychiatry 111:*503–510, 1965.
12. Grinspoon, L., Ewalt, J., and Shader, R. Psychotherapy in chronic schizophrenia. *Am. J. Psychiatry 124:*67–74, 1968.
13. Hogarty, G., Goldberg, S., Schooler, N., and Ulrich, R. Drug and sociotherapy in the aftercare of schizophrenic patients: II. Two year relapse rates. *Arch. Gen. Psychiatry 31:*603–608, 1974.
14. Hogarty, G., Goldberg, S., and Schooler, N. Drug and sociotherapy in the aftercare of schizophrenic patients: III. Adjustment of nonrelapse patients. *Arch. Gen. Psychiatry 31:*609–618, 1974.
15. Klerman, G., DiMascio, A., Weissman, M., Prusoff, B., and Paykel, E. Treatment of depression by drugs and psychotherapy. *Am. J. Psychiatry 131:*186–191, 1974.
16. Weissman, M., Klerman, G., Paykel, E., Prusoff, B., and Hanson, B. Treatment effects on the social adjustment of depressed patients. *Arch. Gen. Psychiatry 30:*771–778, 1974.
17. Group for the Advancement of Psychiatry: *Pharmacotherapy and Psychotherapy: Paradoxes, Problems, and Progress.* New York: Mental Health Materials, 1975.
18. Blackwell, B. Minor tranquilizers: use, misuse or overuse? *Psychosomatics 16:*28–31, 1975.
19. Strachey, J. *(ed.) The Standard Edition of the Complete Psychological Works of Sigmund Freud, Vol. 20.* London: Hogarth Press, 1959, p. 231.

31 | The Placebo

ADOLF PFEFFERBAUM

HISTORY AND DEFINITION

The history of the term "placebo" may trace back to the Hebrew Bible (1). The Latin translation of Psalm 116:9, "I will please the Lord in the land of the living," is *Placebo Domino in regione vivorum*. *Placebo* is the first person singular future of the Latin verb *placere*, meaning "to please, give pleasure, to satisfy." By the fourteenth century "placebo" had already gained a negative connotation, being applied to professional mourners who sang "placebos" at funerals, to relieve the dead person's family of this task, for a fee. Later definitions included "a flatterer, sycophant, parasite." The first medical definition appeared in the eighteenth century as "a common place method of medicine." By 1811, the definition became "any medicine adopted more to please than benefit the patient," and by 1894 the concept of placebo as "a make believe medicine" was added. Modern definitions usually mention the quality of pharmacological inertness and refer to the use of placebos in "double-blind" evaluation of drugs.

Although the definition of the placebo as a pharmacologically inert compound is only about eighty years old, the use of the placebo is one of man's oldest medical practices. Prior to the late nineteenth century, most medications were inert; a few were even toxic. Homeopathy was an interesting system of therapy that was popular in the early nineteenth century. It was based on several fictitious biological "principles" and involved the administration of extremely dilute concentrations of the medicinal compounds then in use. It was probably so popular because reducing the doses of the inert compounds did no harm, while diluting toxic compounds rendered them harmless. However, the development of pharmacologically active medications has not eliminated placebo effects from the medical armamentarium. The modern use of placebos ranges from the deliberate administration of an inert compound or of an active compound which is inactive for the specific disease being treated to the unwitting use of inappropriate medication which, nonetheless, results in a cure.

Placebos are not limited to potions, powders, and pills, although this is what usually comes to mind. For a short time, the surgical procedure of internal mammary artery ligation was used successfully to treat angina pectoris. Then, it was shown that merely putting a suture around the artery but not tying it, i.e., sham surgery, produced equally beneficial results (2). Thus, the surgical procedure was a placebo, having no specific effects on coronary artery pathology and yet relieving the angina. As with other placebos, the surgical placebo is generally more effective when performed by an enthusiast than when provided by a skeptic. Psychotherapy may also have a placebo component, and the demonstration of the effectiveness of psychotherapy over and above the placebo effect is a significant challenge (Chapter 30).

In view of the ubiquity of the placebo effect, a more detailed definition has been proposed (1). In general, a placebo can be defined as any aspect of treatment which is used to relieve a condition for which it has no specific therapeutic value, whether or not the therapist or patient is aware that it is inactive. Placebos can be further described in terms of activity: a "pure placebo" is inert, an "impure placebo" is a sub-effective dose of an active drug, and an "active placebo" is an active drug which is not specific for the disorder being treated.

PLACEBO EFFECTS

Through the course of medical history, virtually every known ailment has been "cured" at least once by a medication or procedure which was later found to be inert or nonspecific for that disorder. Some disorders appear to be more responsive to placebos than others (Table 31-1). Symptoms that are a reaction to physical processes, such as pain, claudication, angina, and headache, or that involve subjective responses, like anxiety, depression, and fatigue, are all mediated by cortical processes and are often relieved by placebos. Symptoms involving the autonomic nervous system, such as migraine, hypertension, nausea, seasickness, colitis, and ulcers also seem to be responsive to placebos. In addition, placebos can be effective in treating several allergic diatheses of dermatitis, rhinitis, and asthma; and in some cases a placebo allergen, like plastic flowers, can induce the allergic symptoms.

TABLE 31-1.

PLACEBO RESPONSE FOR SPECIFIC SYMPTOMS

SYMPTOM	NO. OF STUDIES	NO. OF PATIENTS	PATIENTS RESPONDING TO PLACEBO %
Pain	25	961	28
Headache	9	4588	62
Migraine	5	4908	32
Sleep disturbance	3	340	7
Neurosis	6	135	34
Psychosis	17	828	19
Alcoholism	5	210	22
Seasickness	1	33	58
G.I. disorders	4	284	58
Constipation	3	144	12
Hypertension	9	240	17
Dysmenorrhea	4	88	24
Asthma	2	19	5
Hay fever	1	42	22
Colds	3	246	45
Coughing	2	44	41
Rheumatism	8	358	49
Skin diseases	2	19	21
Angina pectoris	10	346	18
Intermittent claudication	1	6	33
Cerebral infarct	3	57	7
Multiple sclerosis	3	152	24
Epilepsy	1	72	0
Parkinsonism	2	31	19

Data abstracted from Haas et al. (3).

One of the most dramatic reports of a placebo response involves a case of terminal cancer (4). It is summarized as follows:

> The patient described had generalized and far advanced lympho-sarcoma. He eventually became refractory to all known palliative therapies and developed anemia severe enough to preclude further radiation or chemotherapy. He had "huge tumor masses, the size of oranges . . . in the neck, axilla, groins, chest, and abdominal cavity." He was considered terminal by his physicians but remained hopeful of a miracle, when the reports of "Krebiozen" as a cure for cancer appeared in the newspapers. Although he did not meet the research criteria—because of his poor prognosis—he was included in a protocol to test the efficacy of this compound.

He was given the first injection on Friday. His physician arrived to see him the following Monday expecting a "moribund or dead" patient. Instead, the patient was remarkably improved, and the tumor masses were half their original size. While none of the other patients in the study had improved, this patient recovered sufficiently to be discharged within 10 days.

Within two months newspaper accounts of Krebiozen failures began to appear, and the patient "began to lose faith" in this cure. After two months of remission, he relapsed and was readmitted to the hospital in his original condition. At this point his physician "deliberately lied," telling him that the drug was indeed effective and had merely deteriorated in storage. He was given injections of "fresh" drug, which were really only water. "Recovery from his second near terminal state was even more dramatic than the first." Again he remained well for about two months, but then the final AMA announcement about Krebiozen appeared, declaring it to be worthless in the treatment of cancer. Within a few days the patient was readmitted to the hospital and died.

PHYSIOLOGY

Wolf (5) had a unique opportunity to make direct observations of an end organ response to placebos during his studies of Tom, a patient with a gastric fistula. These studies demonstrated clearly that placebo effects can occur at the end organ and are not merely changes in subjective experience of an unchanged physiology. Such end organ changes depend upon the state of the organ prior to administration of the placebo, the setting and route of administration, and the previously established reactions. When Tom's stomach was relatively inactive, urogastrone produced a decrease in stomach acid and turgidity; however, when Tom was upset, this drug had no effect on turgidity and, at times, was actually followed by an increase in stomach acid. Tom disliked hypodermic injections, and even injections of distilled water could produce a significant rise in gastric acid and hyperemia. Occasionally, he received physostigmine, which usually induces gastric hyperactivity, hyperemia, hyperacidity, and abdominal cramps. On those days, trials with any other compound following the physostigmine always produced gastric hyperfunction. This occurred not only with water and lactose tablets but even with atropine, which should have the opposite effect.

Similar paradoxical effects were seen with a twenty-eight-year-old female with hyperemesis gravidarium, who had been vomiting for two days (5). A gastric balloon was used to record stomach activity, which is generally reduced during nausea. The patient then received ipecac, which itself will produce nausea. When she received the drug through a stomach tube and was told that it would relieve her nausea, her stomach contractions returned to normal and her nausea subsided.

PHARMACOLOGY

Placebos appear to have a pharmacology which is similar to that of active drugs (6). Placebos used for analgesia for postpartum pain produced a time-response curve resembling that of aspirin. In a study of patients' reports of their "pep and appetite," placebo effects were cumulative, i.e., pep and appetite increased with each day's medication. Placebos also possessed a carry-over effect, in that the reported levels of pep and appetite remained elevated after the placebo medication was withdrawn (6). Another study demonstrated a dose effect of placebos, showing that four pills a day were more effective than one pill per day in treating depression and anxiety (7).

Like all potent drugs, placebos also have some side effects or undesirable actions. This is sometimes referred to as a "negative placebo reaction." Commonly reported side effects of placebos are drowsiness, fatigue, motor disturbance, headache, nervousness, and nausea—the very symptoms they treat. The reports of minor side effects are as high as 94 percent (8). Occasional major side effects can include overwhelming weakness, rash, diarrhea, urticaria, and even "drug dependence" (9).

MECHANISMS OF ACTION

That placebos do have a significant physiological effect is a fascinating phenomenon. Even more intriguing are the questions of how and why. In early work on placebos, Beecher (10) postulated that increased stress or pain enhanced the effectiveness of placebos. Discriminating between the perception of pain and the reaction to pain perception, he suggested that the reaction to pain perception is influenced by both placebos and stress. To support this hypothesis, he pointed out that only 25 percent of men injured in battle require morphine for pain, while 80 percent of men with similar injuries in civilian life require the drug. Furthermore, in a relatively nonstressful laboratory environment, Beecher could not discriminate between the effects of saline and 15 mg of morphine in relieving brief experimental pain. However, this positive correlation between effectiveness and pain was not confirmed by others, who found that placebos became less effective as pain increased (6).

It is possible, of course, that only certain persons respond to placebos, while others do not. This question of a "placebo responder" is of particular relevance for drug trials, in which it would be advantageous to exclude individuals who regularly respond to a placebo. Many studies have correlated placebo response with personality measures. The results are generally similar to those of Linton and Langs (11), who reported that strong placebo responders are passive, poorly defended, insensitive, and nonintellectual, while weak placebo responders are self-examining, intellectually curious, sensitive to internal and external cues, and better defended. The general tone of these descriptions implies that placebo responders are not as well developed psychologically as are nonresponders. This is consonant with the general clinical folklore that naive, unsophisticated patients can be "fooled" by placebos. Some investigators would add a social-class dimension to the placebo-responder concept, suggesting that lower socio-economic patients with anxiety and depression improve more on placebo than do middle socioeconomic patients, who respond better to psychotherapy (7). Others have even suggested that placebo response should be perceived as an adaptive mechanism for coping with otherwise impossible conditions (12).

In general, the discrimination of a placebo responder from a nonresponder is not maintained across repeated dosages or across different syndromes. Many investigators question the usefulness of the placebo-responder concept, or at least recognize that response to placebo is determined by many interacting variables (8). Although patient personality may be a factor, the physician's personality may be equally important in determining the placebo's effectiveness. Rather than placebo-prone personalities, a more useful conceptualization may be that of functions being placebo prone or resistant (13). This would be consistent with the observation that some pathological disease states respond to placebo with greater frequency than do others.

Conditioned reflex theory suggests a possible mechanism for the placebo response. This would seem to be a plausible explanation for the previously described experiment with Tom and physostigmine. Conditioned reflexes may be responsible for the phenomenon of "expectancy" in humans, and there are studies of conditioned behavior in animals which could be interpreted as demonstrating a placebo effect. In one study, rats were given intraperitoneal injections of saline and then put into a cage where activity was measured (14). Then, with this same design, some rats were given saline injections, while others received amphetamine, which increases activity. After a variable number of trials, all rats again received saline injection and cage exposure. The greater the number of amphetamine trials previously experienced, the higher the rat's activity after the final saline injection; this suggests that there was a conditioned or placebo response to a placebo injection. In a separate experiment, chlorpromazine, which decreases activity, was used in the same paradigm. However, the final placebo response was opposite to that expected, since the activity actually increased rather than decreased. Thus, while the conditioned response theory may provide explanations for some placebo phenomena, it clearly is not the entire answer.

Psychological explanations of placebo effects are also offered. Physicians are the sole prescribers of proprietary drugs, and their social role is that of healer (15). The patient expects the physician to "do something" that will make him better. Indeed, the mere act of handing him a prescription for medication is "doing something." In spite of the inactive or toxic substances administered throughout antiquity, physicians and healers maintained a position of respect in society. Something must have transpired to improve patients after treatment—probably the placebo effect. It is interesting that with ever more "active" drugs, the physician may now be held in less esteem than he was in the past when he relied more heavily on the placebo effect.

Often, the psychoanalytical concept of "transference" is invoked to explain placebo effects. This would involve faith in the doctor as a powerful healer, expectations of being helped, and reaction to the physician as a representative of the potent and effective world body of scientific healing. The concept of regression to the oral dependent phase of development is often cited as a mechanism for this readiness to respond to the physician's administrations. Some have suggested that all forms of psychotherapy rely, in part, upon the mobilization of a patient's expectation of being made better (16). Negative placebo reactions or placebo side effects can also be considered in this light and may correspond to negative transference reactions.

The doctor-patient interaction is affected by more than the patient and his transference. The physician's personality and his attitude toward the patient and the medications also influence the placebo quotient of his prescriptions. In a study using dextroamphetamine or placebo as an anorexogenic agent, different resident physicians were "conditioned to respond to the patients in a similar manner" (17). Treatment modalities included times when the physician was blind to the drugs being given and times when he knew their identity. At the end of one week, there were significant physician, drug, and treatment modality effects on patients' weight loss; these all disappeared by four weeks, when the only significant effect was that of the active drug, dextroamphetamine. Inspection of the data, however, reveals that the results would have been quite different if certain physicians were included and others excluded. The physician's personality and behavior had a significant impact on the patient and on the placebo effect, reflecting that quality often described as "bedside manner."

It should also be remembered that inert and inactive placebos are never totally without effect. Some side effects can be explained by an allergic reaction to the substance used to make the "inert" placebo. Sham surgery, with its anesthesia, incision, and blood loss, is far from inert. Lactose placebo may be a "sweet" pill, while, by comparison, the active compound may be a "bitter" one. The physical properties of the placebo may also be important. One study indicated that phobias respond better to green pills than to red or yellow ones (18). Finally, if everything else is held constant, a 5-grain lactose placebo four times a day for many years could result in a significant weight gain.

INDICATIONS

Leslie (19) has suggested that there are several indications for placebo use. He has included support for strong dependency feelings, substitution for sedative or hypnotic medications, inducement for return visits for more specific psychotherapy, provision of a "gentle sop" while an impatient patient waits for diagnostic procedures to be completed, and use as a research tool. Probably, there are occasions when the deliberate use of placebos as a therapeutic agent is appropriate. However, in some of the above-mentioned situations, the substitution of placebos for active medication may reflect the physician's unwillingness to deal with an unpleasant interpersonal situation (Chapter 30).

The employment of placebos in the evaluation of the effectiveness of other medications is one of their most important uses. The introduction of the *double-blind* paradigm marked a significant advance in the evaluation of all medical treatment and is currently considered to be indispensable in the evaluation of any new treatment. The minimal requirement is that both the patient and the physician be "blind," i.e., unaware of the identity of the medication being administered. Also, those involved in the evaluation of the patient's response must also be blind to the medication's identity. Ideally, everyone who has contact with the patient should be blind, and knowledge of the identity of the medication should be restricted to as few people as practicable. The use of the double-blind technique has greatly relieved problems of unconscious patient and physician bias in evaluating drug effects.

Although double-blind trials are valuable, the use of placebos in such tests of new treatments is not always warranted. If there are known, effective treatments for a given disorder, then new treatments are usually compared to those agents, rather than to placebos. The use of the double-blind technique can also lead to a false sense of confidence in the results. It is difficult, if not impossible, to provide identical matching placebos (20), and both patient and staff may attempt to guess whether the medication is a placebo or the active agent. In one study, 96 percent of the patients believed that they were on the active medication, even though they knew that there was a 50 percent chance that they were receiving a placebo (21). Thus, most patients were convinced that the physician was actively taking care of them. Patients and staff may go to extraordinary lengths to discover the identity of the drug. Even if they fail to identify it, they often form opinions about its identity. Right or wrong, those opinions can influence the response.

CONTRAINDICATIONS

Using placebos as a diagnostic tool must be done with extreme caution. The absence of response to a placebo may suggest an organic basis for the disease, but the presence of a response in no way rules it out. The positive response to placebos may deter the physician from pursuing underlying serious organic pathology.

Finally, the ethics of placebo use must be considered. Deception is certainly a part of the use of placebos, although when the physician and patient are both unaware that the drug is a placebo this may not be an ethical issue. Is it ever appropriate to knowingly use deception in treating a patient? In certain cases the answer must be "yes." For instance, when the angry paranoid patient asks the whereabouts of another person, it may not be wise to reply truthfully. However, the routine, conscious use of placebos can lead to difficulties. It can precipitate loss of the physician's credibility, should the patient find out that he is receiving a placebo. In addition, even knowing better, the physician may come to regard the patient in a less favorable light, because he responds to the placebo. The deception of the patient, no matter how well intentioned, must have some effect on the physician-patient relationship. This is especially true when treating "psychosomatic" disorders, where the use of placebos can be a means of avoiding psychological issues (Chapter 30). Another danger is that the physician may come to believe that the placebo is indeed effective, especially if it is an active compound such as a vitamin. It would seem, therefore, that the potency of placebos should be recognized and considered in the evaluation of any treatment but that the deliberate and deceptive use of placebos should be avoided, except in unique situations.

REFERENCES

1. Shapiro, A. K. Semantics of the placebo. *Psychiatr. Q. 42:653–695*, 1968.
2. Cobb, L. A., Thomas, G. I., Dillard, D. H., Merendino, K. A., and Bruce, R. A. An evaluation of internal-mammary-artery ligation by a double-blind technique. *N. Engl. J. Med. 260:1115–1117*, 1959.
3. Haas, H., Fink, H., and Hartfelder, G. The placebo problem. *Psychopharmacol. Serv. Cent. Bull. 2(8):1–65*, 1963.
4. Klopfer, B. Psychological variables in human cancer. *J. Proj. Tech. 21: 331–340*, 1957.
5. Wolf, S. Effects of suggestion and conditioning on the action of chemical agents in human subjects—the pharmacology of placebos. *J. Clin. Invest. 29:100–109*, 1950.
6. Lasagna, L., Laties, V. G., and Dohan, J. Further studies on the "pharmacology" of placebo administration. *J. Clin. Invest. 37:533–537*, 1958.
7. Rickels, K., Hesbacher, P. T., Weise, C. C., Gray, B., and Feldman, H. S. Pills and improvement: a study of placebo response in psychoneurotic outpatients. *Psychopharmacologia 16:318–328*, 1970.
8. Honigfeld, G. Non-specific factors in treatment. 1. Review of placebo reactions and placebo reactors. *Dis. Nerv. Sys. 25:145–156*, 1964.
9. Vinar, O. Dependence on a placebo: a case report. *Br. J. Psychiatry 115:1189–1190*, 1969.
10. Beecher, H. K. Evidence for increased effectiveness of placebos with increased stress. *Am. J. Physiol. 187:163–169*, 1956.
11. Linton, H. B. and Langs, R. J. Placebo reactions in a study of lysergic acid diethylamide (LSD-25). *Arch. Gen. Psychiatry 6:53–67*, 1962.
12. Shapiro, A. K. Placebo effects in psychotherapy and psychoanalysis. *J. Clin. Pharmacol. 10:73–78*, 1970.
13. Lehmann, H. E. and Knight, D. A. Placebo-proneness and placebo-resistance of different psychological functions. *Psychiatr. Q. 34:505–516*, 1960.
14. Pihl, R. O. and Altman, J. An experimental analysis of the placebo effect. *J. Clin. Pharmacol. 11:91–95*, 1971.
15. Houston, W. R. The doctor himself as a therapeutic agent. *Ann. Int. Med. 11:1416–1424*, 1938.
16. Frank, J. D. *Persuasion and Healing.* Baltimore: Johns Hopkins University Press, 1961.
17. Freund, J., Krupp, G., Goodenough, D., and Preston, L. W. The doctor-patient relationship and drug effect. *Clin. Pharmacol. Ther. 13:172–180*, 1972.
18. Schapira, K., McClelland, H. A., Griffiths, N. R., and Newell, D. J. Study on the effects of tablet colour in the treatment of anxiety states. *Br. Med. J. 2:446–449*, 1970.
19. Leslie, A. Ethics and practice of placebo therapy. *Am. J. Med. 16: 854–862*, 1954.
20. Blumenthal, D. S., Burke, R., and Shapiro, A. K. The validity of "identical matching placebos." *Arch. Gen. Psychiatry 31:214–215*, 1974.
21. Stallone, F., Mendlewicz, J., and Fieve, R. P. How blind is the double-blind?: An assessment in a lithium-prophylaxis study. *Lancet 1:619–620*, 1974.

32 | Methodological Aspects of Psychopharmacology

HELENA CHMURA KRAEMER

INTRODUCTION

Evaluation of scientific studies is a continuing challenge both to the basic scientist and to the clinician. The problem is not merely to distinguish bad research from good research. Often, it is tempting to assume that reports in reputable scientific journals have more scientific validity than those which appear elsewhere. And yet, even the best methodology, applied to a thoughtful and explicit research question, cannot ensure that the interpretation of the results is correct. This chapter describes some ways in which to approach the evaluation of research data. Very little will be said about the actual process of statistical analysis (cf. 1–5). Rather, we will concentrate upon broader issues of experimental design.

To a great extent, the intellectual processes needed to evaluate reports of research findings overlap those required to design and to analyze research data. In one respect, the former process is easier, because the evaluation is retrospective; in another, it is more difficult, since evaluation must be based entirely upon the information presented. Attempts to evaluate a research project presuppose that the essential information is presented in the research report. This includes a description of the specific research question and of the methods used. In addition, the report should specify the population to whom the results apply, the procedure used to obtain a sample of that population, and the basis for believing that this sample represents the specific population. Any measures used should be defined so that no misunderstanding as to the import or significance can ensue, and descriptive statistics should permit an evaluation of the magnitude of the effect. Finally, sufficient information about the statistical analysis should be included so that the basis of the researcher's claim to a true, rather than chance, finding can be evaluated.

RESEARCH RATIONALE

To illustrate the approach to research evaluation, we will focus on one simple research question: does a given treatment (drug) used for a specified type of subject affect a certain outcome measure? The "outcome measure" may be any measurable response of a subject to treatment, ranging from physical measures of weight, blood pressure, or recovery time to psychological measures of mood, alertness, or psychotic state.

POPULATION SPECIFICATION

In evaluating a research report, one should first focus upon the specification of "subject." The totality of subjects to whom the results of the research are relevant is the *population*. Practical considerations dictate that the entire population cannot be studied. Thus, the researcher selects a relatively small subgroup of the population, the *sample*, to represent the population. Whatever is seen in the study of the sample should be typical of what would have happened in the population had it been studied in its entirety.

One can never be absolutely sure that a sample is representative of a population, but elementary methodology textbooks suggest that the best approach is to select a *random* sample, i.e., one in which each member of the population has an equal chance of being selected for study. At this point, theory and reality part company: it is virtually impossible to select a random sample in real applications. To do so, one needs access to the population as a whole. Not only is the researcher usually denied this access, but it is often unclear exactly how to identify the population in its entirety. In reality, a sample is selected, simply enough, because it is accessible to the researcher. The researcher must then delineate the boundaries of the population which is represented by presenting descriptive material about his sample. Since the applicability of whatever other information is contained in the research report depends on a comprehension of the population to which the results apply, this definition is a necessary first step.

EXPERIMENTAL MEASURES

The outcome measure must be defined. If it is objective and well defined, such as weight, blood pressure, or hormone level, little need be said. If, however, the measure is one of mood or affect or if it is a subjective rating, considerably more care should be taken (cf. Chapter 5). A score on a written test labeled "depression" is just a score, unless it has been shown to correlate with behaviors which are acknowledged to constitute depression. Whether or not the researcher develops his own measures, it is his responsibility to present evidence that they are valid indicators of the phenomenon being measured.

DATA PRESENTATION

The essence of a research report must be an accurate and informative description of what happened to the sample subjects and what can be anticipated for other members of the population. If the sample size is very small, data on individual subjects may be presented. For large samples, *descriptive statistics* are used, including means, variances, medians, percentages, and graphical data summaries. Such descriptions should indicate whether the effect being studied is of sufficient magnitude to be of practical or clinical significance. If it is not, attempts to show statistical significance are irrelevant. Statistical tests are of value only in providing an indication of the applicability of specific results to the general population. Totally ineffective treatments can produce the appearance of effectiveness simply by chance.

STATISTICAL ANALYSIS

The choice of particular statistical procedure used to test whether an apparent drug-placebo response difference may be accounted for by chance factors alone depends upon the nature of the response measure being used and the technique for generating responses.

With experimental designs in which subjects are randomly assigned to drug and placebo groups, the statistical significance of a difference between drug and placebo is classically evaluated with a t-test (3). This procedure, however, is valid only if: 1) the response measures are interval scaled and 2) the variability of responses within each group are of similar magnitude. If the two groups are of the same size, the second requirement is not as vital to the validity of the test procedure. Theoretically, one should also require that the measures follow a normal distribution, i.e., the familiar bell-shaped curve, but the t-test is relatively robust with respect to this requirement, generally tending not to mislead when this requirement is violated.

If the response measures are on an ordinal scale or if they are interval scaled but do not satisfy the variance/sample size requirement, an alternative procedure is the Mann-Whitney test (3,4). Not only does this test impose less stringent criteria on the quality of the data, but it tends to be easier to compute and entails no great loss in test power.

Finally, the response measures may be categorical. For example, the response may be in terms of side effects, such as nausea and vertigo which cannot be ordered. In this case, the χ^2 test (3,4) is an appropriate technique to compare drug and placebo response.

The above three procedures are listed in order of their power and, concomitantly, in order of the quality of the response measures. One cannot validly apply a more powerful test procedure than one is entitled to by the nature of those measures without risk of false positive and false negative conclusions. Nor can one apply these procedures when measures are obtained by a repeated-measure design. All three tests require that each observation be on a separate and independent subject.

If each subject contributes both a drug and a placebo response measure which is interval scaled, the most common procedure is use of the "matched pair t-test" (3); for ordinal-scaled data, there is the Wilcoxon Matched-Pairs Signed-Ranks Test (4). Both of these procedures assume that an appropriate measure of change is the difference between drug and placebo response. Why the *difference* between drug and placebo response? Why not *percentage change* or some other more complex change measure? How one assesses change is a very controversial question. One can avoid the issue by using a test procedure which yields the same results whatever the appropriate change measure, e.g., the Sign Test (3,4), which looks only at whether there is or is not a change in a given direction, rather than at the magnitude of that change.

More elegant procedures, such as regression analyses and anlysis of covariance, can be used in certain of these situations; and improved techniques are currently being evolved (5).

DATA EVALUATION

The *significance level* of a statistical test is an evaluation of the probability that the result is due simply to random or chance effects. If we define as a "positive result" the conclusion that the drug affects the outcome measure, the significance level is the risk of a false positive result (a Type I error). Scientific convention decrees that this risk be kept small, usually to less than 5 percent or 1 percent. There is also the risk of a false negative result, so that an effective treatment appears to be ineffective (Type II error). The *power* of a statistical test is the complement of this risk, i.e., the probability of a true negative result. There are no set standards for minimal test power. Generally, the power of the test depends upon the effort put into the research as reflected by sample size, research design, reliability of measurement, and choice of statistical test procedures. The confidence engendered in the validity of the conclusion depends upon an understanding of the factors which may lead to both types of errors.

False Positive Results

Even a perfectly executed research project has a chance of a false positive result, as defined by the significance level. This is, however, a minimal risk. A greater risk occurs when the significance level does not define the risk, because there are basic design errors which introduce extraneous factors that obscure or distort the treatment effect.

The researcher needs to demonstrate that the reaction of a subject is changed by the drug or treatment being studied. The simplest way of accomplishing this task is to split the sample into two groups, one being given the drug—the "experimental group"—and the other being treated similarly but with no drug—the "control group." The difference between the response of the two groups should be a measure of drug effectiveness. Unfortunately, any nonrandom assignment of subjects to experimental and control groups may produce differences which are due to selection bias rather than to treatment. Subtle and unconscious biases on the part of the researcher or subject may produce false positive results. For example, the enthusiastic researcher may unconsciously choose slightly healthier or younger subjects for the "experimental group." An intriguing example of potential bias is that introduced by the use of the consent form for human subjects. The factors which determine whether a person will agree to participate in a research project are not well understood; nor is it obvious that there is any uniform set of such factors for all research interventions. If a person is randomly assigned to experiment or control group and, when approached for consent, is then informed of his assignment, his decision to participate may depend on the assignment. If the decision process were in some way correlated with the outcome measure, false positive results might arise.

In general, one must have confidence that any differences between test groups are related solely to treatment effect. If assignment is random, there is some assurance that the groups at least start the same. However, any subsequent differential treatment of groups may produce differences which are not related to drug effect. Thus, if one group is monitored, given pills or injections, or counseled, while the control group has literally no intervention, apparent differences may be induced by the process, not the drug. It is essential that, as far as possible, the one and only difference is the drug itself. If a subject is informed as to which group he is in, his expectations may produce group differences. Similarly, if researchers know which subjects have been exposed to the drug, their treatment of subjects or evaluation of response may be affected. These considerations have led to the "double-blind" design for experiments, in which neither subject nor investigator knows the design until the experiment is over (Chapter 31). Anything which is not essential to the definition of the treatment should be uniformly administered to both groups. If the treatment is a medication, a similar, but inert, substance—placebo—should be administered to the other group, since the process of administering medications may itself produce a response known as the placebo effect (Chapter 31).

Individual differences among subjects also have a major impact upon scientific studies (Chapter 5). The behavioral response of a subject to administration of a drug depends, first, on his normal base response; second, on his reaction to the experimental situation (placebo response); and third, on his reaction to the drug itself. Subjects may differ substantially at all three of these levels. In the type of study described above, one can assert that the drug is effective only if the between-group differences are large relative to within-group differences. The effect of substantial individual differences is to make within-group differences very large, so that the behavioral effect of the drug must be concomitantly larger.

Baseline response and placebo response can themselves be of importance (Chapter 31). In addition, their presence weakens the ability to identify a real drug effect. To overcome this problem, one can use the same subjects for both control and experimental groups. In such a design, each subject is given a placebo trial at one time and a drug trial at another. The placebo response would reflect that subject's baseline and placebo reaction; the drug response would indicate the additional effect of the drug. The difference between the two should reflect pure drug response, with variability among subjects arising only from individual differences in the reaction to the drug. Thus, at least in theory, the research question is asked more directly, so that the outcome will be clearer, the tests more powerful, and the subjects fewer.

Precautions must still be taken in designs in which the subject serves as his own control. Subjects must be treated identically under experimental and control conditions. Each subject must be informed that, in the course of the experiment, he will be given both placebo and drug; but no subject should be informed explicitly or implicitly when or in what order these will be given him. Otherwise, any observed drug effect may, in fact, be strictly due to subject or evaluator expectations and perceptions, rather than to the drug itself.

The time factor itself may also produce false positive results. Over time, subject cooperation and compliance may diminish, evaluator competence may change, or the subject response on the behavioral variable may vary. If every subject were given drug and placebo in the same order, a detected difference might arise from these time-related changes, with no relation to the drug. For this reason, it is advisable to randomly assign the order of treatments for each subject or to randomly divide the sample into two halves, one half to be given placebo first, the other, drug first (cross-over design). Such designs are not without ethical ramifications. Often, researchers are loath to risk using a new drug except for a patient who seems to be unresponsive to conventional treatments. If the "placebo" is the conventional treatment to which the subject already failed to respond, a serious bias may have been introduced into the study.

Even if time effects are absent, a false positive result may result because of *regression to the mean*. Virtually all measurements of subject response, particularly of behavioral response, are unreliable to some extent. As a result, those who give an abnormal response on the "placebo" test comprise two subgroups: those who are indeed abnormal and those who are inappropriately classified as abnormal because of measurement errors. Upon retest, a few of the truly abnormal subjects would inappropriately be classified as normal and most of the false-abnormal subjects would also fall within the normal range. Thus, a sample which initially had 100 percent in the abnormal range would now have a substantial proportion in the normal range, giving the appearance of a drug-induced change, even though no such change actually occurred.

The above considerations were deliberately restricted to a research project studying a single behavioral parameter. Typically, however, several parameters are studied simultaneously. Investigation of a large number of parameters can create insoluble problems of interpretation. To illustrate the difficulty, suppose one replaced all the data with random numbers. It would be comforting to believe that no significant drug effects would then be found. When only one behavioral parameter is being studied, the probability of a significant result would be the significance level, e.g., 5 percent. However, as the number of behavioral parameters increases to 5, 10, 50, or 100, the probability that one or more of these parameters would be found, by chance, to be significantly affected by the drug increases from 5 percent to 22.6 percent, 40.1 percent, 92.3 percent, and 99.4 percent, respectively. That is, of the total number of behavior parameters, 5 percent would be expected to be found to be significantly affected by the drug, even with totally random data. This phenomenon makes it difficult to interpret the results of a multiparameter study. For pilot studies, this research approach is of tremendous value. Not only does it provide an empirical basis for selection of behavioral variables, but it also helps to identify unforeseen sampling and measurement difficulties and to provide a statistical basis for sample-size selection and analytical decisions. However, as a basis for clinical decisions, the results from such studies must be validated by additional investigation of a particular parameter of interest.

False Negative Results

False negative results, too, can arise by chance; but, unlike false positive results, there is usually no indication of the magnitude of this risk. With small sample size the risk may be greater than 50 percent. For this reason alone, one should treat negative results more tentatively than one would deal with positive results. By far the most common reasons for false negative results are: too small a sample size, insensitive or unreliable measures, and inadequate statistical analysis. One other reason deserves specific mention.

For the reasons already mentioned, cross-over designs are deservedly favored in pharmacological research. However, evaluation of the resulting data should be tempered with the understanding that carry-over effects can produce false negative results. Thus, multiple treatments in close temporal sequence may mean that the response to a treatment is affected not only by the treatment itself but by the preceding treatments. If response to a particular treatment is assessed on the basis of the sample as a whole, true drug responses may be masked by carry-over effects. This interference can be minimized by expanding the time sequence, so that response returns to baseline levels after each treatment. Alternatively, one can take sequence effects into account in analysis. In either case, separate descriptive statistics of drug responses for each subgroup permit an evaluation of the impact of carry-over effects on the outcome, at least on a superficial level.

CONCLUSION

Statistical analysis is not designed to unearth effects where none apparently exist. It should, instead, be used to minimize the chance of error. Ultimately, if one is convinced of the clinical significance of the results, statistical consideration provides an additional measure of assurance that comparable results can be expected for other population members. In the face of apparent clinical importance, a lack of statistical significance should motivate a search for further verification of the result. Conversely, if one does not accept the clinical significance of the results, statistical significance is irrelevant.

REFERENCES

1. Chasson, J. B. *Research Design in Clinical Psychology and Psychiatry.* New York: Appleton-Century-Crofts, 1967.
2. Dixon, W. J. and Massey, F. J., Jr. *Introduction to Statistical Analysis.* New York: McGraw-Hill Book Company, 1969.
3. Siegel, S. *Nonparametric Statistics for the Behavioral Sciences.* New York: McGraw-Hill Book Company, 1956.
4. Goldstein, A. *Biostatistics.* New York: The Macmillan Company, 1964.
5. Klein, D. F., Ross, D. C., and Feldman S. Analysis and display of psychopharmacological data. *J. Psychiatr. Res. 12*:125–147, 1975.

513

33 | Convulsive and Coma Therapies and Psychosurgery

GEORGE GULEVICH

INTRODUCTION

In psychiatry, "somatic therapies" refer to physical treatments of psychiatric disorders in which drug use is either absent or secondary to the primary therapeutic modality. Modern somatic therapies include convulsive and coma therapies and psychosurgery. It is of interest that the major modern somatic therapies were all introduced in Europe between 1933 and 1938. The prevailing orientation of European psychiatrists during that decade was decidedly organic; and the major mental disorders, including schizophrenia, depression, and mania, were presumed to have biological origins. These attitudes may have been influenced by the earlier success of malaria therapy for general paresis, as described below. The treatments described in this chapter reflect some of the first attempts to treat psychiatric disorders by deliberately altering brain chemistry. Although many of these treatments have subsequently been replaced by psychoactive drugs, they still are of great importance in the history of psychiatry.

MALARIA THERAPY

The first successful biological treatment in Western medicine for any mental illness may have been the malaria therapy for general paresis, or tertiary syphilis. In the early 1900's, general paresis accounted for about 50 percent of the patients in mental hospitals. In view of the sanitary standards of those institutions, it is not surprising that the Austrian psychiatrist von Jaurreg had opportunities to observe the effects of severe febrile illness in psychotic patients. He noticed that some patients were less psychotic after they recovered from their fever. In 1917, von Jaurreg decided to see if the deliberate induction of a febrile illness might be of value in treating psychotic patients. He elected to use malaria for this purpose, because it could be controlled with quinine. Von Jaurreg took blood from patients with malaria and injected it into patients with "chronic psychosis." After ten to twelve bouts of fever, the patients were treated with quinine. This treatment was tried on patients with many psychiatric disorders but worked only for those with tertiary syphilis. Subsequent investigations have demonstrated that the high temperatures produced by the fever immobilized the syphilis spirochetes in the brain. Naturally, the introduction of powerful antibiotics such as penicillin have obviated the need for malaria treatments (1).

INSULIN COMA THERAPY (ICT)

Shortly after the discovery of insulin, several psychiatrists began to prescribe it to psychiatric patients who needed to gain weight. An Austrian, Manfred Sakel, noted that the occasional schizophrenic patient who inadvertently developed insulin coma would often emerge from the coma with an improved mental state. In 1933, Sakel described the use of insulin coma for treating schizophrenia. Insulin coma therapy was somewhat cumbersome, often protracted, and required a special unit with well-trained medical personnel. Over a period of two to four weeks, patients were given incremental doses of insulin, until they developed a hypoglycemic coma. Treatment then consisted of repeated induction of insulin coma. A full course of therapy often entailed induction of one hundred or more comas, requiring hospitalization for four to five months, even when treatments were given six times a week. Insulin coma therapy now enjoys only limited use throughout the world, having been replaced primarily by drug therapies. The treatment process is difficult, potentially dangerous, and expensive. Thus, this decline in popularity is understandable. However, some proponents still regard insulin coma as the most effective available means for treating schizophrenia. The mechanism by which insulin coma produces its therapeutic effects is unknown (2).

PHARMACOLOGICAL CONVULSIVE THERAPIES

METRAZOL

The convulsive therapies were introduced by von Meduna on the basis of two observations. Along with other psychiatrists of that time, the Hungarian noted that many patients, including schizophrenics and severe depressives, would lose their psychotic symptoms after a spontaneous convulsion. On the basis of the statistics which were available at that time, von Meduna also concluded that epilepsy and schizophrenia rarely occurred together. Thus, he hypothesized that by inducing convulsions in schizophrenic patients, he might ameliorate their schizophrenic symptomatology. Von Meduna first attempted to produce convulsions with intramuscular injections of camphor and oil. The toxic properties of this combination produced difficulties, however, and he eventually used a soluble synthetic camphor derivative, pentylenetetrazol (Metrazol). Pentylenetetrazol can be injected intravenously and produces seizures within approximately thirty seconds (3–5).

Initially, Metrazol convulsive therapy was used for the treatment of schizophrenia. It was later recognized that the affective psychoses responded better to convulsive therapy than did schizophrenia. However, Metrazol never became a widely accepted treatment modality. Patients were extremely reluctant and fearful of this treatment, since the seizure would frequently precede the loss of consciousness. Prior to the seizure, patients would often have a sense of extreme foreboding, precordial pains, and a feeling that they were going to die. The introduction of electroconvulsive therapy (ECT) in 1938 practically eliminated the use of this particular somatic therapy.

INDOKLON

The only other pharmacological agent now used for convulsive therapy is hexafluorodiethyl ether (Indoklon). It was discovered by the American pharmacologist Kranz in 1957, and can be applied as an inhalant by means of a mask and vaporizer. After inhaling hezafluoro-diethyl ether, patients lose consciousness, have some mild clonic movements, and finally develop a tonic clonic convulsion similar to that resulting from other forms of convulsive therapy. Indoklon therapy uses essentially the same techniques employed with ECT, and the indications for and effectiveness of the two treatments are similar. However, unlike ECT, Indoklon therapy frequently causes nausea and may cause liver damage. Indoklon therapy has never achieved the•popularity of ECT as a treatment modality for severe depression (3–5).

ELECTROCONVULSIVE THERAPY (ECT)

Two Italian psychiatrists, Cerletti and Bini, introduced ECT in 1938. The standard technique that they devised is still rather extensively used, although different types of current have been recommended. The effects of ECT on brain function are unclear (3–5). However, it is known that ECT markedly alters the turnover of several neurotransmitters, including norepinephrine (cf. Chapter 10).

Technique
The proper preparation of the patient for ECT is essential and should include a complete physical and psychiatric examination. The physical examination should focus in particular on the cardiovascular and neurological functioning of the patient. A pre-ECT electrocardiogram (ECG) is required. X-rays of the dorsal, thoracic, and lumbar vertebrae are also needed to permit detection of spinal osteoporosis or of old spinal fractures. The patient should also be counseled about the results to be expected from ECT and about possible side effects. Counseling is also extremely important in helping to allay any unrealistic fears that the patient may have about ECT. These counseling sessions should include appropriate family members, so that they may continue to be supportive to the patient during the treatment period. This approach to pre-ECT counseling enhances the rapport both between the therapist and the patient and between the therapist and the patient's family.

In most institutions, ECT is administered in the morning, three times per week, with at least one day intervening between each treatment. The patient is instructed to take nothing by mouth from the preceding midnight. Approximately fifteen minutes prior to the treatment, the patient is given atropine intramuscularly to decrease salivation and respiratory secretion. Alternatively, atropine can be given intravenously immediately before the treatment. After he receives the atropine, the patient is made comfortable and asked to remove any dental prostheses which might be aspirated during the administration of ECT. It is valuable to have staff members present who have established some positive rapport with the patient. This appears to facilitate the reduction of pre-ECT anxiety and helps to orient the patient to his surroundings following ECT.

Once the patient is comfortable, he is anesthetized with a short-acting barbiturate. In most cases, sodium methoxehital (Brevital) is given intravenously in a dosage level of 30–100 mg. Sodium methoxehital has largely replaced sodium thiopental, because the former is shorter acting, is less likely to produce cardiac arrhythmias, and seems to have less hypotensive effect. Sodium methoxehital should be administered only by qualified personnel who are skilled in all aspects of cardiopulmonary resuscitation. Usually a muscle relaxant drug is also administered, to prevent fractures and muscle ruptures during the convulsion. This modification of ECT was first introduced by Bennett, in 1940, who used curare to paralyze the muscles. Currently, the electrically induced seizure is modified with succinylcholine (Anectine), a neuromuscular depolarizing agent. A dosage of 30–80 mg of succinylcholine will attenuate the seizures, so that only minimal clonic movements of the fingers and toes are apparent. Manifestations of succinylcholine action begin as fasciculations in the various muscles, followed by loss of knee and other reflexes, and finally by muscular paralysis.

As the succinylcholine produces paralysis, the patient is preoxygenated with an air bag. Moistened electrodes are then placed bitemporally, and electric current is applied as prescribed for the particular machine being used. A soft bite-block is used to prevent injury to the patient, and the jaw is held shut. Following administration of the current, a tonic phase ensues which is quickly followed by peripheral clonic movements that may last from several seconds to one minute. Following the clonic phase, the patient is again oxygenated and then allowed to recover. Performed in this manner, ECT produces no pain and no awareness of the seizure. Succinylcholine is hydrolized within one to three minutes, and the effects of sodium methoxehital are usually over in two to four minutes. Upon awakening—usually within a matter of one to two minutes—the patient will experience post-ictal confusion for up to thirty minutes. During this recovery period, the patient should have vital signs monitored and be given supportive reassurance by a member of the staff who is known to him. Some patients become very confused and agitated during this period. This post-ECT excitement state can usually be managed with 5 mg of intramuscular chlordiazepoxide (Librium) (3–6).

Unilateral electrostimulation was introduced in 1956, as a method which might produce less confusion and memory impairment. In this technique, one temporal electrode is placed on the nondominant side. Presently, the general consensus is that unilateral ECT does produce less confusion and memory loss than does bilateral stimulation; however, the therapeutic effects also appear to be somewhat less. To achieve desired results, workers preferring the unilateral method often give a few more treatments than might be necessary with the bilateral method (5,6).

Complications

To the prospective patient, the fear of complications or of adverse side effects are often the most distressing aspect of ECT. It is mandatory that the psychiatrist be fully aware of complications and adverse effects, so that he can help the patient to make a suitable judgment regarding the administration of ECT. Prior to the introduction of muscle relaxant drugs, the most frequent complications in convulsive therapy were fractures. The fractures were of two main types: those in the dorsal spine, generally between the fourth and eighth vertebrae, and those in the long bones, generally in the head of the humerus and the head of the femur. Occasional ruptures of muscle groups were also noted in unmodified ECT. Although these particular problems were alleviated with the introduction of anesthetics and muscle relaxants into the ECT procedure, cardiovascular and pulmonary complications became more common. Thus, clinicians must be aware of possible effects these drugs might have on a patient with a history of myocardial disease, hypertension, or other serious medical disorders.

With ECT, fatalities generally result from cardiac arrest, respiratory arrest, or myocardial infarction. Even with unmodified ECT, fatalities were extremely rare. Many workers believe that the electrically induced convulsion does not differ from a spontaneous one, and the extensive literature on seizure disorders has amply demonstrated that the occurrence of spontaneous seizures need not affect other aspects of an epileptic's health.

The most common side effects of ECT are memory loss and confusion. Memory loss is characterized by a combination of anterograde and retrograde amnesia. Amnesia generally becomes noticeable after the third or fourth treatment and worsens as the number of treatments increases. Normally, older people exhibit more memory loss with ECT, although the extent of memory loss varies widely among patients. Following cessation of treatment, memory gradually returns over three to six weeks, depending upon the number of treatments given. Post-ECT confusion is an acute organic brain syndrome with disorientation, memory impairment, euphoria, and affective dullness. The intensity of the organic reaction depends upon both the number and the temporal spacing of the treatments. Again, elderly patients tend to become more confused than do younger patients, although there are wide individual variations. A reduction in treatment frequency will ameliorate the confusional state. Since almost all patients receiving ECT will develop memory loss and some degree of confusion, it is important for the psychiatrist to be aware of the impact of these changes upon the patient's family. Often, family members become extremely concerned and fearful, when the patient fails to recall their name or, perhaps, even to recognize them. Prior development of therapeutic rapport between the psychiatrist and the family can help the family through this difficult time (3–6).

Indications

ECT was originally introduced as a treatment for schizophrenia. Shortly after its introduction, however, it became obvious that the best results were obtained in severe depressions. For many years, ECT was the overwhelming treatment of choice for severe depression and for various forms of schizophrenia. More recently, with the development of effective psychopharmacological agents and with increased public concern about the effects of ECT, its use has declined.

Severe depressions continue to be the primary indication for ECT (3–7). The effect of ECT on severe endogenous depressions can be one of the more spectacular therapeutic responses that psychiatrists are likely to see. Recurrent unipolar depression, the depressed phase of bipolar affective illness, involutional depression, postpartum depression, and depression of later life all respond well to ECT. Both retarded and agitated depressions respond well to ECT, often evincing dramatic improvement after three to five treatments. The target symptoms of depression which generally respond to ECT include suicidal ideation, anorexia, weight loss, constipation, early-morning awakening, decreased sexual functioning, low self-esteem, feeling of worthlessness and hopelessness, and pronounced guilt feelings. Usually, six to twelve treatments are required. The number of treatments must be determined empirically, since patient response varies markedly. Most clinicians agree that it is advisable to give two to three treatments after depressive symptoms have improved. Cessation of treatments at the first sign of the clearing of depression may result in quicker relapse, although this has not been demonstrated conclusively.

There is considerable evidence that ECT is at least equal to and perhaps superior to antidepressant drugs in the treatment of depression (7). In addition, the speed of action of ECT is somewhat faster than that of the tricyclic antidepressants (tricyclics). This may be an important fact to consider when treating the acutely suicidal patient. However, since such patients require hospitalization, the suicidal risk of using antidepressants may be obviated. On the negative side, the relapse rate following ECT treatment is considerably higher than that with tricyclics. Thus, depressed patients treated with ECT should subsequently receive maintenance therapy with tricyclics. Memory loss and confusion are also negative consequences of ECT. Obviously, these symptoms make the patient much less accessible to ongoing psychotherapy and to examination of those psychosocial factors which led to or aggravated the depression. Generally, depression should be treated with an adequate trial of antidepressants (Chapter 11). ECT should be considered as a treatment modality if drug therapy fails. ECT may also be appropriate for patients who present so severe a suicide risk that even hospitalization offers less than adequate security or for patients who previously have had good responses to ECT and poor responses to antidepressants.

ECT is also indicated for treating catatonic stupors and catatonic excitement (3–6). For these states, treatments are generally given on a daily basis. In fact, treatments may be given several times a day, to help calm the extremely agitated patient. Thus, for exceptionally difficult manic patients, ECT may be valuable during that period before lithium carbonate becomes effective (Chapter 12). Similarly, ECT should be considered as an adjunct for the antipsychotic drugs in treating the excited state of catatonic schizophrenia (Chapter 9). There is little or no evidence that ECT is useful in treating the primary symptoms of characterological disturbances, psychoneurotic disorders, or addictions.

Contraindications

Administration of ECT in its modified form is considered to be a safe procedure and is appropriate for a wide variety of patients. Many clinicians believe that there are virtually no absolute contraindications for ECT. It has been used successfully on a large number of patients who had prior histories of myocardial infarction, coronary artery disease, and other serious medical problems. However, increased intracranial pressure is a definite contraindication for ECT, since treatment elevates cerebral spinal fluid pressure and could increase the possibility of tentorial herniation in such patients. A recent history of myocardial infarction with continuing ECG changes and elevated enzymes is also a contraindication for ECT. Treatments can be resumed once the enzymes and the ECG have stabilized, but the patient should be treated with great caution. ECT can be administered in the presence of old or healed vertebral fractures or of vertebral osteoporosis. The use of muscle relaxants can minimize the possibility of exacerbating any spinal pathology. ECT has been administered to patients with major medical problems such as peptic ulcer, subdural hematoma, aortic aneurysm, and congestive heart failure, without aggravating any of these pre-existing conditions. In addition, it has been used successfully in pregnant women, with no apparent sequelae to mother or fetus. Thus, when ECT is strongly indicated, the presence of physical illness rarely appears to preclude its use. The clinician must weigh the possible advantages of ECT against the possible risks, explain the risks to the patient, and proceed accordingly (3–7).

Current Status of ECT

ECT has been beset by controversies ever since its introduction. These controversies have taken on moral, legal, ethical, and legislative overtones. When antidepressants became available in the early 1950s, the use of ECT diminished dramatically. However, as the limits of antidepressant medications have become clear, ECT use has gradually increased. More recently, legislative, social, and legal developments have placed constraints on the use of ECT. Several states have proposed legislation which would significantly delimit the clinician's discretion in using ECT. Much of the support for this type of legislation comes from groups who believe that ECT has been abused in its administration, to the serious and permanent detriment of patients. Many complain that ECT produces permanent damage to the brain, as reflected in memory loss and other sustained changes of affect. Others argue that it has been used for behavior control and punishment, rather than as a therapeutic measure.

Concern about sustained brain damage from ECT is one with which most clinicians are quite familiar. Available data reveal no decrement in cognitive tests given to patients before and after short-term ECT (3–8). However, this may be more indicative of the inadequacy of cognitive test procedures than of a lack of cerebral deficit due to convulsive therapy. Some clinicians report that patients who have received many ECT treatments can suffer cognitive impairment. However, evidence of such an effect in systematic, controlled studies is lacking. How is the patient who needs help and the psychiatrist who wishes to provide help to proceed through this current dilemma? Obviously, no definitive answers are yet available. Perhaps the best approach involves an open exchange among the physician, the patient, and the patient's family, so that treatment modalities can be selected in a rational, therapeutic environment.

PSYCHOSURGERY

Psychosurgery may predate written history, as demonstrated by the presence of trephine holes in prehistoric skulls. In early historic times, trephination was widely prescribed to relieve both physical and psychological distress. The modern method of psychosurgery was described in 1933 by Egas Moniz of Portugal, for which he won a Nobel Prize. Almedia Lima performed the first operation in 1935. Moniz argued that the fixed ideas and repetitive behavior seen in certain psychoses were accompanied by abnormal stabilization of cellular connections, particularly in the frontal lobes. He reasoned that psychotic patients might be cured, therefore, if these fixed arrangements of cellular connections were destroyed. Moniz reported that of his first twenty patients, one-third completely recovered, one-third improved, and one-third were unchanged. Freeman and Watts modified the original surgical procedure of Moniz and introduced psychosurgery to the United States in 1942 (9,10).

Moniz and Lima performed a bilateral prefrontal lobotomy by making several spherical cuts in the white matter of both hemispheres. The more widely used standard lobotomy by Freeman and Watts was a bilateral blind operation in which the white matter was cut in the plane anterior to the horns of the lateral ventricles. Most lobotomies sever tracts between cortex, subcortex, and basal ganglia. "Lobotomy" refers specifically to removal of cortical tissue, while "leukotomy" indicates that only white fibers have been severed (8–10). Lobotomy has a fatality rate of 2–4 percent, with frequent postoperative complications such as cerebral hemorrhage and convulsive seizures. In addition, it produces personality changes such as tactlessness, insensitivity, crudeness, sloppiness, irresponsibility, and a general disregard for social relations. As more experience was gathered with a variety of techniques and as data about the long-range consequences of such procedures accumulated, there was a trend toward smaller operations. Stereotactic operations in discrete brain areas were introduced in 1952 and included such procedures as thalamotomy, with destruction of the dorsal medial nucleus of the thalamus.

Psychosurgery was never intended as a specific treatment for any individual mental illness. It was used primarily to reduce disturbed behavior in schizophrenic patients. Currently, psychosurgery is scarcely used in the United States. However, in England, psychosurgery continues to have proponents, who use a variety of stereotactic procedures in selected psychiatric patients. Generally, these patients have suffered from their psychiatric disorder for many years and have been unresponsive to other treatment modalities. Best results seem to be obtained in obsessive-compulsive neurotics, who often report relief from their symptoms after years of suffering. In the United States, psychosurgery has recently been used in an effort to control aggressive individuals, frequently on individuals who were incarcerated for violent acts. Serious ethical, legal, and medical implications of using these procedures to control aggressive behavior in incarcerated individuals have sharply curtailed this practice.

The chemical mechanisms and balances which are altered by psychosurgery are not understood, and it is not yet possible to relate the effects of this procedure to those of any chemical mode of therapy. If

the treatment is of value in obsessive compulsive patients, an understanding of the underlying mechanism might be of immense value in
developing an effective pharmacological treatment for this intensely
disabling disorder, without the dangers and problems of psychosurgery.

REFERENCES

1. Kalinowsky, L. B.   Biological psychiatric treatments preceding pharma-cotherapy. *In: Discoveries in Biological Psychiatry.* F. J. Ayd and B. Blackwell, *eds.,* Philadelphia/Toronto: J. B. Lippincott, 1970, pp. 59–67.
2. Kalinowsky, L. B.   Insulin coma treatment. *In: Comprehensive Textbook of Psychiatry, II.* A. M. Freedman, H. I. Kaplan, and B. J. Saddock, *eds.,* Baltimore: Williams & Wilkins, 1975, pp. 1976–1979.
3. Kalinowski, L. B. and Hipius, H.   *Pharmacological, Convulsive, and Other Somatic Treatments in Psychiatry.* New York: Grune & Stratton, 1969.
4. Sargant, W., Slater, E., and Kelly, D.   *An Introduction to Physical Methods of Treatment in Psychiatry.* Edinburgh: Churchill Livingstone, 1972.
5. Kalinowsky, L. B.   The convulsive therapies. *In: Comprehensive Textbook of Psychiatry, II.* A. M. Freedman, H. I. Kaplan, and B. J. Saddocks, *eds.,* Baltimore: Williams & Wilkins, 1975, pp. 1969–1976.
6. Saltzman, Carl.   Electroconvulsive therapy. *In: Manual of Psychiatric Therapeutics.* R. I. Shader, *ed.,* Boston: Little, Brown, 1975, pp. 115–125.
7. Klein, D. F. and Davis, J. M.   *Diagnosis and Drug Treatment of Psychiatric Disorders.* Baltimore: Williams & Wilkins, 1969.
8. Redlich, F. C. and Freedman, D. X.   *The Theory and Practice of Psychiatry.* New York: Basic Books, Inc., 1966.
9. Freeman, W.   Psychosurgery. *In: American Handbook of Psychiatry.* S. Arieti, *ed.,* New York: Basic Books, 1959, pp. 1521–1541.
10. Kalinowsky, L. B.   Psychosurgery. *In: Comprehensive Textbook of Psychiatry. II.* A. M. Freedman, H. I. Kaplan, and B. J. Saddock, *eds.,* Baltimore: Williams & Wilkins, 1975, pp. 1979–1982.

34 | Promise and Limits of Psychopharmacology

JACK D. BARCHAS, PHILIP A. BERGER,

ROLAND D. CIARANELLO, and GLEN R. ELLIOTT

In his volume *The Structure of Scientific Revolutions*, Kuhn attempts to identify the changes which lead to a major shift in theoretical constructs in a scientific field, i.e., a scientific revolution. Included among the important developments are the discovery of empirical data which cannot be explained by previous conceptualizations and the appearance of new information which lies beyond the scope of earlier theories. Clearly, these and other processes were operative in the scientific revolution which has followed the development of potent psychopharmacological agents for treating mental illness. Cumulatively, the discovery and study of these agents have substantively changed the treatment of psychiatric patients and have provided a set of admittedly incomplete, but nevertheless powerful, conceptualizations about psychiatric disorders. To effectively examine future developments in psychopharmacology, we must consider its impact upon treatment practices in psychiatry, the current limits of such treatments, the problems arising from the availability of psychoactive drugs, and the ethical issues of deliberately manipulating mental function (1). Ultimately, we will need to integrate the information coming from psychopharmacology with that arising from analytical, behavioral, sociological, and other approaches to psychiatry.

CONDITIONS IN THE PRE-DRUG ERA

To comprehend the extent of the revolution which occurred in the treatment of the mentally ill after the introduction of pharmacotherapies, one must recall the conditions which existed before these therapies were introduced. Many psychiatrists who are still active can re-

527

member both the pre- and postdrug era, so that firsthand descriptions are relatively easy to obtain.

Before drug therapies became available during the mid-1950's, the primary treatment center for the mentally ill was the state mental hospital. Few outpatient clinics existed for psychiatric patients. Most general medical hospitals would not admit severely ill psychiatric patients; those which did often kept them only briefly, before transferring them to a state mental hospital. These state mental hospitals more closely resembled custodial institutions than treatment facilities.

Generally, the fate of the mentally ill was viewed pessimistically during this period. Each year the population in mental hospitals increased, since patients continued to be admitted but very few were discharged. Typically, patient living areas were crowded and poorly furnished. Schizophrenic patients with paranoid delusions could be found crouched in corners, living in constant fear. Catatonic patients might maintain the same rigid posture for prolonged periods, developing swollen legs and pressure sores. Hallucinating patients would pace the floor, talking to their voices and apparently unaware of their environment. Violent patients might attack staff members or other patients for reasons known only to themselves, leading to hostility and suspicion on both sides.

The psychiatrists charged with the care and treatment of psychiatric patients just described were baffled. Causes of and therapy for such disorders were unknown, and the illnesses were largely ignored in medical education. Before World War II, these patients were cared for mainly by physicians whose primary orientation was neurologic. After World War II, much of the responsibility was taken by physicians trained in psychoanalytic psychotherapy. However, neither neurological diagnosis and treatment nor psychoanalytic psychotherapy were effective in treating chronic schizophrenia or severe mania, so that the physician's primary functions became defined as administrative and custodial. Most patients could be expected to sit around on benches or floors, as their physical health gradually deteriorated over the years. Manic patients would laugh, joke, and maintain constant activity for days at a time until they collapsed, exhausted by the frenetic pace. Combative patients were secluded in rooms without furniture or strapped to beds which were bolted to the floor to prevent injury to the patients and others. Agitated patients were often placed in warm baths or tied in wet sheets in an effort to calm their frenzy (2).

Unpleasant as these conditions are to recall, their widespread existence generally did not result from deliberate actions of inhumane individuals. Many decent, well-meaning people endeavored to improve conditions in public mental hospitals. Their efforts were frustrated by public apathy, by the social stigma of mental illness, by lack of funds, and especially by the nonexistence of effective treatments.

ASPECTS OF THE IMPACT OF PSYCHOPHARMACOLOGY

As already mentioned, until the mid-1950's, most patients with severe mental illness were hospitalized in state and county mental hospitals. The population in these facilities had increased for many years, reaching a peak of over 500,000 by 1955; it then began to decrease, coinciding with increasing utilization of psychopharmacological therapies and other treatment changes. As therapy has improved, this decrease in the hospitalized patient population has continued, despite increases in the general population and in the face of a steadily increasing admission rate. By 1973, the number of patients in mental hospitals had fallen to 250,000.

In one sense, the above statistics are misleading. Naturally, many of the patients who leave the mental hospitals still have symptoms of mental illness. However, most can be treated in outpatient clinics and transitional facilities, enabling them to return to work, to reestablish family ties, and to participate in community life. Even patients who remain in the mental hospitals encounter a markedly different environment, with emphasis on milieu therapy and upon improving coping and adaptational mechanisms. Clearly, the treatment of severe mental illness has undergone profound and dramatic changes. These changes probably resulted from the interaction of numerous factors; but it is more than chance that they coincided with the development of effective pharmacological treatments for severe psychiatric illness.

In addition to improving the prognosis for psychiatric patients, effective psychopharmacological agents have had significant impact on basic and clinical research in psychiatry (3). Clinical research was stimulated as investigators attempted to confirm the effectiveness of these medications for treating mental illness. Such studies emphasized the need to precisely define mental disorders and their subtypes. In addition, they stimulated the development of new methods for evaluating the improvement or worsening of psychiatric symptoms, including the double-blind and crossover research designs (Chapter 32).

Basic research on brain function has also been promoted and influenced by the promise of drug treatments for mental illness. As emphasized throughout this text, much of this research is directed toward either explaining why available psychopharmacological agents are effective or discovering biological bases for the development of newer, more effective drugs. Basic science investigations have provided a set of hypotheses about severe psychiatric disorders which have permitted increasingly definitive biochemical and pharmacological studies of such states. Progress in these areas has been remarkable and hopefully will continue to yield substantive improvements in treatments of the mentally ill.

PROBLEMS ASSOCIATED WITH THE DEVELOPMENT OF PSYCHOPHARMACOLOGICAL AGENTS

Although psychopharmacological agents have many positive features, their use has led to some difficult clinical and social problems. Areas which have received particular attention include: side effects of psychopharmacological agents, abuse potential of some psychoactive drugs, and value conflicts which arise from attempts to treat mental illness.

SIDE EFFECTS

As with all drugs in medicine, psychopharmacological agents do produce undesired effects (Chapter 17). The antipsychotic medications are remarkably safe, but some patients who use them do develop serious side effects, including tardive dyskinesia. Although antidepressant drugs generally have fewer long-term side effects, they are considerably more toxic than the antipsychotics. Thus, it is unfortunately true that the tricyclic antidepressants are often the instrument used by depressed patients who wish to commit suicide. Many of the psychopharmacological drugs are surprisingly safe during chronic use, although their possible teratogenic and carcinogenic activities require further evaluation. However, even relatively mild side effects, such as nausea, dry mouth, or sedation, can profoundly compromise the effectiveness of psychopharmacological agents, since patients may prefer to avoid these symptoms by not taking their medications. Naturally, efforts to reduce unwanted effects of such drugs continue to be an important component of research.

SUBSTANCE ABUSE

Abuse of psychoactive substances predates written history and is found in most human cultures. However, many of the newly discovered psychoactive agents developed for psychopharmacological treatment or research have particularly potent effects on mood, thinking, and behavior. The ready availability of substances like LSD, amphetamines, and short-acting barbiturates have greatly increased the incidence of drug abuse, resulting in a significant public health and legal problem (Part III). Occasionally, drug abusers will harm themselves or others because the hallucinogens have distorted their perceptions or beliefs. For example, aggressive acts are probably more common with abusers of certain stimulants, such as amphetamines, which facilitate paranoid ideation. Although Part III concentrates primarily upon the clinical and basic science aspects of these drugs, an improved understanding of their actions will undoubtedly lead to better approaches to the problems they pose.

INVOLUNTARY TREATMENT

The existence of effective psychopharmacological agents naturally raises the possibility of providing treatment for patients against their wishes. This problem is part of a larger philosophical issue—informed consent—which is the center of increasing debate both within and outside of psychiatry (4). Although the exact legal mechanism varies, most states permit treatment of highly disturbed psychiatric patients without their consent. In California, these patients must be gravely disabled or demonstrably dangerous to themselves or others as a result of mental illness. In practice, the law is applied to depressed patients who are suicidal or to schizophrenic patients who are unable to care for their bodily needs.

Some people argue that involuntary treatment is never acceptable, since individuals should always have the right to reject efforts to alter their behavior by external means (4). For example, Szasz (5) has suggested that the government and psychiatry have joined together, as did the state and the church previously, to compel individuals to conform to certain patterns of behavior and belief. Szasz argues that individuals have the right to determine their own behavior, beliefs, and future, even if some consider those actions to be potentially harmful. He states that should a given belief actually lead to criminal behavior, the individual can be tried and punished for breaking the law, irrespective of issues about the presence or absence of mental illness. Although Szasz offers an attractive interpretation of civil liberties, his viewpoint has logical consequences which are difficult for us to accept. For example, it implies that a depressed patient should be allowed to commit suicide or that paranoid schizophrenics who believe that their food is poisoned should be allowed to starve. In addition, it assumes that the current beliefs of an individual are inviolate and ignores the possibility that aberrant biological or pharmacological processes might temporarily preempt normal thought processes.

Some patients receive treatment regardless of their expressed wishes. Those who attempt suicide may subsequently regret their action and respond to treatment; they may never try to kill themselves again and may be grateful for help given. Similarly, schizophrenics commonly are thankful to be able to resume their former lives and relationships after they received involuntary treatment for their bizarre behavior. Thus, some argue that if it produces such responses, involuntary psychiatric treatment can be viewed as liberating and humane, rather than restrictive and dehumanizing. To the extent that treatment permits patients to return to society and to be free from disturbing thoughts or self-destructive impulses, legal mechanisms for involuntary treatment will probably continue to be available.

Clearly, simple solutions to the philosophical dilemma of involuntary treatment for patients with severe mental illness do not exist. Like other medical advances, such as organ transplants and artificial kidneys, effective psychopharmacological medications pose serious questions for society. Perhaps ethical considerations should become a more explicit part of health care than they have been in the past. This would require that biomedical sciences more effectively integrate their methods with those of the social sciences and philosophy in tackling difficult health problems. Ethical considerations cannot be dealt with through the scientific method. Although science can provide information which is useful in reaching an ethical decision, there will always be a point at which individual judgment must be exercised.

Still another problem is raised by the patient who wants and needs hospital treatment and does not receive it. In too many areas, hospitals have discharged patients whose needs for treatment are too great for the usual outpatient facility. Frequently, this has been done in the name of economy, depending upon the ease of writing a prescription for medication. Whether the patient actually takes the medication and receives proper follow-up, including psychotherapy and vocational aid, becomes of secondary concern in such cases. For acutely ill patients who are released too rapidly and for some chronically ill patients, such a course of events can have tragic consequences. Many patients still need humane and appropriate long-term treatment facilities.

Within that setting, whether voluntary or involuntary, patients should receive careful and appropriate treatment; and drugs should not be used beyond that level which is specifically helpful to the patient. As in all other areas of psychiatric treatment, patient confidentiality is an important consideration (6). Particular care needs to be asserted in order that the drugs are used for therapeutic rather than patient control purposes in such institutions. Drugs cannot substitute for adequate staffing.

INAPPROPRIATE USE OF PHARMACOLOGICAL KNOWLEDGE

In one sense, involuntary treatment may be viewed as a special case of the general problem of determining when psychopharmacological agents can be used appropriately. Two issues illustrate the potential difficulty of deciding when to use drugs which are intended for a highly specific population. The first involves the widespread use of amphetamines for treating hyperactive children (Chapter 26). Frequently, children are treated without being appropriately diagnosed, and the effects of such treatment on the overall pattern of mental and physical growth may be ignored. The second issue involves the pharmacological treatment of aggressive disorders (Chapter 17). Many individuals are concerned that such treatments will be used for social control, rather than for specific aggressive disorders. They suggest that this is an example of the potential misuse of psychoactive substances to quell troublesome behavior patterns. Certainly, it is important to ask when an intervention is in the service of society, rather than for the benefit of the individual. Scarce and unequal resources are powerful determinants of aggressive behavior and probably account for more aggressive behavior than do the psychiatric aberrations.

Unquestionably, drugs can be used inappropriately. So too can any other resource. We believe that the suffering of psychiatric patients is as intense as any known. If we are to relieve that pain, it is important to continue to gain knowledge, even as we strive to create a climate which resists misuses of this or any other resource. Humans have always found ways to influence the actions of others—often unfairly and inappropriately. However, such behaviors arise from social processes which are essentially independent of the means employed and must be addressed in those other contexts.

FUTURE DIRECTIONS IN PSYCHOPHARMACOLOGY

Despite impressive strides in the pharmacological treatment of psychiatric disorders, much remains to be done. Antipsychotic drugs reduce symptoms of schizophrenia but do not provide a cure. In addition, they sometimes have adverse side effects which themselves decrease the patient's ability to function. Antidepressants require weeks to produce their effects and are completely ineffective against some forms of depression. In addition, there are disorders, such as infantile autism and senility, for which we can offer painfully little. Thus, we must continue not only to improve upon existing pharmacological agents but also to expand the scope of our pharmacological armamentarium. Beyond that, we must continually strive to uncover the etiologies of these disturbances.

Development of More Effective Pharmacological Agents

Drug treatments for depression and mania appear to be without major long-term side effects, but they lack universal efficacy. As already mentioned, antidepressants are sufficiently toxic to be used in suicide attempts. Ideally, the margin between the helpful and harmful dosage should be much greater. The discovery of more effective psychopharmacological treatments for schizophrenia, mania, and depression will require continued collaboration among laboratory scientists, animal pharmacologists, and clinical researchers.

Discoveries of new psychoactive agents will undoubtedly continue to involve both empirical and theoretical research. Many of the newer medications in use today were developed by systematic modification of existing drugs, and this will continue to be an important source of compounds. However, other pharmacological agents may result from an increased understanding of brain functions, as basic research uncovers the biochemical factors which predispose to psychiatric symptoms. Knowledge of the mechanisms controlling synthesis, release, receptor interactions, and inactivation should suggest new classes of drugs which selectively interfere with these processes. Extensive studies of the relationships between behavior and biochemistry will be essential (Chapter 1). Basic research into the pharmacological actions of psychoactive drugs should also yield information about the mechanisms by which they produce side effects. This knowledge should aid in efforts to systematically modify available agents to reduce such unwanted effects.

One possible approach to reducing unwanted effects of drugs entails placement near the desired site of action (7). For example, small plastic membranes placed in the conjunctival sac of the eye are currently used to release medication for the treatment of glaucoma. Local placement of the medication permits dramatic reduction of circulating concentrations, thus avoiding unwanted effects in other areas of the body. Unfortunately, local placement of psychoactive medication would require application to specific areas of the brain. The practical and philosphical problems of such a technique are formidable, and efforts to develop drugs which would be taken up or act only at specific sites are still in their infancy. Still, here, as elsewhere, anticipation of possible developments will permit advance analysis of probable social implications. Already we need to begin technological and ethical assessments of this area of biomedical research.

IMPROVEMENT OF MODELS OF PSYCHIATRIC DISORDERS

A crucial aspect of drug testing is the availability of good models upon which to study drug effects. For obvious reasons, these preliminary screenings must be performed in animals. A number of existing animal models are believed to predict antidepressant and antipsychotic activity of new medications in man. Generally, these tests were developed empirically by examining the actions of available medications on numerous animal behavioral paradigms. As discussed in Chapter 1, such animal paradigms may or may not bear a direct relationship to human mental illness, even though they can be useful in predicting some drug actions in humans. Unfortunately, they lead to a circular process, since new drugs will necessarily have actions that resemble those of the drugs upon which the animal tests were based. As a result, a drug which might be extremely effective in reducing the symptoms of mental illness could be missed by animal screening tests, if it acts through different biochemical mechanisms.

One promising approach to developing better animal models for testing new pharmacological agents involves efforts to more closely approximate human mental illness. For example, nonhuman primate models of behavioral disorders are being developed and evaluated. Several of these models not only permit tests of individual animals in isolation but also allow studies of these animals in social groupings (8).

PHARMACOLOGICAL TREATMENT OF OTHER DISORDERS

There are still an impressive number of serious psychiatric disorders for which we lack effective treatments. Striking examples such as infantile autism and senility have already been mentioned. In addition, there are the various drug dependencies, including those to alcohol and nicotine. Substance abuse and its consequences are important health problems for which we currently have only palliative therapy. Other serious and disabling illnesses, such as the obsessive-compulsive and sociopathic disorders, require further investigation of biological mechanisms which may be involved and of pharmacological agents which may alleviate the distressing symptoms they produce.

We hope that further investigation will provide a better means of identifying those patients whom we can help and those drugs which should be used. For example, it seems reasonable that some patients would actually do better without any of our current therapies, while others should be treated rapidly and vigorously. Differentiation of such patients would not only improve therapy but would also provide better incorporation of psychopharmacological agents into treatment plans involving other modes of therapy, including various psychological and sociological approaches.

SUMMARY

The development of effective pharmacological treatments has had a profound impact upon psychiatry. Psychoactive agents which decrease the symptoms of psychiatric disorders have significantly improved the prognosis for patients with mental illness. In addition, the development of such substances has stimulated and directed basic research into brain physiology and pharmacology. Furthermore, the need for precise testing of new medications has led to improved clinical research methodology.

Future research in psychopharmacology will necessarily involve both laboratory and clinical studies. Efforts should be directed toward developing an understanding of the mechanisms of disease and improving the efficacy and specificity of the medications which have already produced a revolution in the treatment of severe mental illness. Such studies will link biological science, social science, and clinical medicine into a unit which has tremendous potential for reducing human suffering.

REFERENCES

1. Berger, P., Hamburg, B., and Hamburg, D. Mental health: progress and problems. *Daedalus*, 261–276, 1977.
2. Ayd, F. J., Jr. The impact of biological psychiatry. *In: Discoveries in Biological Psychiatry*. F. J. Ayd and B. Blackwell, *eds.*, Philadelphia: Lippincott, 1970. pp. 230–243.
3. Hamburg, D. A., *ed. Psychiatry as a Behavioral Science*. Englewood Cliffs: Prentice-Hall, 1970.
4. Gonda, T. A. and Waitzkin, M. B. The right to refuse treatment. *Curr. Conc. Psychiatry*, 5–10, 1976.
5. Szasz, T. *Law, Liberty, Psychiatry*. New York: Macmillan, 1963.
6. Grossman, M., Johnson, R. G., Satten, J., Krueger, A. L., and Barchas, J. D. Report of APA task force on confidentiality as it relates to third parties. *Amer. Psychiat. Assn. Report No. 9*, June, 1975.
7. Brodie, H. K. H. and Sack, R. L. Promising directions in clinical psychopharmacology. *In: American Handbook of Psychiatry*, 2nd ed., Vol. 6. D. A. Hamburg and H. K. H. Brodie, *eds.*, New York: Basic Books, 1975. pp. 533–551.
8. Hamburg, D. A., Hamburg, B., and Barchas, J. Anger and depression in perspectives of behavioral biology. *In: Emotions—Their Parameters and measurement*. L. Levi, *ed.*, New York: Raven Press, 1975, pp. 235–278.

Index